HANDBOOK OF
INTERVENTIONAL RADIOLOGY
AND ANGIOGRAPHY

HANDBOOKS IN RADIOLOGY SERIES

Other Volumes in This Series

HANDBOOK OF INTERVENTIONAL RADIOLOGY AND ANGIOGRAPHY

MYRON WOJTOWYCZ, M.D.
Professor
Department of Radiology
Angiography and Interventional Radiology Section
University of Wisconsin at Madison Medical School
Madison, Wisconsin

SECOND EDITION

with 103 illustrations

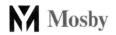 Mosby

St. Louis   Baltimore   Boston
Carlsbad   Chicago   Naples   New York   Philadelphia   Portland
London   Madrid   Mexico City   Singapore   Sydney   Tokyo   Toronto   Wiesbaden

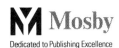

Dedicated to Publishing Excellence

A Times Mirror
Company

Executive Editor: Susan M. Gay
Senior Developmental Editor: Elizabeth Corra
Project Manager: Linda Clarke
Senior Production Editor: Patricia C. Walter
Designer: Nancy McDonald
Electronic Production Coordinator: Christine Poullain
Manufacturing Supervisor: Karen Lewis

SECOND EDITION
Copyright © 1995 by Mosby–Year Book, Inc.

Previous edition copyrighted 1990

Printed in the United States of America
Composition by Mosby Electronic Publishing, Philadelphia
Printing/binding by Maple Vail–York

Mosby–Year Book, Inc.
11830 Westline Industrial Drive
St. Louis, Missouri 63146

Library of Congress Cataloging in Publication Data
Wojtowycz, Myron
    Handbook of interventional radiology and angiography / Myron
Wojtowycz. -- 2nd ed.
       p.   cm. -- (Handbook in radiology series)
    Rev. ed. interventional radiology and angiography.   c1990.
    Includes bibliographical references and index.
    ISBN 0-8151-9440-4 (alk. paper)
    1. Radiology, Interventional--Handbooks, manuals, etc.
2. Angiography--Handbooks, manual, etc.   I. Wojtowycz, Myron.
Interventional radiology and angiography.   II. Title. III. Title:
Interventional radiology and angiography.   IV. Series.
    [DNLM: 1. Radiography, Interventional--handbooks. 2. Angiography-
-handbooks. WG 39 W847h 1995]
RD33.55.W64   1995
617'.05--dc20
DNLM/DLC
for Library of Congress   95–172
                                                  CIP

95 96 97 98 99 / 9 8 7 6 5 4 3 2 1

To Stefan and Olena. Persecuted by the Nazis and driven from your native land by the Bolsheviks, you lived not with bitterness, but in hard work and love. From you I gained an appreciation for liberty, tolerance, justice, and compassion—and very much more.

Preface to the Second Edition

Five years have passed since the publication of the first edition, and we have reached the mid-point of the 1990s. Some techniques, such as laser angioplasty and percutaneous placement of stainless steel Greenfield filters through 30 Fr sheaths, have faded into deserved oblivion. Others, particularly TIPS and the insertion of expandable biliary endoprostheses, have entered wide application. Disposable biopsy guns are now routinely employed in our department and across the country. Vascular stenting, catheter atherectomy, and local thrombolytic enzyme infusion are among the various treatments undergoing continued investigation without yet having many indications firmly established. Spiral computed tomographic angiography, spiral computed tomographic arterial portography, and magnetic resonance angiography are enjoying rapid development and they may further displace conventional diagnostic arteriography from everyday practice.

In this edition I have attempted to provide an updated overview of angiography and interventional radiology, at least as it is practiced at the University of Wisconsin–Madison (needle localization of breast lesions, prostate biopsies, and fallopian tube recanalizations are among the methods omitted for lack of my personal experience). It is hoped that the new figures and tables included will be helpful to the reader. With over 500 new references cited, this book is also meant to serve as a bibliographic source for those who find specific topics discussed to an insufficient degree.

I am grateful to Joan Kozel for her creative contributions in illustrating the work. I also thank my colleagues, Drs. Andrew Crummy, John McDermott, and Ian Sproat, for their support and forbearance during the manuscript revision.

Myron Wojtowycz, M.D.

Preface to the First Edition

Over the past decade, cross-sectional imaging has revolutionized the practice of radiology. One consequence of cross-sectional imaging has been the contraction of the indications for diagnostic angiography. At the same time, a broad range of percutaneous interventions has been made possible. Catheter and wire technologies have advanced, and the refined instruments have been applied to novel purposes. Baskets, balloons, needles, thrombolytic drugs, lasers, fiberoptics, and lithotriptors of various shapes and sizes have become available, creating a bewildering array of options for treating conditions once requiring open surgery. Even more bewildering can be the enormous amount of information pertaining to radiologic diagnosis and percutaneous interventions.

The aim of this book is to provide residents with a quick and coherent introduction to the field of vascular radiology and percutaneous interventions as it stands on the threshold of the 1990s. It may also serve as a convenient review for those about to take their radiology board examinations. This text is not meant to be used alone; rather, it should supplement the many distinguished and more encyclopedic books that have been published recently. In addition, I hope general radiologists will find this handbook a useful reference.

Aside from relying on my personal experience over the past seven years in vascular and interventional radiology, I have attempted to integrate a great deal of information recently presented in medical, surgical, and radiologic publications. It is inevitable that some of the information will soon be outdated in the more rapidly progressing areas such as caval filters, biliary stone removal, vascular stenting, laser angioplasty, and percutaneous atherectomy. One can only ask for the reader's understanding.

It should be acknowledged what this book is *not*. Although basic techniques are presented, the gamut of "tricks of the catheterization trade" is not addressed. Neither is the institution and management of an admitting interventional radiology service (although it must be emphasized that with the proper collegial environment, percutaneous angioplasty and other interventions can be performed safely on patients referred directly from primary care physicians). Pediatric conditions and procedures are not specifically addressed. Perhaps the most important omission is a directed discussion of cardiopulmonary resuscitation, and the treatment of serious contrast medium reactions. Rather than superficially treat a vital topic, I direct the reader to the recommendations of the American Heart Association and the American College of Radiology.[1-3] *Anyone engaging in invasive and angiographic procedures must be versed in resuscitation and life support!*

With a recognition of these limitations, I hope this book will meet the reader's approval. I owe a great debt to Holly Jackson and Joan Kozel for assistance in preparation of the manuscript and illustrations. I also wish to thank Drs. Andrew Crummy, John McDermott, and Phil Carlson for their review of the manuscript and helpful suggestions. I alone am responsible for any defects that remain.

Myron Wojtowycz, M.D.

1. American Heart Association: Standards and guidelines for cardiopulmonary resuscitation and emergency cardiac care. *JAMA* 1986; 255:2841–3044.
2. Albaran-Sotelo R, Atkins JM, Bloom RS, et al: *Textbook of Advanced Cardiac Life Support.* Dallas, American Heart Association, 1987.
3. Commission on Public Health and Radiation Protection, Committee on Drugs, with the cooperation of the Committee on Professional Liability (Commission on Standards in Radiologic Practice), American College of Radiology: *Prevention and management of adverse reactions to intravascular contrast media.* Chicago, American College of Radiology, 1977.

Contents

1

Basic Principles of Arteriography

KEY CONCEPTS

1. Know before starting what questions are to be answered or aims are to be achieved by angiography.
2. Essential preangiographic information includes history of hypersensitivity to contrast media, presence of coagulopathy or use of anticoagulant medications, and signs of renal insufficiency.
3. Catheters and wires should not be advanced against resistance.
4. A test injection by hand should precede any angiographic run to confirm that the proper vessel is selected and the catheter tip is free in the lumen.
5. Low-osmolality contrast media are better tolerated by patients and are associated with fewer adverse reactions and possibly less nephrotoxicity, but cost considerably more than conventional ionic media.
6. Good hydration is the most important factor for preventing contrast material–induced renal dysfunction.

Catheter angiography has been a valuable diagnostic tool for decades. Now, as a purely diagnostic measure, its scope has become limited, and magnetic resonance angiography may further constrain its application. Even so, with percutaneous angioplasty, local thrombolytic infusion, and therapeutic embolization, its applications have expanded in a therapeutic role. This chapter is meant to acquaint the reader with some techniques and instruments commonly used in arteriographic procedures as well as hazards of the procedures. Many of the principles described apply equally to selective venous catheterizations.

ARTERIAL ACCESS

The Seldinger Technique

Selective catheter angiography became possible on a wide scale only after Sven Ivar Seldinger described a method of puncturing an artery and introducing a catheter safely without the need for surgical exposure of the vessel.[1] His technique remains the basis for arteriography today.

After the arterial pulse has been identified and the proper site for puncture chosen, the skin over the vessel is shaved, scrubbed with povidone iodine, and draped; lidocaine 1% is injected for local anesthesia (8 to 10 ml usually suffices). A small skin incision is made to allow easy entry of the needle and catheter. In thin individuals, care must be taken to prevent the scalpel from injuring the vessel.

An 18-gauge hollow needle with a sharp stylet (Seldinger needle, or one of its many variations) is advanced into the vessel, and the stylet is removed. If the needle tip is in the arterial lumen, a stream of pulsating blood is seen. If there is no blood return, the needle is slowly withdrawn until it is removed completely or until pulsatile blood is encountered (Fig. 1-1). When blood returns, a guidewire is passed through the needle and into the arterial lumen. With a good length of wire in the vessel, the needle is removed and the artery compressed while the diagnostic catheter is threaded onto the wire. As the wire is held taut ("clotheslined"), the catheter is advanced into the vessel under fluoroscopic control.

If any resistance to wire introduction is noted, it is best to remove the wire from the needle to see if pulsatile blood continues to return. Should backflow be absent, the needle must be repositioned or removed and a new needlestick performed. When a needle is removed after successful arterial puncture but a guidewire is not introduced, compression of the artery for 5 to 10 minutes is required. The presence of a hematoma not only makes repeated arterial puncture more difficult but also affords less control for manipulations of the catheter and makes effective arterial compression after catheter removal more difficult.

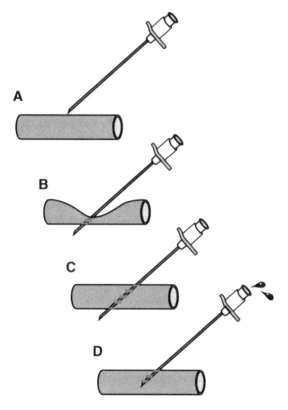

Fig. 1-1   **A,** Blood may not return during advancement of a hollow needle. **B,** The arterial wall is compressed by the needle, **C,** which then passes through the far wall. **D,** Pulsating arterial blood passes through the needle when its tip has been pulled back into the vessel lumen.

If blood continues to flow through the needle after the wire is withdrawn, the angle of the needle may be adjusted and another attempt at wire introduction made. When there is good backflow of blood but continued difficulties with wire insertion, injection of a small amount of contrast material through the needle (most easily performed through a plastic connecting tube) during fluoroscopy is often revealing. The needle tip may be in a small branch artery, it may be angled against the wall of the vessel or only partially within the lumen, or it may be against an atherosclerotic plaque. Appropriate adjustments can then be made.

Needles without Stylets
Alternatives to Seldinger-type needles are sharp, hollow needles lacking stylets. When these needles are advanced into an artery, tip entry can be

recognized immediately. One variation has a short Teflon sheath that can be slipped directly into the vessel. A disadvantage of hollow needles is that small pieces of tissue or clot may occlude the needle and prevent blood return. For this reason, such needles must be flushed before repeated puncture attempts. Also now available are needle systems with contained blood return that minimize the operator's risk of exposure to blood while they allow recognition of the intraluminal position of the needle tip.

Angle of Entry

For entering an artery, the direction of the needle should match the palpated or expected course of the vessel as much as possible (Fig. 1-2). The actual angle of incidence is best at about 45°. Too steep or too shallow an angle can cause problems in catheter exchanges and other manipulations. However, if they anticipate that the direction of entry might be switched during the procedure (as in balloon angioplasty of the superficial femoral artery after bilateral runoff arteriography from the ipsilateral femoral approach), some angiographers prefer to come straight down with the needle, making a 90° angle of entry. Subsequently, catheters can be used to reverse the direction of wire placement.

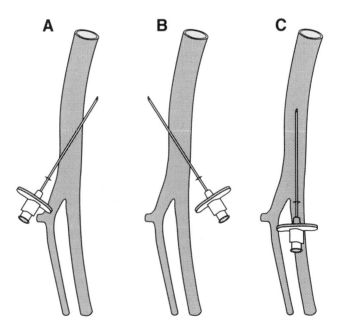

Fig. 1-2   Aligning the needle with the course of the artery improves the odds of successful entry (**C**). A needle angled medially (**A**) or laterally (**B**) may cross in front of or behind the vessel.

Use of Dilators

If a wire is securely in the vessel but catheter introduction is difficult, use of one or more Teflon dilators is recommended. The tapering and stiffness of dilators allow their introduction when other catheters cannot be passed, such as in groins scarred from previous surgery or angiographic procedures. It may be necessary to "overdilate," that is, to pass a 6 Fr* dilator before inserting a 5 Fr catheter. This is often the case when entry is obtained through a synthetic vascular graft. If a dilator can be inserted but problems with catheter passage continue, a heavier, stiffer wire can be placed through the dilator.

Sheaths

A vascular sheath is recommended when multiple changes of catheters are anticipated, when manipulation of the catheter is difficult because of obesity or other local factors, or when bleeding occurs about a catheter in place. Sheaths are supplied fitted over short dilators. Most sheaths have hemostasis valves and flushing sideports. If a sheath does not enter the artery easily, it must be removed and inspected to ensure that crimping or tip flaring has not occurred.

Puncturing Grafts

Catheters can be safely introduced through synthetic graft materials, such as Dacron or Gore-Tex, as long as the grafts have been in place for at least 2 months.[2] In fact, the rate of major complications from femoral graft puncture is no greater than that from puncture of the native artery and substantially lower than that associated with catheterization from an axillary artery approach.[3] Catheter introduction tends to be more difficult because of local scarring from the surgical procedure, as well as the toughness of the graft material. Overdilation of the tract by 1 Fr or 2 Fr may be needed, and use of a low-friction Teflon catheter or sheath is recommended. If no sheath is used, manipulations and removal are best performed with a guidewire through the catheter. Catheter separation occurs with extreme rarity but is possible if proper care is not taken.[3]

Passing Obstructions

If an obstruction is encountered during wire placement, a catheter should be advanced to the vicinity of the obstruction. The catheter is then used to inject contrast material to delineate the nature and severity of the obstruction. At times, use of digital subtraction "roadmap" angiography can be extremely helpful.[4] A hooked-tip catheter, such as a Berenstein or H1H

---

*French is a measure of circumference, translating to 3 French/mm diameter for round tubes.

shape, can direct the guidewire through tortuous vessels and past eccentric plaques. When a hooked-tip catheter is used, a soft-tip straight or steerable guidewire is often the most appropriate choice for successful negotiation of the vessel. The patient should be given 5000 units of heparin intravenously or intraarterially to prevent acute occlusion if a very tight stenosis is catheterized. If an intimal flap is raised during passage attempts, access from that site should be abandoned for all but the most exceptional of circumstances.

Catheter Removal and Hemostasis

At the close of a procedure, pigtail catheters and those catheters with back curves, such as Simmons or sidewinder catheters, should be straightened before removal. This usually requires passage of a guidewire beyond the tip of the catheter. A guidewire should be used for withdrawal of any multi-sidehole catheter in order to prevent blood-splash exposures.[5] As the catheter is removed, firm pressure is placed over the site of arterial puncture (not necessarily at the site of skin incision itself) with compression of the proximal vessel as well. Pressure should not be so firm as to obliterate distal pulses, but there should be no bleeding or oozing from the incision or hematoma formation in the soft tissues. Compression is maintained continuously at least 10 minutes before pressure is gingerly released to check for effective hemostasis. A longer period of compression is prudent if manipulations are difficult, if large catheters are used, or if a hematoma is present. If bleeding recurs, compression must be reinstituted for a similar time period. Any hypertension should be controlled by nifedipine or other medications before an arterial catheter is removed.

Universal Precautions

Anyone performing arteriography or other invasive procedures must be versed in universal precautions and the particular policies in place at one's institution. In a review of more than 500 consecutive invasive procedures, Hansen and associates documented skin exposure to the patient's blood in 3% of the procedures.[5] Fortunately, needlestick injuries and parenteral exposure to blood were much less common. Careful handling and prompt proper disposal of needles, scalpels, and other sharp instruments must be part of the training and practice of all operators. Needles should never be recapped. Masks and face shields must be employed during any angiographic procedure. All angiographers should be vaccinated against hepatitis B.

Common Femoral Artery Puncture

The vessel most commonly used for arterial access in angiography is the common femoral artery. The pulse is palpated below the inguinal ligament (which courses between the pubis and the anterior superior iliac spine). The inguinal crease is *not* a reliable marker for the location of the ligament! In obese individuals the inguinal crease may be as much as 11 cm caudal to the inguinal ligament.[6] If the patient is heavy or if the pulse is not easily palpable, it is useful to check the site fluoroscopically before administering local anesthesia. For retrograde catheterization, the skin incision can be made over the inferior margin of the femoral head, with the intention of entering the artery no higher than the midfemoral head. The position of the inguinal ligament averages 1.5 cm cephalad to the mid-femoral head, and puncture at or below this level virtually guarantees infrainguinal vessel entry.[7] If an antegrade puncture is required, skin entry can be made at the level of the acetabulum, again aiming to enter at or immediately distal to the mid common femoral artery.[8]

It is important to puncture the artery over the femoral head, for the common femoral artery is larger than its branches, the superficial femoral and profunda femoris (deep femoral) arteries, and it is thus less prone to injury. Also, manual compression of the puncture site is more effective over the femoral head. Low puncture with larger catheters has been implicated in pseudoaneurysm formation.[9] Then again, puncture above the inguinal ligament prevents effective compression and exposes the patient to an elevated risk of major, life-threatening hemorrhage.[10] Still, a point to remember is that infrainguinal puncture is no *absolute* guarantee against retroperitoneal hemorrhage.[7]

Puncture of the femoral limb of an aortobifemoral graft can sometimes be perplexing. If a Seldinger double-wall technique is employed, one may enter the native femoral artery deep to the end-to-side graft insertion. In such a case, the guidewire meets resistance in the vessels of the pelvis or near the aortic bifurcation. Injection of contrast medium through the needle or through an inserted dilator confirms that the diseased native vessel has been entered. The needle or dilator is then slowly withdrawn until pulsatile blood no longer returns. If the limb of the graft has been traversed, a second squirt of pulsatile blood is noted with further withdrawal. The guidewire is then inserted into the graft and advanced into the aorta.

When a femoral pulse is poorly palpable and there is no feasible alternate access site, fluoroscopy may detect mural calcification. If present, calcium can guide needle passage. Otherwise, real-time sonography can be used to mark the course of the vessel and to exclude the possibility of occlusion. (Ultrasound should also be used to examine the femoral artery if there is any question of aneurysm or pseudoaneurysm.) If the artery is not entered but venous blood returns through the needle, passage of a guidewire into the vein (coursing medial to the artery) can serve as a marker for further needle placements. In exceptional cases, a venous catheter can be used to inject contrast material for a digital subtraction roadmap of the artery. Another approach has been recently described by Millward and colleagues.[11] A finger is placed immediately lateral to the pubic tubercle and 3 cm caudal to the palpable inguinal ligament to feel the point allowing the most posterior depression (between the iliopsoas muscle laterally and the pectineus muscle medially). The femoral vein lies in the floor of this depression, and 1.5 cm lateral to the depression lies the femoral artery. Using these landmarks, Millward and colleagues have been able to puncture pulseless femoral arteries quite consistently.

A question that often arises in the presence of peripheral vascular disease is which side should be chosen for femoral artery puncture. Does one enter the artery in the more symptomatic leg, or should access be obtained on the less symptomatic or asymptomatic side? In many cases, the less symptomatic side presents a stronger pulse and easier access, but, should a local complication arise, the patient now has bilateral problems. If entry is gained through the more ischemic limb, there may be greater risk of causing dissection or occlusion, and many surgeons may be discomfitted by the presence of a hematoma at the site of a planned operation. Even so, there is no evidence that arteriography predisposes to subsequent graft infection at the puncture site chosen.[12] Choosing the symptomatic side for access does allow measurement of any pressure gradient in the iliac arteries, and it facilitates balloon angioplasty if a lesion amenable to treatment is uncovered. The choice of side is basically a matter of judgment, and it should be made on an individual basis for each patient.

Axillary or Brachial Artery Puncture
The only other arteries used routinely for selective catheterization studies are the axillary and brachial arteries. Upper extremity arterial access is necessary in the face of bilateral femoral or iliac artery or aortic occlusion, as well as for certain selective arterial studies most easily approached from above. Among the latter are celiac, mesenteric, or renal artery catheterizations in severely angled vessels. Entry through the left upper extremity is preferred to minimize the possibility of stroke. A catheter placed from the right exposes both carotid and vertebral arteries to potential emboli; a left-sided catheter crosses only the left vertebral artery origin. Care should be taken that a catheter placed down the descending aorta does not buckle into the ascending aorta and form a loop in the left ventricle during manipulations.

Besides the risk of cerebral embolization, upper extremity arterial puncture poses problems with needle entry (owing to the greater mobility and smaller size of the vessels in comparison to the common femoral artery), effective compression of the artery (especially for "high" axillary punctures), and patient discomfort from the prolonged immobilization in abduction needed after angiography by way of axillary artery puncture.

Neural injury can arise from needle puncture or from compression by hematoma. The complication rate of axillary puncture is at least twice as high as that of common femoral catheterization.[3,13] Placement of even 4 Fr and 5 Fr catheters through the brachial artery can result in major complications in 11% of patients, mostly from spasm or arterial thrombosis.[14,15] For this reason, upper extremity access should be used only if femoral artery catheterization is not possible.

Translumbar Aortography

If no femoral pulse is palpable, but abdominal aortography and runoff angiography are needed, translumbar puncture remains a valuable option. A special 18-gauge needle bearing a 6 Fr sheath is placed directly into the abdominal aorta from a left flank approach. It is *critical* that the patient have normal coagulation status and no problems with hypertension to be a candidate for this approach. A certain degree of retroperitoneal hemorrhage is expected after translumbar aortography, and a large amount of blood may extravasate before such hemorrhage becomes clinically evident.[16] For this reason, translumbar aortography is not performed on outpatients, and serial hematocrit determinations can be used for early detection of bleeding.

For translumbar study, the patient is placed prone on the angiography table, and a skin entry site is chosen approximately one handbreadth to the left of the spinous process, below the level of the twelfth rib. Local anesthesia is administered superficially, and lidocaine is also injected into the deeper soft tissues with a 20-gauge spinal needle. The sheath needle is advanced under fluoroscopic guidance to the appropriate level (see the next two sections, Low Translumbar Approach and High Translumbar Approach). If the needle is placed too horizontal, vertebral body is encountered. When this happens, the needle must be withdrawn almost completely from the patient and redirected in a slightly more vertical angle until its tip passes anterior to the vertebral column. Often the pulsatile wall of the aorta can be felt as the needle tip comes in contact with it. The operator then advances the needle 1 to 2 cm by a quick jab to pierce the wall, with care taken not to cross the midline.

If the sheath has only an endhole, both the trocar and the metal cannula of the needle are removed; if there are sideholes in the sheath, only the trocar is removed. The sheath (with or without cannula) is slowly withdrawn until pulsatile blood returns. A short J-tip guidewire is then inserted and monitored fluoroscopically to ensure that it passes easily into aortic lumen, and the sheath is introduced over the wire. After the sheath is in place, it is flushed, and a small amount of contrast material is injected to confirm proper positioning. The sheath is secured by sterile tape or towel clips to prevent inadvertent withdrawal. No more than 15 ml/second must be injected through an endhole-only sheath because the high-velocity jet formed at the tip can injure endothelium.

The potential of major unrecognized hemorrhage dictates that catheter exchanges not be performed through an aortic puncture. If arterial blood returns through the needle but wire placement is unsuccessful, a separate puncture may be attempted. However, multiple repeated aortic entries are dangerous.

Low Translumbar Approach
For low puncture, the sheath needle is directed in the axial plane, 35° to 45° from the horizontal, toward the level of L3. Low entry has the advantage of providing better opacification of the lower extremity runoff vessels, particularly if the sheath tip can be directed caudally during placement. However, the infrarenal abdominal aorta can be variable in location because of tortuosity, sometimes actually lying to the right of the midline. Also, with the L3 approach there is a higher likelihood that the needle might enter an aneurysm or an occluded aorta. Preangiographic examination with ultrasound can alert one to the necessity for high translumbar puncture.

High Translumbar Approach
If aortic occlusion or aneurysm is suspected, a high translumbar route is the appropriate choice. The needle is directed cranially toward the pedicle of T12, again making a 35° to 45° angle with the horizontal (coronal) plane. The L1 level or T12-L1 interspace must be avoided to prevent injury to the renal artery. Because of the steep angle of entry with respect to the course of the aorta, direction of the sheath tip caudally is rarely possible, and injection must be made into the descending thoracic aorta. Because much of the injected contrast enters the mesenteric circulation and the renal arteries, opacification of distal vessels tends to be worse than that provided by the low lumbar approach. One particular risk of high translumbar puncture is pneumothorax, especially in patients with obstructive lung disease.

CENTRAL VENOUS ACCESS

Selective central venous studies can be performed by way of the upper extremity or right jugular veins, but most are approached from the common femoral vein. The femoral vein is posteromedial to the artery, so the skin medial to the femoral pulse is anesthetized. Puncture technique is identical to that employed for arterial studies, except that a syringe containing saline should be used for gentle aspiration. When central catheters are placed (particularly if the tip is positioned in the chest or right atrium), the lumen must not be exposed to atmospheric pressure. Carelessness may result in air embolism.

GUIDEWIRES

Guidewires are designed to allow the safe introduction of the catheter to the vessel and selective positioning of catheters within the vascular system. Most conventional wires are composed of a stainless steel coil of wire supported by a stiff inner mandril running the length of the coil and tapering over 5 to 15 cm to a soft tip. There is also another fine supporting wire in the core, joining both ends of the coil; this wire is meant to prevent complete transection of the guidewire, should the coil break. Standard wires have a soft leading end and a stiff trailing end that is not ordinarily inserted into a catheter.

In the United States, wire sizes are usually expressed as diameter in inches. The wires most commonly used in adult angiography have 0.035- or 0.038-inch diameters. Much finer wires, such as 0.018-inch guidewires, are used in special applications, including percutaneous angioplasty of small vessels. Some angiographers now use 3 Fr catheter systems for lower extremity arteriography, and such catheters are inserted over 0.025-inch stiff mandril wires placed through 20-gauge needles.[17] When finer wires are employed, a very stiff shaft is needed; otherwise, difficulties are encountered with coiling or kinking of the wire in the extravascular soft tissues.

Standard wires are 145 cm long, allowing insertion of 100-cm catheters without difficulty. Exchange wires up to 300 cm long are used when a selectively placed catheter must be exchanged for another without losing access to the vessel of interest. The wire must be long enough for the catheter to be completely removed without withdrawal of the wire tip from its selective position.

Wires are further characterized by the length of taper to the inner mandril, tip configuration (straight, 1.5 mm-, 3 mm-, and 15 mm-diameter J), stiffness (standard, heavy-duty, "coat hanger"), and coating. J-tip wires are valuable in atherosclerotic vessels, because straight wires tend to catch on the edge of plaques with the attendant danger of producing arterial dissection. J-tip wires are more likely to deflect from obstructions. Heavy-duty or extra-stiff wires may be needed to traverse scarred puncture sites or very tortuous vessels. Steerable wires are designed for efficient transmission of torque to a flexible curved or angled tip; they may be employed to traverse tight, eccentric stenoses. Teflon and heparin coatings decrease the friction and thrombogenicity of guidewires. Coating with hydrophilic polymers has produced wires with extremely low coefficients of friction. Special deflecting systems are available for directing catheter tips. The ends of deflecting wires are quite stiff, and they should not be passed beyond the tip of the catheter being deflected (see Chapter 14, entitled Pulmonary Angiography). One should become familiar with a variety of wires and develop preferences on the basis of experience.

CATHETERS

As with guidewires, angiographic catheters come in a range of shapes and sizes. Catheter size is conventionally designated in "French," in which 3 Fr is equal to a 1 mm diameter. Packaging labels list the size, shape, material, length of the catheter, presence of sideholes, and maximum diameter of the guidewire that can be used with the catheter. Among the materials used are polyethylene, polyurethane, nylon, and Teflon, and the catheter-handling characteristics vary accordingly. For example, Teflon is smooth and stiff and has a relatively low coefficient of friction. It is useful when insertion of other catheters through a graft or scarred puncture site is difficult. Other polymers are designed to accommodate high injection rates through a thin-walled tube. Some catheters are constructed with a steel mesh incorporated into the wall to provide ready translation of torque to the catheter tip. Review of manufacturers' catalogues, discussion with other angiographers and manufacturers' representatives, and experience can provide an idea of which catheters are most useful for a given indication.

For flush aortography, a pigtail tip is recommended. Pigtail catheters contain multiple sideholes, permitting dispersal of contrast medium in a relatively compact bolus while preventing a strong jet effect from producing injury or perforation of a vessel. Pigtail catheters must be removed over a guidewire.

Selective catheterization requires a shaped tip to engage the orifice of the artery being selected. A Cobra (C2) catheter has an angled tip joined to a gentle curve, making it suitable for selection of many renal and mesenteric arteries (see Fig. 1-3). Brachiocephalic vessels approached from the femoral artery are often easily engaged by a Headhunter (H1) tip. Highly curved catheters, such as Simmons or sidewinder catheters, must have their primary curves reconstituted by manipulation in the aortic arch or brachiocephalic arteries. They are most useful in hooking sharply angled vessels (celiac axis, renal artery to a ptotic kidney, and so forth). For secure positioning of a selective catheter, it is often necessary to pass a guidewire well into the vessel and advance the catheter over the wire.

Most catheters presently in use are available in 5 Fr to 7 Fr sizes. The 5 Fr catheters are more flexible and tend to advance better over a wire coursing through tortuous vessels. Larger catheters allow better control of torque and movement in patients whose size or anatomy makes selective angiography difficult.

Once a catheter is introduced into a vessel and the guidewire removed, the catheter must be immediately flushed with a solution of heparinized saline (2000 units of heparin in 500 ml 0.9 N saline). Allowing blood to remain stagnant within a catheter for any length of time invites thrombosis. Flushing should be repeated every 2 to 3 minutes throughout the procedure. Before each flush, a small amount of blood should be freely aspirated into the syringe.

H1   Simmons   C2   Pigtail   Berenstein

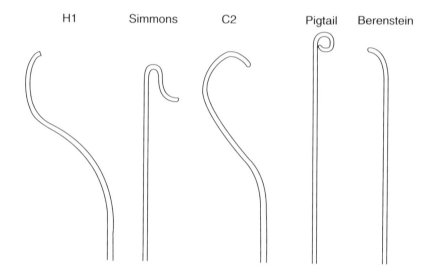

Fig. 1-3   Various catheter shapes useful in arteriography.

If a catheter has no sideholes, the tip of the catheter may sometimes rest against the vessel wall, and no blood can be aspirated. In such a situation, the catheter must be slowly withdrawn until blood does freely return through the lumen. Placement of one or two sideholes near the catheter tip may prevent this problem, as well as decrease the intensity of the tip jet created with injection. However, sideholes should not be placed in catheters used in the brachiocephalic vessels. There is a small but finite risk that thrombus may form in a sidehole (due to the relative ineffectiveness of flushing in keeping sideholes clear). Embolization of such a thrombus is commonly inconsequential but can be disastrous in the coronary or cerebral circulation. For the same reason, "double-flushing" (forceful aspiration with one syringe followed by forward flushing with a different syringe) is advised in the brachiocephalic vessels.

An occluded catheter *must not* be opened by forward injection of fluid or by passage of a guidewire. This turns the occluding material into emboli. Instead, the catheter hub may be cut and a vascular sheath of appropriate size slipped over the catheter into the site of entry. In this manner the catheter can be removed without loss of vascular access.

Whenever a wire is inserted into a catheter, the first few millimeters of wire exiting catheter tip behave as a stiff instrument, no matter how soft the guidewire tip actually is. Therefore, if the catheter endhole is wedged against an atherosclerotic plaque or other obstruction, the catheter should be slightly withdrawn. In small vessels it is prudent to form the tip of a tight J wire by advancing the wire just to the end of the catheter and then withdrawing the catheter to unsheath the wire.

FILMING

Conventional Film Angiography

Basic Equipment

The type of equipment available in a given department dictates the form of the angiographic images obtained. Conventional films may be individual "cut" sheets or continuous rolls placed in special magazines and rapid film changers. These devices permit up to six films per second to be obtained. For lower extremity runoff angiography, special long-leg films and ceiling-mounted tubes have been used in some institutions. Alternatively, moving step-tables can be used to shift the patient position over several stations during a single injection, in essence "following" the opacification of vessels after contrast medium injection. Newer angiographic units may be supplied with tables permitting continuous or variable-speed motion, extending "bolus chasing" to digital studies.

Spot films using 70-mm or 100-mm cameras are sometimes used in angiography, but the small size of the frames makes the appreciation of fine detail difficult. Cineradiography is customarily performed in cardiac angiography, but the high radiation doses and cumbersome film viewing make this technique unpopular for noncardiac applications. Most peripheral arteriograms do not call for extremely rapid frame rates.

Setting Up

After the catheter is placed, a test injection under fluoroscopy must be performed prior to filming to ensure that the tip is free (not wedged) and in the correct vessel. Selective catheter placement assures the best opacification of vessels with the least amount of contrast medium, and it minimizes confusion from the undesired filling of other overlapping vessels. The rapidity of blood flow in the artery can be gauged by the test injection, and injection parameters are set to nearly match that flow. Injection rates of 20 ml/second and 30 ml/second are typical for abdominal and thoracic aortography, respectively. Selective renal and mesenteric studies usually call for rates of 6 to 10 ml/second. Inferior mesenteric artery injection is commonly performed at 2 to 3 ml/second. Duration of injection is at least 2 seconds and may be up to 10 or 15 seconds, depending on whether step-table angiography is being employed or dense organ opacification is required (see Table 1-1).

With conventional film angiography, a scout film is obtained to check positioning of the patient and exposure factors. The catheter is attached to a power injector and the injection parameters are set. If the need for subtraction (analog) films is anticipated, the first exposure occurs before the injection of iodinated contrast material. Exposures must be made at a frame rate and duration appropriate to the problem at hand. For rapid flow of blood through an arteriovenous fistula, rates of three or more frames per second are needed for evaluation. For flow through aneurysmal vessels in patients with poor cardiac output, one exposure every 2 to 3 seconds for a protracted period may be needed. Delayed films (through 20 to 40 seconds) are necessary for assessing venous opacification or extravasation in cases of trauma or gastrointestinal bleeding.

In some settings, flow can be manipulated by medications or other means. Distal extremity vessel opacification is enhanced by warming of the extremity, reactive hyperemia after release of pressure cuffs, or direct injection of nitroglycerin or tolazoline.[18] Tolazoline can be injected into the superior mesenteric artery immediately prior to angiography to improve visualization of the portal venous system. Dilute epinephrine has been administered into renal arteries to decrease flow through normal vessels and make abnormal vessels more conspicuous.

A single projection is often insufficient for diagnostic angiography. The position of atherosclerotic plaques cannot be anticipated, and use of two orthogonal projections can improve detection of stenosis in 30% to 40% of patients.[19,20] Two or more projections are mandatory for the proper evaluation of aortic aneurysms or thoracic aortic trauma. If the angiography suite is equipped with only one radiographic tube, a separate injection of contrast material must be performed for each projection. However, if two tubes are available, simultaneous biplane filming can be performed, and the total dose of contrast medium injected is minimized.

All studies obtained must be developed and reviewed before the termination of angiography. Conventional films give one the advantages of a large field of view, high spatial resolution, and the ability to use a step-table and simultaneous biplane filming. Disadvantages include relatively low contrast resolution, inability to view images immediately, and the large number of superfluous films usually exposed.

Digital Angiography with or without Subtraction

Digital subtraction angiography (DSA) stores images electronically and uses a dedicated computer to subtract images in real time, ideally showing nothing but those vessels filled with contrast medium.[21] The resultant angiogram can be reviewed without delay. The high contrast resolution of DSA allows dilute contrast medium (diluted 1:1 with saline) to be employed. Another advantage is that the images can be electronically manipulated to change the contrast and window level, integrate frames, and compensate for a certain amount of motion. Other special features, such as "bolus chasing," are available on various imager models. One recent technical innovation is the active

Table 1-1 Suggestions for Peripheral and Mesenteric Angiography

Study	Catheter	Positioning	Injection	Projection	Filming	Comments
Thoracic aortogram						
Trauma	6 Fr pigtail 110 cm	Aortic root	25–35 ml/sec for 2 sec	45° RPO + lateral (additional, if needed, by DSA)	2 per sec each projection (biplane) for 4–6 sec	Include from lower great vessels (thoracic inlet) to diaphragm.
Aneurysm	6 Fr pigtail 110 cm	Aortic root	20–30 ml/sec for 2–3 sec	30° RPO + lateral (additional, if needed, by DSA)	1–2 per sec projection (biplane) for 6–10 sec	For very large aneurysms slow injection rate, increase volume, and prolong filming.
Arch (before selectives)	5 Fr pigtail 100 cm	Aortic root	15–20 ml/sec for 2 sec	30° RPO	2–6 frames per sec by DSA	
Abdominal aorta						
For AAA or suspected mesenteric ischemia	5 Fr pigtail 65 cm	About T12	15–25 ml/sec for 2–3 sec	Biplane filming	2 per sec for 4 sec (each projection), then 1 per sec to 10 or 12 sec	For AAA a slower, longer injection may be optimal (15 ml/sec for 3 sec) but if good filling of mesenteric vessels is desired, 25 ml/sec for 2 sec may be better.
For IMA origin +/or body of AAA	5 Fr pigtail 65 cm	L2-3	5 ml/sec for 3 sec	DSA with 20° LPO	1–2 per sec frame rate	
As part of aorta/iliac femoral runoff study	5 Fr pigtail 65 cm	L1-2 (at renals)	10–12 ml/sec for 2 sec	DSA—AP	At least 2 frames per sec carried through nephrogram phase	
Distal abdominal aorta for runoff						
For iliac/distal runoff	5 Fr pigtail 65 cm	About L3 (sideholes above bifurcation)	6–8 ml/sec for 2–3 sec	DSA—bilateral 30° oblique pelvis (including femoral bifurcations) and AP runoff	DSA frame rate according to flow	Frame rate faster for pelvis—for vessels below knee, longer injection and slowed frame rates are appropriate. Obtain additional projections where needed
Unilateral lower extremity runoff						
Iliac/distal runoff	4–5 Fr straight flush cathether or dilator (ipsilateral) or 5 Fr Simmons 1 or 2 (contralateral)	Common or external iliac artery	3–4 ml/sec for 2–4 sec	DSA—bilateral 30° oblique pelvis (including femoral bifurcations) and AP runoff	DSA frame rate according to flow	Frame rate 4–6 per sec for AVMs or AV fistulae and obtain multiple projections. If looking for posttraumatic flaps or other fine detail, do cut films and inject 5–6 ml per sec for 3–5 sec.

	Catheter	Tip position	Injection	Projection	Filming	Comments
Pelvis (internal iliac)						
For trauma, tumor or impotence workup	5 Fr Simmons 1 or 2 (ipsilateral) 5 Fr H1H or Berenstein (contralateral)	Tip in main trunk of internal iliac	2–4 ml/sec for 25–40 ml total	AP +/or obliques per inclination	1 per sec for 12–15 sec	For impotence, do contralateral posterior oblique with penis placed over contralateral thigh (after IC papaverine). For trauma, late films may be needed to detect extravasation.
Upper extremity						
For subclavian/axillary	5 Fr H1H, Berenstein, Simmons 1 or 2	Tip just past vertebral origin	3–4 ml/sec for 12 ml total	AP	DSA or film 2–3 per sec for 4 sec, then 1 per sec for 6 sec	
For brachial	Same as above	Tip in midaxillary	3–4 ml/sec for 3 sec	AP	DSA or film 1–2 per sec for 8 sec	Be aware of possible high brachial bifurcation at the axillary level.
For forearm and hand	Same as above	Tip in distal brachial	1–3 ml/sec for 10–20 sec	AP (hand supinated)	DSA (or film) 1–2 per sec for 10–20 sec, according to flow	Make sure hand is maximally vasodilated (body and extremity warming is best).
GI/mesenteric						
Celiac	Cobra or Simmons 5 Fr	Tip proximal to bifurcation	6–10 ml/sec for a total of 40–60 ml	AP	1 per sec for 5 films, then every other sec for 5 films, then every third sec for 5 films	Smaller injection volumes for arterial anatomy only: larger, if portal study is desired. May need lateral aorta first.
Common hepatic	Cobra or Simmons (or H1H or Berenstein, over an exchange wire after celiac engaged)	Well seated in CHA	4–8 ml/sec for a total of 30–50 ml	AP	1 per sec for 8 films, then every other sec for 7 films	Normally inject about 6 ml for total of 30 ml, but may do a slow, long injection for "infusion" study of possible mets.
Splenic	Cobra or Simmons	Proximal splenic	6–8 ml/sec for a total of 60–80 ml	AP	As for celiac	If patient has little gas and can suspend breathing, sometimes DSA can be done.
LGA	Simmons 1 or 2 (place in celiac and pull back to "hook" LGA)	Proximal LGA	2–3 ml/sec for a total of 15–20 ml	AP	As for celiac	Select if gastric bleeding source present or suspected. Most bleeds from LGA respond to embolization.
SMA	Cobra or Simmons	Proximal SMA	6–8 ml/sec for a total of 60–80 ml	AP	As for celiac	SMA is at level of L1—may need lateral aorta first.
IMA	Simmons 1 or 2	Proximal IMA	2–4 ml/sec for a total of 16–30 ml	AP	As for celiac	IMA is at L3—may need lateral aortogram or LPO distal aortogram to show patency.

Table continued on p. 18

Table 1-1—Cont'd   Suggestions for Peripheral and Mesenteric Angiography

Study	Catheter	Positioning	Injection	Projection	Filming	Comments
Renal	5 Fr Cobra or Simmons	Proximal or mid main renal artery	6–8 ml/sec for 3 sec	AP or 30° contralateral posterior oblique	DSA or film 2–3 per sec for 3 sec followed by 1 per sec for 6–10 sec	For renal tumor workup, more contrast (up to 30–35 ml total) and delayed filming +/or DSA may show renal vein.
Pulmonary	7–8 Fr Grollman or pigtail catheter (placed with the aid of a deflecting wire)	Main left or right pulmonary artery (or in lobar arteries as guided by perfusion scan)	20–30 ml/sec for a total of 40–60 ml	30° ipsilateral posterior oblique (other projections as necessary—at least 2 per lung studied)	3 per sec for 3 sec, followed by 1 per sec for 6 sec	Always check pressures *first.* Gauge flow rate by hand injection. Lower rates/volumes for superselective injections. DSA may be used (4–6 frames per sec) to "fill in" projections or to check questionable areas.

These are but guidelines; the rest is common sense. If you are looking for tumor blush, extravasion, or portal filling, use longer, higher-volume injections and film late (to at least 25–30 sec). If a focal abnormality is present, the more selective your catheter placement, the better your chance of defining it. For high-flow situations (e.g., AVM, AV fistula, pulmonary artery), increase the injection rate and filming rate. Hand inject before power injecting, to ensure that you are where you think you are, that the catheter is not under a plaque or dug into intima, and that the catheter is not likely to flip out of a selected vessel during injection. Sideholes are recommended for selective catheters (aside from those used in brachiocephalic arteries) to minimize the risk of intimal dissection and to diminish the jet effect, which may flip the catheter out of the vessel. We use low-osmolality contrast media exclusively for vascular studies (300 mgI/ml for DSA, 360 mgI/ml for cut film angiography). Conventional film angiography is preferred for studies needing high spatial resolution or delayed filming (if motion is likely) or in the presence of bowel gas (as in an arteriogram for active GI bleeding).

AAA, abdominal aortic aneurysm; AP, anteroposterior; AV, arteriovenous; AVM, arteriovenous malformation; CHA, common hepatic artery; DSA, digital substraction angiography; GI, gastrointestinal; IC, intracutaneous; IMA, inferior mesenteric artery; LGA, left gastric artery; LPO, left posterior oblique; RPO, right posterior oblique; SMA, superior mesenteric artery.

rotation of a C-arm gantry (up to 30° per second) during contrast medium injection, thus providing multiple projections from a single angiographic run. The results may be displayed with or without subtraction, depending on the feasibility of a separate "mask" run of exposures.

High contrast resolution is valuable in the study of the vessels of the ankle and foot.[22] In upper extremity angiography, use of dilute contrast material decreases the considerable discomfort that has been associated with conventional angiography in the past. In many applications DSA can be used interchangeably with conventional film angiography according to the discretion of the angiographer, and many of the procedures outlined earlier (see Setting Up) also apply for DSA studies. However, if a patient is uncooperative or unable to remain motionless for the duration of exposures, conventional filming is preferred. Digital *subtraction* angiography is inappropriate in viewing the abdomen if a large amount of bowel gas is present, especially if delayed exposures are needed, and should not be employed in the search for a gastrointestinal bleeding source. However, present-day systems allow high-quality, high-resolution *unsubtracted* digital images to be obtained, and studies using undiluted conventional doses of contrast medium may be quite adequate for diagnosis in such situations.

Originally, DSA used intravenous injection of contrast medium, but it soon became apparent that intraarterial injection overcame many of the problems encountered.[23] Intraarterial studies are much less subject to motion artifact, smaller doses of contrast medium can be used, and the study is much less dependent on cardiac output. Arterial injections are routinely performed through 4 Fr or 5 Fr catheters, minimizing the risk of postangiographic bleeding. In our department, intravenous DSA has virtually disappeared, but it does remain an option if no arterial access site is available

CONTRAST MEDIA

Conventional Ionic and Low-Osmolality Iodinated Media

Vessels subjected to angiography must be rendered radiopaque by injection of iodinated contrast medium. For many years the prime agents in use were ionic derivatives of fully substituted triiodobenzoic acid, namely, diatrizoate and iothalamate. The ions released in solution by these compounds are meglumine and/or sodium cations and the radiopaque anions. Over the past decade intravascular contrast agents have become available in the United States that are either dimeric ionic compounds (ioxaglate) or nonionic derivates of triiodobenzoic acid (iohexol, iopamidol, ioversol). The newer agents, by virtue of their lower osmolality at diagnostic concentrations, cause fewer physiologic alterations during injection, produce less pain or discomfort, and are associated with fewer adverse reactions than the conventional ionic contrast media.

Individual agents are often referred to in terms of concentration (percentage weight per volume), for example, Renografin 76 (diatrizoate sodium and diatrizoate meglumine). Perhaps a better term for comparison is iodine content (in milligrams per milliliter). "Full-strength" agents for angiography typically range from 300 to 370 mg/ml iodine content. Contrast media of lower concentration may be employed for DSA.

Conventional ionic contrast media are usually five to seven times the osmolality of blood in the concentrations injected.[24] Following contrast media injection, most patients report a transient sensation of heat that can be quite painful with selective arteriography of the extremities. Lidocaine has been added to ionic contrast material for lower extremity arteriography in the past. Use of lower osmolar ionic or nonionic media (one third to one half the osmolality of conventional ionic contrast media) makes patient discomfort much less of a problem, and lidocaine is not combined with the newer media. Lidocaine should never be injected into the brachiocephalic vessels.

Iothalamate and diatrizoate have anticoagulant properties that are not shared by the new nonionic agents.[25] It has been common practice to leave ionic contrast material in a catheter during manipulations. However, because the margin of safety with respect to thrombus formation is decreased, catheters containing nonionic agents should be flushed with heparinized saline immediately after contrast injection.

There is little question that low-osmolality agents decrease adverse reactions, and mortality rates are also lower (see the section on Risks Related to Contrast Media, later in this chapter). However, their use has elicited great controversy at present because of their cost, 12 to 15 times higher than that of conventional ionic media.[26] If the new agents are adopted universally for all vascular contrast studies in the United States, it has been estimated that fatalities might be prevented at the cost of about $3.4 million per life saved![26] Scoring systems or other methods of high-risk patient selection have been proposed to limit use of the new, expensive agents to those individuals most likely to benefit.[24,26] However, malpractice issues make it unlikely that such proposals will be widely accepted. No doubt these issues will take years to be settled. At the University of Wisconsin–Madison our department switched to low-osmolality agents for all intravascular injections several years ago, but cost factors may force a change in that policy. The expiration of patents on low-osmolality contrast media may lead to a drop in price in the near future.

Carbon Dioxide

Not all angiographic examinations have utilized iodinated contrast material. Carbon dioxide has seen limited application as a vascular contrast agent, and the advent of DSA has enhanced its use.[27] Prototype gas delivery systems are now undergoing evaluation. Carbon dioxide injection can be considered for selected patients with a history of prior life-threatening reaction to iodinated media or very marginal renal function.

PATIENT PREPARATION AND MONITORING

Routine Measures

At the time of consultation by the patient's clinical service, the precise indications and aims of angiography should be elicited. If the same diagnostic information can be gained by less invasive, less expensive means, or if angiographic study is unlikely to yield the information sought, this subject should be thoroughly discussed with the referring clinician. Before angiography is scheduled, pertinent history—including use of anticoagulants or presence of bleeding tendency, status of renal function, and prior reactions to contrast media administration—must be obtained. These data are especially important if the patient will be examined on an outpatient basis or if admission is to occur on the same day as the arteriogram.

When possible, the patient is seen the evening before angiography. The radiologist explains the purpose, nature, and risks of the study in order to obtain informed consent and establish rapport with the patient. History of symptoms, previous pertinent surgical procedures (such as bypass graft placement), and allergies is obtained. Physical examination includes assessment of peripheral pulses to determine if a conventional common femoral artery approach is possible or if alternative arterial access must be pursued.

Orders are written for intravenous hydration and restriction of oral intake to clear liquids or nothing by mouth for at least 6 to 8 hours prior to the procedure. In most cases no routine premedications are given on the ward. When the patient is brought to the angiography suite on a cart, the peripheral pulses are checked and marked, and premedication is given at that time. Benzodiazepines are highly effective at relieving anxiety and are quite safe. Diazepam can be slowly given intravenously at a total dose of 5 to 10 mg. Midazolam is a shorter-acting drug that can be administered either intravenously or intramuscularly; the usual dosage is 2 to 4 mg. Both drugs should be administered in small increments to avoid oversedation, and particular care must be exercised in elderly patients. Fentanyl is a short-acting (30 to 60 minutes) synthetic opiate that can be given in 50-μg increments for pain. However, respiratory depression can occur at doses as low as 50 to 100 μg.[28]

Physiologic monitoring is mandatory for those undergoing arteriography. Electrocardiography, automatic blood pressure measurement, and pulse oximetry are highly recommended. Oxygen, intubation equipment, and medications for treating possible life-threatening reactions (such as atropine, diphenhydramine, epinephrine, phentolamine, naloxone) must be at hand. Examining physicians must be familiar with cardiopulmonary resuscitation, as well as with treatment of more common untoward reactions.[29]

After arteriography the catheter is removed, and hemostasis is achieved by manual compression. It is sometimes useful to move the patient onto the transporting cart or bed prior to catheter removal, for any extra patient motion can cause puncture site bleeding. Any hematoma present should be noted in the chart and outlined in ink on the skin. The patient is instructed to remain at bedrest with the relevant extremity immobilized for a minimum of 4 hours. During this time the patient's vital signs are monitored frequently, and the peripheral pulse and puncture site are checked (e.g., every 15 minutes during the first hour after arteriography, and decreasing in frequency over the course of several hours). Intravenous hydration is continued, and oral intake is encouraged. The patient is later visited on the ward by the angiographer at the end of the working day.

Selected Problems

If a patient has a history of hypersensitivity to contrast media, one must ascertain the nature of the previous episode. Although repeated reactions do not always occur, such patients are at increased risk from contrast medium exposure.[30] Nonionic or reduced-osmolality agents are less likely to produce adverse reactions, but fatal events have also occurred with these agents.[26] For this reason, 1 to 3 days of premedication with oral corticosteroids and use of low-osmolar contrast media are advised for those patients with previous serious reactions (see the section on Risks Related to Contrast Media).[31,32]

Patients on heparin should have its administration stopped prior to arterial puncture. The effective half-life of heparin is about 90 minutes, so that active reversal of anticoagulation may not be needed in many cases.[33] Otherwise, protamine sulfate can be given by slow intravenous injection at a dose of 10 mg protamine/1000 units of heparin being neutralized.[33] The effects of heparin are reflected by prolongation of the activated partial thromboplastin time (PTT). Heparin anticoagulation should not be reinstituted for at least 1 hour after the completion of angiography.

Reversal of warfarin (Coumadin) anticoagulation is more of a problem, for the effective half-life is measured in days. If immediate arteriography is needed, fresh frozen plasma can be used to replenish the hepatic coagulation factors affected by warfarin. The prothrombin time (PT) reflects the efficacy of warfarin anticoagulation. As a rule of thumb, arteriography should be avoided if PT or PTT is more than 150% of control, or if a patient has fewer than 50,000 platelets/mm^3.

Outpatient Arteriography

Arteriography can be performed on an outpatient basis as long as the patient has no attendant major medical problems, is cooperative and reliable, and has a companion for transportation and overnight assistance, should problems arise after discharge. Standard evaluation and monitoring procedures must be arranged in a dedicated area, for example, through an ambulatory surgery service. Patients are kept supine and immobile for at least 4 hours and then engage in limited ambulation before being discharged by the angiographer. Instructions are provided for controlling recurrent bleeding and obtaining assistance for emergency problems. The patient's phone number is recorded for a follow-up call the next day. Necessity for hospital admission has been reported in 3% to 6% of those undergoing outpatient angiography.[34,35] Use of a 3 Fr catheter system may enhance safety, for Reidy and Ludman have found no significant puncture site bleeding in any of nearly 300 patients studied as outpatients.[17]

RISKS OF ARTERIOGRAPHY

The safety of arteriography has been well documented over its many years of use, but because of the invasive nature of the study and exposure of the patient to iodinated contrast media, there are real risks of major complication. The incidence of problems requiring directed therapy has been reported as 1.7%, 2.9%, 3.3%, and 7% after femoral, translumbar, axillary, and brachial artery punctures, respectively.[13,14] The 0.025% mortality rate described in the survey by Hessel and Adams resulted from arterial dissection, aneurysm rupture, vasovagal reactions, cardiac and neurologic complications, and renal failure.[13] If more than 800 arteriograms are performed annually in an institution, the rate of nonfatal complications is significantly lower than if fewer studies are performed.[13]

Direct Injury

The most common problem related to catheterization is puncture site bleeding, which may require surgical repair or transfusion. Intervention for local bleeding should be necessary in less than 1% of studies.[36] Major hematomas are more likely to occur in hypertensive patients, those undergoing catheter interventions, and patients maintained on full anticoagulation. When problems with hemostasis are anticipated, a tailored arterial compression device, such as the FemoStop (Bard, Murray Hill, N.J.), may be applied at the time of catheter removal. Such a device has also been found useful in obliterating postangiographic pseudoaneurysms using ultrasound to guide the positioning, degree, and location of compression.[37] Another hemostatic device undergoing clinical trials is an applicator that fills the subcutaneous needle tract with bovine collagen plugs prior to wire withdrawal. Early experience has shown it to be quite effective in the prevention of major bleeding.[38] Subintimal passage of the catheter or wire can produce vascular occlusion. Local endothelial trauma or catheter-related thrombi can do the same. One potentially fatal but fortunately rare complication is cholesterol embolization, which results in widespread small vessel occlusion from a shower of cholesterol crystals in patients with severe atherosclerotic disease.[39] Repeated angiography through a site recently used for catheterization (within 7 days) or leaving a sheath in place for more than 24 hours following arteriography may dispose to sepsis.[40] Thresholds for catheter-associated complications recently suggested by the Standards of Practice Committee of the Society of Cardiovascular and Interventional Radiology (depending on the specific patient populations at risk) are as follows: significant puncture site hematoma, 3%; puncture site occlusion, 0.5%; pseudoaneurysm, 0.5%; arteriovenous fistula, 0.1%; distal emboli, 0.5%; arterial dissection or subintimal passage, 2%; and subintimal injection of contrast media, 1%.[41]

Risks Related to Contrast Media
Idiosyncratic Reactions
Idiosyncratic or hypersensitivity reactions to iodinated contrast media are unpredictable and vary from sneezing, nausea and vomiting, or urticaria to laryngeal edema, cardiovascular collapse, and death. The great majority of reactions are mild and require no treatment, but severe reactions complicate about 1 study per 1000, and the risk of death ranges from 1 per 12,000 to 1 per 75,000.[31] Mild reactions can be expected in about 2% to 4% of patients exposed to conventional ionic media, with urticaria accounting for more than two thirds of the reactions.[42,43]

A history of any allergy approximately doubles the risk for adverse reaction to the contrast medium and increases the chance of severe reaction fourfold.[30] No definite dose-response effect to contrast media has been demonstrated, but there may be a positive correlation between the dose administered and severe and fatal reactions.[31] Repeated exposure in those with documented reactions to contrast produces another reaction 15% to 60% of the time, but premedication with corticosteroids and diphenhydramine can decrease this rate to less than 10%.[30]

A controlled study by Lasser and colleagues confirmed that premedication with oral methylprednisolone 32 mg given the evening before and repeated the morning of contrast injection decreased by 33% to 62% the incidence of reaction to ionic contrast agents administered intravenously.[31] Limiting premedication to a morning dose of methylprednisolone alone did not show a protective effect. A comparable reduction in risk can be produced by use of nonionic contrast media instead of the conventional ionic agents. Addition of steroid premedication for patients receiving low-osmolality contrast media has produced an even further reduction in adverse reactions.[32]

If a patient gives a history of severe hypersensitivity to contrast media, a 3-day course of premedication with oral corticosteroids is prudent. If prolonged premedication is not possible, at least one dose given 6 to 12 hours before angiography is recommended, together with use of low-osmolality contrast agents. However, one must be prepared to treat any and all reactions that might occur (Table 1-2).

Nephrotoxicity
Risk factors for renal failure after contrast administration include preexisting renal insufficiency, dehydration, diabetes mellitus, hyperuricemia, and multiple myeloma. Those patients at particular risk are diabetics with renal disease (especially if serum creatinine exceeds 3.5 mg/dl) and those with combined hepatic and renal dysfunction.[30,44,45] The reported incidence of renal dysfunction after arteriography has varied greatly, from 0.5% to 38%, reflecting differences in patient selection and criteria for renal dysfunction.[44–47] Few of those with disturbances of function have overt oliguria, and fewer still need support by hemodialysis. Any creatinine rise becomes apparent within 24 hours, peaks in several days, and usually reverses completely by 2 weeks. Nevertheless, permanent loss of renal function is a small but real risk.

Injection of contrast medium produces an initial vasodilatation that is followed by a reactive vasoconstriction in the renal circulation, an effect implicated in renal toxicity. These physiologic changes are less marked with nonionic media.[48] A drop in creatinine clearance after arteriography has been shown to be less severe and shorter in duration in patients receiving iopamidol.[49] Early clinical studies did not show any clear decrease in nephrotoxicity with the use of low-osmolality media.[44,46] However, Barrett and Carlisle have performed a metaanalysis of 31 randomized trials, and they conclude there is a significant renal protective effect of low-osmolality contrast media, particularly in patients with preexisting renal insufficiency.[50]

What is undoubtedly the most important protective measure is patient hydration. Liberal administration of intravenous and oral fluids is highly recommended unless specifically contraindicated by cardiac or other disease.[51] The amount of contrast material administered during a single study is not related to renal complications in those without underlying disease, but a dose limit of 4 ml/kg body weight is commonly observed by angiographers.[52] Furosemide and mannitol infusion have been proposed for maintaining renal blood flow and preventing toxicity, but benefit from either medication remains to be established in practice.[53] There is evidence

Table 1-2   Guide for the Treatment of Acute Reactions to Contrast Media

| Signs and Symptoms | Treatment | Treatment Dose/Route of Administration | | Treatment Interval | Treatment Precautions |
		Adults	Children		
Nausea/vomiting					
Transient	Supportive				
Severe, protracted	Prochlorperazine injectable (Compazine)	5–10 mg/IM, IV	>2 years old: 0.13 mg/kg/IM <2 years old: not recommended	Every 3–4 hr	Observe patients IV—administer slowly; drowsiness
Urticaria					
Scattered, transient	Supportive				
Scattered, protracted	Diphenhydramine injectable (Benadryl)	25–50 mg/IM, IV	1.25 mg/kg/IM, IV	Every 2–3 hr	Observe patients Drowsiness
Profound	Cimetidine injectable (Tagamet) **or**	300 mg (diluted—10 ml)/IV	5–10 mg/kg (diluted)/IV	Every 6–8 hr	Administer slowly; drowsiness
	Ranitidine injectable (Zantac)	50 mg (diluted—10 ml)/IV	Use not established	Every 6–8 hr	Administer slowly
Bronchospasm	Oxygen	3 L/min	3 L/min		
Mild–moderate	Subcutaneous epinephrine 1:1000	0.1–0.2 mg (0.1–0.2 ml)/subcutaneous	0.01–0.02 mg/kg to 0.2 mg maximum/subcutaneous	Every 10–15 min	Noncardioselective β-blockers
Accelerating, severe	IV epinephrine 1:10,000	0.1 mg (1 ml)/IV	0.01 mg/kg to 0.1 mg maximum/IV	Every 2–3 min	Administer slowly; β-blockers (especially noncardioselect)
Wheezing—protracted, isolated	Metaproterenol (Alupent) **or** Terbutaline (Brethaire) **or** Albuterol (Proventil)	2 deep inhalations (all)/ metered dose inhaler	If possible: 1 to 2 deep inhalations (all)/ metered dose inhaler	Every 4–6 hr	Proper inhalation technique (use of insert)

Hypotension					
Normal sinus rhythm, tachycardia	IV fluids (e.g., normal saline, Ringer's solution)	1–2 L/IV (rapid)	10–20 ml/kg/IV (rapid)	As per blood pressure, urine output	Fluid overload
Bradycardia	IV fluids (e.g., normal saline, Ringer's solution) **plus**	1–2 L/IV (rapid)	10–20 ml/kg/IV (rapid)	As per blood pressure, urine output	Fluid overload
	Atropine injectable	1 mg/IV (push)	0.02 mg/kg to 0.6 mg (maximum)/IV	Every 3–5 min to total 3 mg for adults or 2 mg for children	Monitor pulse rate
Seizures/convulsions					
Isolated	See hypotension				
Multiple, continuous	Diazepam injectable (Valium)	5–10 mg/IV	0.2–0.5 mg/kg/IV	Every 20 min	Respiratory depression

Reproduced with permission from Bush, WH, Swanson, DP: Acute Reactions to Intravascular Contrast Media: Types, Risk Factors, Recognition, and Specific Treatment. *Am J Roentgenol* 1991; 157:1153–1161.

36. Waugh JR, Sacharias N: Arteriographic complications in the DSA era. *Radiology* 1992; 182:243–246.
37. Trerotola SO, Savader SJ, Prescott CA, Osterman FA: US-guided pseudo-aneurysm repair with a compression device. *Radiology* 1993; 189:285–286.
38. Schräder R, Steinbacher S, Burger W, et al: Collagen application for sealing of arterial puncture sites in comparison to pressure dressing: A randomized trial. *Cathet Cardiovasc Diagn* 1992; 27:298–302.
39. Fine MJ, Kapoor W, Falanga V: Cholesterol crystal embolization: A review of 221 cases in the English literature. *Angiology* 1987; 38:769–784.
40. McCready RA, Siderys H, Pittman JN, et al: Septic complications after cardiac catheterization and percutaneous transluminal coronary angioplasty. *J Vasc Surg* 1991; 14:170–174.
41. Standards of Practice Committee of the Society of Cardiovascular and Interventional Radiology: Standard for diagnostic arteriography in adults. *J Vasc Interv Radiol* 1993; 4:385–395.
42. Shehadi WH, Toniolo G: Adverse reactions to contrast media: A report from the Committee on Safety of Contrast Media of the International Society of Radiology. *Radiology* 1980; 137:299–302.
43. Sigstedt B, Lunderquist A: Complications of angiographic examinations. *Am J Roentgenol* 1978; 130:455–460.
44. Parfrey PS, Griffiths SM, Barrett BJ, et al: Contrast material–induced renal failure in patients with diabetes mellitus, renal insufficiency, or both: A prospective controlled study. *N Engl J Med* 1989; 320:143–149.
45. Swartz RD, Rubin JE, Leeming BW, Silva P: Renal failure following major angiography. *Am J Med* 1978; 65:31–37.
46. Gomes AS, Lois JF, Baker JD, et al: Acute renal dysfunction in high-risk patients after angiography: Comparison of ionic and nonionic contrast media. *Radiology* 1989; 170:65–68.
47. Mason RA, Arbeit LA, Giron F: Renal dysfunction after arteriography. *JAMA* 1985; 253:1001–1004.
48. Golman K, Almén T: Contrast media–induced nephrotoxicity: Survey and present state. *Invest Radiol* 1985; 21:S92–S97.
49. Katholi RE, Taylor GJ, Woods WT, et al: Nephrotoxicity of nonionic low-osmolality versus ionic high-osmolality contrast media: A prospective double-blind randomized comparison in human beings. *Radiology* 1993; 186:183–187.
50. Barrett BJ, Carlisle EJ: Metaanalysis of the relative nephrotoxicity of high-osmolality and low-osmolality iodinated contrast media. *Radiology* 1993; 188:171–178.
51. Eisenberg RL, Bank WO, Hedgock MW: Renal failure after major angiography can be avoided with hydration. *Am J Roentgenol* 1981; 136:859–861.
52. Miller DL, Chang R, Wells WT, et al: Intravascular contrast media: Effect of dose on renal function. *Radiology* 1988; 167:607–611.
53. Cruz C, Hricak H, Samhouri F, et al: Contrast media for angiography: Effect on renal function. *Radiology* 1986; 158:109–112.
54. Hans B, Singh HS, Mittal VK, et al: Renal functional response to dopamine during and after arteriography in patients with chronic renal insufficiency. *Radiology* 1990; 176:651–654.

2

Angiography of the Abdominal Aorta, Pelvis, and Lower Extremities

KEY CONCEPTS

1. Arteriography remains the simplest, most reliable examination for precisely defining the extent of aortic and lower extremity vascular disease.
2. Digital subtraction angiography, intraarterial injection of vasodilators, reactive hyperemia, and distal catheter placement are used to optimize distal vessel filling.
3. Abdominal aortic aneurysms are studied preoperatively to establish the relationship of renal arteries to the aneurysm, the state of the mesenteric circulation, and involvement of the iliac or common femoral arteries.
4. Aneurysms are prone to rupture, occlusion, and distal embolization.
5. Vascular grafts should be studied at the first sign of any problem.
6. Arteriography is highly accurate for study of traumatic vascular injury but is rarely needed in the absence of specific signs.

INDICATIONS

Abdominal aortography and lower extremity runoff arteriography are the "bread and butter" of the peripheral angiographer. Despite recent improvements and innovations in the noninvasive evaluation of lower extremity vascular disease, angiography with contrast material remains the definitive diagnostic measure before surgery or transluminal intervention. Symptomatic peripheral vascular disease, whether occlusive or aneurysmal, continues to afflict 2% to 3% of men and 1% of women above the age of 60.[1] Aside from this large population of patients, arteriography of the lower extremities is often needed in evaluation of severe pelvic or extremity injuries, both penetrating and nonpenetrating, and a variety of less common disorders such as tumors, arteriovenous malformations, thromboangiitis obliterans, frostbite, popliteal entrapment syndrome, and cystic adventitial disease.

ARTERIAL APPROACH

Common Femoral Artery

The standard approach for abdominal aortography and lower extremity angiography is common femoral artery catheterization. Assuming femoral pulses are present, the femoral approach has the advantage of providing optimal opacification of vessels at lowest risk. After abdominal aortography, the flush catheter is withdrawn to the aortic bifurcation so that injection of contrast material fills the runoff vessels bilaterally, with little of the injected volume diverted to the kidneys or viscera outside the field of interest. In general, the side with the strongest femoral pulse is chosen for arterial catheterization, but there are certain advantages to entry in the more symptomatic side (see the section on Common Femoral Artery Puncture in Chapter 1 entitled Basic Principles of Arteriography).

Alternatives in the Face of Occlusive Disease

When femoral pulses are lacking, catheterization may be attempted through an axillary artery or a brachial artery or by a translumbar approach. Upper extremity arterial access allows catheters to be placed selectively when needed. However, in older patients with tortuous vessels, it may be very difficult to direct a catheter into the descending thoracic aorta. The left upper extremity should always be preferred, to minimize the possibility of embolic stroke. Translumbar aortography does not allow selective placement of the catheter, but it is a reliable method that has a somewhat lower complication rate than upper extremity arterial puncture.[2] Both approaches are fraught with hazard in the presence of poorly controlled hypertension or coagulation disorder. Because major hemorrhage can occur without early warning signs, particular care must be taken in selecting patients for translumbar study (for more details about arterial access, see Chapter 1 entitled Basic Principles of Angiography).

When a vascular bypass graft is present, direct entry should be avoided if there is a pulse in the opposite groin. However, grafts may be punctured at no great risk as long as dilators are used and the catheter is manipulated and removed over a guidewire.[3] Among those needing direct graft entry are patients with aortobifemoral or axillofemoral bypasses.

Obtaining Optimal Distal Vessel Opacification

With the increased use of saphenous vein bypass grafting for disease below the knee (which marks the practical limit for the use of synthetic materials), there is need to obtain good preoperative definition of the runoff vessels in the distal calf, ankle, and foot.[4,5] Patency of the distal vessels is predictive of subsequent graft patency.[6] Conventional filming and contrast medium injections at the aortic bifurcation yield inadequate images in approximately one quarter of distal arterial examinations.[7] For this reason various techniques have been used to improve filling of distal arteries in the face of occlusive disease.

Digital Subtraction Angiography

One of the simplest measures to apply is digital subtraction angiography (DSA). When conventional films are insufficient, the foot (or the fluoroscopy C-arm) can be rotated into a lateral projection and a 6-inch or 10-inch fluoroscopic field centered over the talus. A total injection of 20 to 25 ml of contrast material (300 mg iodine/ml) usually provides the arterial detail needed. Digital subtraction has been shown to be superior to conventional film angiography in this clinical setting.[7,8]

Reactive Hyperemia

If DSA alone fails to demonstrate distal anatomy, vasodilatation may be produced by various means. Placement of an occlusive cuff on the thigh with inflation above arterial pressure for 7 minutes produces a reactive hyperemia immediately after cuff deflation. Flow becomes more rapid, and vascular opacification improves in nearly 90% of patients.[9] Although this technique is quite safe, it lengthens the procedure, can be quite uncomfortable for the patient, and does carry a finite risk of producing vascular occlusion. Compression of a bypass graft must be avoided.[10]

Vasodilators and Other Measures

Tolazoline has long been used as an adjunct to arteriography. It is a potent vasodilator with a duration of action of several minutes when injected intraarterially. It is customarily given at a dose of 25 to 50 mg diluted in 10 ml of saline, and injected slowly through the catheter immediately prior to filming. The presence of heart disease is a contraindication to the use of tolazoline, for the drug has the potential of inducing hypotension, tachycardia, arrhythmias, and myocardial infarction.[11]

A safe alternative medication is dilute nitroglycerin. Injected into the arterial catheter as a bolus of 200 µg in 10 ml of saline just prior to contrast material injection, nitroglycerin is more effective than tolazoline in producing vasodilatation, and it is approximately equivalent in effect to reactive hyperemia.[12] Extrinsic warming of the feet and legs is also valuable in obtaining distal vascular opacification.[11]

When all other measures fail and the decision must be made to amputate or place a graft, antegrade catheterization of the superficial femoral artery with injection of contrast material directly into the popliteal artery may be appropriate.[11] If long occlusions are present in the iliac arteries with poor collateral flow through the pelvis, puncture of the common femoral artery on the symptomatic side allows a greater concentration of contrast medium to reach the distal arteries. Failure to show arterial fill despite all these measures generally means the distal vessels are occluded. However, there are preliminary indications that magnetic resonance arteriography (MRA) may be more sensitive for defining distal runoff vessels, and MRA may supplement or replace some conventional arteriographic studies.[13] As a last resort, arteriography can be performed during surgery, with the advantages of direct vascular access and higher-dose injection while the patient is heavily sedated or under general anesthesia.[6]

Proper length of filming time is important when evaluating distal disease by catheter arteriography, up to 50 or 60 seconds in extreme cases. When reactive hyperemia or vasodilatation is used, contrast material injection rates should be increased, and any filming delay must be shortened; the time needed for contrast medium to appear in the distal vessels may be substantially decreased with these techniques.[9]

FILMING ALTERNATIVES

Step-Table Angiography

Step-tables have been widely employed in lower extremity arteriography. When conventional films are used, contrast material injections and table steps can be combined in a variety of ways. One may choose to use the table step during the abdominal aortic run to also obtain views of the pelvis. The runoff vessels may then be filmed over three or four stations during a subsequent injection of contrast medium. During translumbar angiography, a single injection may be made with filming at four different stations, from the abdominal aorta to the level of the knees. Filming routines may be easily adapted to suit the particular patient or the angiographer's preference.

A technique that has led to satisfactory results—with repeated injections (for failure in filling or film timing) needed in fewer than 10% of patients examined—starts with a single-stage set of exposures of the abdominal aorta. The pigtail catheter is placed at the level of the renal arteries in order to prevent major reflux into celiac or superior mesenteric artery branches. Contrast medium is injected at 20 ml/second for 2 seconds, while films are obtained at a rate of two exposures per second for 3 seconds, followed by one exposure per second for 6 more seconds. This program allows the kidneys to be evaluated through their nephrographic phase.

After aortic filming is complete, the catheter is withdrawn to the distal abdominal aorta, which leaves the sideholes superior to the aortic bifurcation. A long injection of a large volume of contrast medium is programmed, with the flow gauged by a hand test injection under fluoroscopic guidance. A typical injection in a 60-year-old man might be 7 ml/second for a total of 12 seconds. After a filming delay of 3 seconds, the first three exposures are obtained at the pelvis at one exposure per second. The table moves and two films are exposed at the level of the thighs, followed by a second step and four film exposures at the knees. After the third step, filming is slowed to one exposure every 2 seconds for six films at the level of the calf. If the very distal vessels of the ankle and foot must be imaged (as in the case of diabetics, patients with rest pain, or those with ulceration or gangrene), a fifth station can be added to the run.

With a step-table angiogram, timing is critical. A long, high-volume injection provides a good margin for error. With this program, it is impossible for the injected contrast medium to "get ahead" of filming, because the injection finishes only at the time exposures are being made at the popliteal level. A filming delay is set to allow adequate pelvic arterial opacification. A longer delay may be needed for patients with severe occlusive disease, poor cardiac output, or large aneurysms.

While the films are being developed, DSA may be used expeditiously to "fill in" regions of interest. Areas that often merit imaging in more than one projection include the iliac arteries, the common femoral bifurcations, renal artery origins, and graft anastomoses.

Digital Subtraction Runoff Technique

If a large image intensifier (14-inch diameter) is available, DSA may be used for complete lower extremity arteriography. For most systems presently installed, only a single field may be imaged during one injection. A DSA study has the advantage that one may observe in real time the arrival of contrast medium and the adequacy of filling. Because table position does not change during a run, individual injection volumes may be kept to a minimum (for example, 14 ml injected over 2 seconds for popliteal filming).

Because of edge cutoff with the round field of view of DSA, it is sometimes advisable to examine the lower extremities separately in larger patients. A greater segment of the leg can be imaged, limiting the amount of overlap necessary between fields. Also, it is easier to set proper exposure factors when examining a single leg than if both legs (including a radiolucent gap) are viewed together. Exposure factors can also constrain DSA study of the abdomen or pelvis in large patients, limiting the degree of obliquity or the frame rate that can be achieved.

Although individual injection volumes are smaller with DSA, the total amount of contrast medium used does not differ greatly from that given during step-table film runoff angiography. Because of the multiple table positionings and repeated injections of contrast material needed, the duration of a DSA study is also not substantially different. In lower extremity angiography the technique chosen depends on the equipment installed, preference of the angiographer, and acceptability of images to referring clinicians.

The newly introduced technique of digital "bolus chasing" available on some of the newer angiographic units being sold combines the advantages of digital angiography and step-table methods.[14] Table movement can be modified during the angiographic run, while the arterial advance of contrast medium is continuously observed on the fluoroscopic monitor. In some patients masks can be obtained either immediately before or immediately after the contrast images are obtained, allowing the generation of subtraction images.

Use of Multiple Projections

Atherosclerosis does not produce uniform concentric stenoses. If a plaque is located on the posterior wall of the aorta or common iliac artery, it may be poorly appreciated on the anteroposterior (AP) projection. Biplane aortography is absolutely necessary in cases of lower extremity embolization or abdominal aortic aneurysm (AAA). In suspected embolization, an irregular or ulcerated plaque can be the source of embolized clot, and such a plaque must be diligently sought. The lateral projection is invaluable in evaluating aneurysms, for it most easily demonstrates the neck of the aneurysm, as well as its relationship to the renal arteries.

Use of both oblique views for pelvic angiography improves detection of plaque and the grading of stenosis severity in more than a third of patients with significant atherosclerosis.[15] The right posterior oblique projection best profiles the origin of the right internal iliac artery and left deep femoral artery. The left posterior oblique does the same for the contralateral vessels (Fig. 2-1). Multiple views must absolutely be obtained whenever symptoms or noninvasive pressure measurements indicate more severe disease than that apparent on AP angiography. Some newer angio-

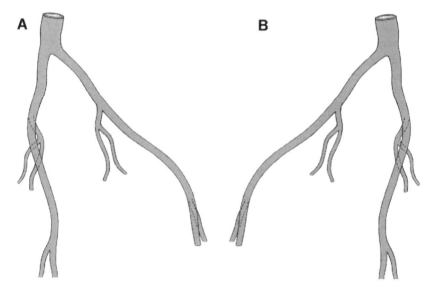

Fig. 2-1 **A,** In the left posterior oblique view of the pelvis, the left common iliac and right common femoral artery bifurcations are displayed without overlap. **B,** The right posterior oblique view is best for observing the bifurcations of the opposite vessels.

graphic units allow continuous gantry rotation and acquisition of digital images (with or without subtraction). Such rotational angiography has obvious advantages in the evaluation of pelvic arteries.

POINTS OF ANATOMY

The abdominal aorta bifurcates at the level of L3, and its branches, the common iliac arteries, are of variable length (Fig. 2-2). The internal iliac (hypogastric) artery divides into a posterior trunk, which gives off the superior gluteal, iliolumbar, and lateral sacral arteries, and an anterior trunk, which supplies the pelvic viscera, including urinary bladder, rectosigmoid colon, and uterus. The external iliac arteries have no major branches except in the region of the inguinal ligament, where the inferior epigastric and deep circumflex iliac arteries arise.

The common femoral artery (Fig. 2-3) normally bifurcates near the inferior margin of the femoral head, but occasionally the point of division is several centimeters more cephalad. The profunda femoris (deep femoral artery) provides major branches about the femoral neck (medial and lateral femoral circumflex arteries) as well as large muscular branches to the upper and middle thigh. The superficial femoral artery (SFA) extends to the adductor canal, at which point it becomes the popliteal artery. The SFA has no major branches in the absence of obstructive disease.

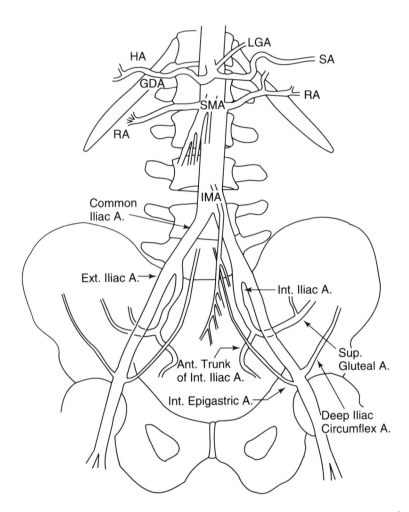

Fig. 2-2 Anatomy of the abdominal aorta and iliac arteries. *GDA,* gastroduodenal artery; *HA,* hepatic artery; *IMA,* inferior mesenteric artery; *LGA,* left gastric
artery; *RA,* renal artery; *SA,* splenic artery; *SMA,* superior mesenteric artery.

The popliteal artery gives off the anterior tibial artery near the head of
the fibula, as well as the tibioperoneal trunk. The latter vessel divides into
the posterior tibial and peroneal (fibular) arteries. The anterior tibial artery
angles laterally and then curves inferiorly to cross the interosseous membrane, forming a characteristic "knee." The vessel gradually swings medially near the ankle and continues into the foot as the dorsalis pedis. The
tibioperoneal trunk continues the axis of the popliteal artery, and the peroneal artery is the more lateral of its branches. The posterior tibial artery

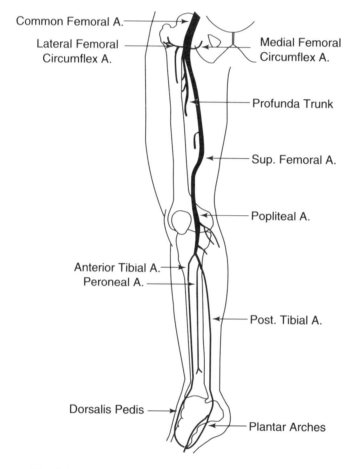

Common Femoral A.

Lateral Femoral Circumflex A.

Medial Femoral Circumflex A.

Profunda Trunk

Sup. Femoral A.

Popliteal A.

Anterior Tibial A.

Peroneal A.

Post. Tibial A.

Dorsalis Pedis

Plantar Arches

Fig. 2-3 Anatomy of arterial supply to the lower extremity.

courses into the foot, where it becomes the plantar arch. The peroneal artery is not directly continuous with any major pedal vessel, but it supplies lateral and medial malleolar arteries, which may become important collateral pathways.

Major Collateral Pathways

In the face of abdominal aortic occlusion, the lower intercostal and lumbar arteries dilate and supply blood to the pelvis and lower extremities by way of internal iliac branches (iliolumbar and superior and middle gluteal arteries) or over the abdominal wall by way of the inferior epigastric and deep iliac circumflex arteries. The inferior mesenteric artery, by virtue of the anastomoses between its superior hemorrhoidal (rectal) branches with the inferior hemorrhoidal arteries, can be a major source of collateral perfusion. In some cases, distal flow is maintained by way of the anterior abdominal wall through internal thoracic (mammary) artery–inferior epigastric artery communications.

In iliac or common femoral artery occlusive disease, the internal iliac branches often play a crucial role. The gluteal and obturator arteries serve as bridges connecting with the lateral and medial femoral circumflex arteries. In unilateral obstruction there are multiple pathways through pelvic branches of the internal iliac.

Perhaps the single most critical vessel for the preservation of distal perfusion in the leg is the profunda femoris. Muscular branches provide fill of the distal SFA or popliteal artery in the presence of SFA obstruction. Because the origin of the profunda femoris is prone to stenosis and this area is poorly seen on an AP projection, the femoral bifurcation should be studied in more than one view.

Geniculate branches form a frame about the knee joint and are important pathways when popliteal flow is obstructed. At the ankle, the three runoff arteries communicate through malleolar vessels. Additional distal anastomoses connect the dorsalis pedis to the plantar arch.

Variants

The sciatic artery, a rare and sometimes perplexing variant, represents the failure of regression of a primitive fetal vessel.[16] The proximal portion of the sciatic artery normally is incorporated into the inferior gluteal artery. More distal segments become parts of the popliteal and peroneal arteries. The external iliac, common artery, and SFA may be occluded, small, or normal in size when a persistent sciatic artery is present. The internal iliac artery is large and does not taper in a normal fashion, and a large branch takes a lateral course at the femoral head. The persistent sciatic artery tends to be ectatic, and it joins the distal SFA by taking a medial bend near the adductor canal. Patients with a sciatic artery often present with claudication, but nearly half of those with symptoms have aneurysmal dilatation in the gluteal segment of the vessel.[16] Because flow is typically slow, care must be taken to extend filming for a sufficient duration if the diagnosis is suspected.

Both the branching and the size of the trifurcation vessels of the calf are subject to variation. Occasionally, a true trifurcation is present, and all three vessels arise from the terminal popliteal artery. In other individuals the anterior tibial artery may originate above the knee from the proximal popliteal. Rarely, the posterior tibial may be the first terminal branch of the popliteal, with the peroneal and anterior tibial arteries sharing a common trunk. Although the posterior tibial artery is the primary runoff vessel in most adults, either of the other calf arteries may be dominant on a congenital basis.

MANIFESTATIONS OF ATHEROSCLEROSIS

Atherocclusive Disease

Patients with signs of peripheral atherosclerosis have a 24% risk of developing critical lower limb ischemia within 5 years.[17] However, because atherosclerosis is a systemic disease, death from myocardial infarction or cerebrovascular accident is more likely than limb loss. Many patients with symptomatic claudication benefit from a structured exercise program. It is those with persistent limiting symptoms, rest pain, or nonhealing ulcers who require runoff arteriography to define the precise morphology of disease prior to surgical or percutaneous transluminal revascularization.

Occlusive atherosclerotic disease tends to follow characteristic patterns. It may primarily affect the infrarenal abdominal aorta and common iliac arteries, sparing more distal vessels. In men this is manifested by the classic Leriche's syndrome of thigh and buttock claudication accompanied by impotence. A similar distribution of lesions may be seen in relatively young women who smoke and have small aortoiliac vessels.[18] The greatest danger of aortic occlusion is from thrombus extension above the level of the renal arteries, which can lead to renal failure and even mesenteric infarction.

In other patients the vessels affected most severely are the SFA or the more distal arteries in the calf. Diabetics tend to have disease involving medium and small arteries, but they are subject to severe diffuse atherosclerosis of larger vessels as well.

Atherosclerotic plaques are characteristically irregular and eccentric; however, short, smooth, concentric lesions and membranes are also seen. Ulceration may be suspected by an excavated appearance to a plaque, but this is more properly a histologic diagnosis. Uncommonly, lesions may grossly project into the vessel lumen, simulating clot or another filling defect. By contrast, thrombus may form either upstream or downstream of a significant stenosis. Atherosclerosis is likely to produce diffuse plaque, and arteries in the vicinity of occlusions or stenoses rarely have entirely smooth lumens of normal caliber.

A positive diagnosis of arterial embolus is possible only when an intraluminal thrombus is uncovered in an otherwise unremarkable vessel. A convex margin to a vascular occlusion is not alone sufficient to make the diagnosis of embolism because in situ thrombosis can have an identical appearance. Most peripheral emboli arise from the heart, but aortic, iliac, and femoral plaques may also be to blame. One should also not forget the (unlikely) possibility of paradoxic venous embolization through a patent foramen ovale. Patients with paradoxic embolization tend also to have symptoms of pulmonary embolism and elevated right-heart pressures.[19] Echocardiography and lower extremity duplex sonography are useful for detection of right-to-left shunting and lower extremity venous thrombosis.

No matter where they originate, arterial emboli tend to lodge at arterial bifurcations, where the vessel lumen tapers. "Blue toe" syndrome is one manifestation of peripheral embolization.

Aneurysms

The second major manifestation of atherosclerosis is aneurysmal disease, and the most common site of involvement is the infrarenal abdominal aorta. Such AAAs are typically fusiform, have a well-defined neck arising distal to the origin of the renal artery, and often extend directly into the common iliac arteries. Aortoiliac aneurysms sometimes are continuous with internal iliac aneurysms. Extension into the external iliacs is distinctly unusual.

Risks of Abdominal Aortic Aneurysm

The overriding concern with aneurysms of any sort is rupture. Distal embolization is a serious complication that occurs less frequently. An unusual form of rupture is development of an aortocaval fistula. Such patients may present with lower extremity edema and high-output cardiac failure.

The risk of AAA rupture is estimated to be 10% for those up to 4 cm in diameter, 25% for those between 4 and 7 cm in diameter, and even higher for those larger than 7 cm.[20] Elective surgery is generally recommended for all symptomatic aneurysms and for asymptomatic aneurysms larger than 6 cm in diameter, because the mortality of elective repair is under 5% but emergency surgery for rupture carries a 50% risk of death.[20] Standard treatment involves resection and graft replacement. Nonresective treatment, ligation with extraanatomic bypass, is an option for high-risk patients, but it can result in severe late morbidity.[21]

Role of Aortography

The role of angiography has been curtailed in establishing the diagnosis of AAA. Because many aortic aneurysms are lined by mural clot, aortography is not especially useful for showing the true size of a lesion. Ultrasonography, computed tomographic scan, and magnetic resonance imaging (MRI) are superior in this regard, and ultrasound is the procedure of choice for following aneurysm growth. However, study with contrast material continues to have certain advantages over cross-sectional imaging. Aortography more precisely defines the relationship of the renal arteries to the aneurysm, delineates mesenteric perfusion, and is considered essential for preoperative planning by many surgeons. The newer techniques of spiral computed tomography (CT) angiography and magnetic resonance angiography show promise, and they may soon replace conventional preoperative aortography for some patients.[22,23]

The surgical approach may be modified by angiographic findings. Rösch and colleagues determined that important surgical decisions were made on the basis of aortography in 75 of 100 patients studied.[24] Particular problems are posed by aberrant renal arteries, suprarenal aneurysm extension, renal or mesenteric artery stenosis, and continued patency of the inferior mesenteric artery (IMA). The IMA is occluded in the great majority of AAAs, but failure to recognize that the vessel is patent may result in failure to reimplant it surgically, with consequent mesenteric ischemia. Postoperative visceral infarction complicates fewer than 3% of aneurysm repairs, but when it does occur, mortality is high.[20,24]

Technique of Examination
When examining an AAA, biplane aortography must be performed. The catheter should be placed above the level of the celiac axis in order to fill all abdominal visceral arteries. The lateral projection is essential for demonstrating the celiac axis, as well as the proximal superior mesenteric artery and IMA (Fig. 2-4). It is also useful for showing the number and location of renal arteries. Filming is extended through at least 12 seconds to allow renal perfusion and possible mesenteric collateral circulation to be assessed. The pelvic arteries and common femorals should also be studied in two planes to exclude aneurysms or occlusive disease in these vessels.

If the renal arteries are not delineated or the IMA is not filled, the catheter may be withdrawn into the neck or body of the aneurysm itself and the study repeated. Injection proximal to a large aneurysm often results in dependent layering of contrast medium, and the catheter may appear to be extravascular on the lateral projection. Power injection into an aneurysm does not pose undue risk to the patient, while it does provide the best opportunity to show small aberrant renal vessels and a patent IMA.

Aortic Ulcers, Inflammatory and Mycotic Abdominal Aortic Aneurysms
Penetrating aortic ulcers are characterized by a discrete ulcer crater and thickened aortic wall. They may be present within an aneurysm at the time of detection. Even when they are not, aneurysmal disease may be present in other segments of the aorta. The natural history of these lesions is one of progressive aortic enlargement resulting in either saccular or fusiform aneurysm.[25] Distal embolization may occur, but dissection is rare.

Inflammatory aneurysms are associated with marked mural thickening of the aorta and retroperitoneal adhesions. Up to 10% of AAAs may show inflammatory components, but the diagnosis cannot be made angiographically.[26] Computed tomographic scan is capable of showing retroperitoneal fibrotic plaque in this condition and is also useful in cases of suspected

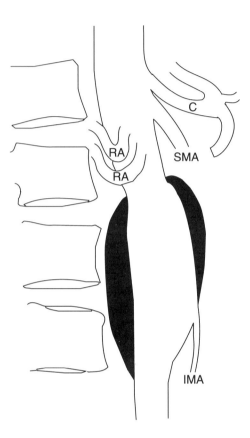

Fig. 2-4 Lateral view of an abdominal aortic aneurysm. Shaded portion repre-sents mural thrombus. *C*, celiac axis; *IMA*, inferior mesenteric artery; *RA*, renal arteries; *SMA*, superior mesenteric artery.

leaking aneurysm because it can demonstrate periaortic or retroperitoneal hematoma. It is extraordinarily rare to show leakage by means of an aor-togram. If brisk bleeding is suspected, a patient is best taken immediately to the operative suite without expending time for diagnostic imaging.

Mycotic aneurysms are distinct from inflammatory aneurysms. When they involve the abdominal aorta, the clinical presentation may include fever and back pain. Nevertheless, blood cultures are often negative. Angiographically, mycotic aneurysms are typically eccentric, irregular, and arise from an otherwise nondilated segment of aorta.[27] On CT or MR studies, a noncalcified mass with an enhancing rim may be present. Mortality is high, and surgical resection is indicated, even for small lesions.

Iliac and Peripheral Aneurysms
Aneurysms of the iliac arteries constitute about 2% of all intraabdominal aneurysms and are usually associated with aortic aneurysms.[28] One third of iliac lesions are isolated, and because they tend to be asymptomatic or produce nonspecific complaints, many are not found until rupture. For this reason, some surgeons recommend repair of any lesion larger than 3 cm in diameter.[28]

Atherosclerotic aneurysms also frequently affect the common femoral and popliteal arteries. Less common sites include the SFA and adductor canal. Diffuse vascular ectasia (arteriomegaly) is another unusual expression of aneurysmal disease. When a large aneurysm or diffuse ectasia is present, contrast medium injection and filming must be prolonged because of the extremely slow flow that may be encountered.

A particular risk of popliteal artery aneurysm is repeated embolization to the small vessels of the calf. Such emboli often lead to amputation if their source is not recognized and treated. Although only 18% to 31% of patients with popliteal aneurysms ever develop symptoms, surgery is advocated for even asymptomatic lesions because of high morbidity and limb loss in patients presenting with acute complications.[29] Local thrombolytic infusion may improve outcome in those with acute thrombosis of a popliteal aneurysm and no visible runoff vessels.[29] More often than not, popliteal lesions are bilateral, and an AAA is commonly present; ultrasonography is recommended to assess possible multivessel aneurysmal disease.

Bypass Grafts
Autologous vein, umbilical vein, and synthetic bypass grafts have become mainstays of vascular surgery. Common types of grafts seen in the abdomen, pelvis, and lower extremities (described by proximal and distal anastomoses) include aortic tube, aortobiiliac, aortobifemoral, axillofemoral, femorofemoral (crossover), femoropopliteal, and femorodistal bypasses. Each graft has an expected long-term patency, which depends on location, graft material, and certain host factors (e.g., patency of distal vessels).

Graft Stenosis and Thrombosis
Acute graft thrombosis can be approached by infusion of thrombolytic enzymes, aspiration thrombectomy, or surgical thrombectomy (see Chapter 11 entitled Local Thrombolytic Infusion). In most cases an underlying abnormality also needs correction by surgical revision or percutaneous angioplasty. However, detecting and repairing an abnormality before occlusion occurs can substantially improve subsequent patency of a graft.[30] For this reason, angiography is indicated as soon as noninvasive

studies or symptoms indicate a problem. Because many potential problems can be uncovered soon after surgery, some advocate routine postoperative intravenous DSA for patients undergoing graft placement.[31] A less invasive study that would likely be more acceptable to patients is duplex ultrasonography. It can detect the majority of graft stenoses even before they become evident by segmental blood pressure measurements.[32,33] At the University of Wisconsin–Madison magnetic resonance angiography has also been used to monitor bypass grafts, but its role in follow-up remains to be established. Early graft occlusion (within 30 days) is commonly due to a problem in surgical technique, and surgical revision is indicated. Later graft stenoses are typically the result of fibrointimal hyperplasia, which tends to occur at anastomoses, and many such stenoses can be treated by percutaneous balloon angioplasty.[34]

Other Complications
Other assorted complications of bypass graft include infection (of prosthetic grafts), pseudoaneurysms, and, in the case of in situ saphenous grafts, arteriovenous fistulas due to unligated perforating veins. In situ saphenous vein grafts, unlike reversed saphenous grafts, are not completely mobilized. Rather, only the ends of the vein are freed and anastomosed to donor and recipient arteries, their valves are disrupted by a valvulotome, and communicating perforators are ligated. An in situ graft is more technically demanding for the surgeon, but there have been reports of improved patency and limb-salvage rates for femorodistal grafts.[35] However, an ongoing cooperative study by Veterans Administration hospitals has failed to confirm any advantage to in situ grafts thus far.[4]

Leaking Anastomoses and Arterioenteric Fistulae
A serious problem with infected grafts is the development of an arterioenteric fistula. It is most likely to affect the third portion of the duodenum and an adjacent infected aortic graft.[36] The most direct diagnostic study is endoscopy, but if endoscopy is impossible or inconclusive, aortography may sometimes demonstrate focal irregularity or ulceration at the anastomotic site. Unfortunately, angiography is usually not helpful in detecting a fistula or an anastomotic disruption. Computed tomography is a more productive examination, for it may uncover retroperitoneal hemorrhage or an abscess adjacent to or surrounding the graft.

Special Examination Techniques
If a failing femoropopliteal or femorodistal graft cannot be visualized by conventional arteriography, the patient may be given heparin, and a catheter is positioned at the proximal anastomosis. Sprayregen and associates found that a number of grafts were obstructed, but not actually throm-

bosed, when they were injected directly.[37] For grafts that cross the knee joint, examination of the patient in a lateral projection with the knee extended, partially flexed, and fully flexed has been recommended.[38] Kinks or loops found in flexion have been correlated with subsequent graft occlusion. Axillofemoral grafts are most easily examined by direct puncture. The proximal anastomosis can be demonstrated by either retrograde catheter placement to the anastomosis or brief manual compression of the graft during contrast material injection.

OTHER CONDITIONS

Thromboangiitis Obliterans and Various Lesions

Thromboangiitis obliterans or Buerger's disease is an uncommon inflammatory vasculitis of unknown cause, usually limited to the small and medium-sized vessels of the extremities.[39] It is an obliterating process that produces intimal hyperplasia and thrombosis. There is a strong association with smoking, and those affected are predominantly men 30 to 50 years of age. Patients may complain of claudication, thrombophlebitis, acral ulceration, and intense pain. The condition is characterized by exacerbations and remissions, and the upper extremities are frequently involved. Raynaud's phenomenon is commonly observed. Many eventually need amputation to some extent, but mortality is not increased. Thromboangiitis obliterans is distinctive in sparing the coronary and cerebral circulations.[39] Acute episodes are treated by antiinflammatory medications and anticoagulation. Bypass surgery has disappointing long-term results in these patients.[40] The most important factor in effective long-term treatment is cessation of smoking by the patient.

The majority of cases show bilateral lower extremity involvement with segmental occlusions, sharp cutoffs, tortuous (corkscrew) collateral vessels, and, at times, vasospasm and arteriovenous shunting. Recanalization may produce "direct collaterals." Unlike atherosclerotic disease, thromboangiitis obliterans shows relatively normal vascular segments between areas of disease ("skip" lesions). Occasionally the iliac arteries and aorta may be affected, and the angiographic findings may be equivocal. The diagnosis is best made histologically by punch biopsy, but biopsy itself may initiate ulceration.

The use of ergot alkaloids for migraine headache or poisoning with the toxin of the fungus *Claviceps purpurea* can produce diffuse or segmental arterial spasm and lower extremity ischemia.[41] The narrowing seen on arteriography is smooth and may reverse with time. Takayasu's arteritis may compromise the abdominal aorta and is usually confined to its proximal portion.[42] Fibromuscular disease has been found in the iliac arteries, the third most common site of involvement.[43] The angiographic appearance is similar to that of lesions in the renal or carotid arteries. Frostbite or electrical injury can cause vascular occlusion, and angiography may be necessary to select a level for amputation.

Popliteal Entrapment Syndrome

The popliteal artery normally courses between the medial and lateral heads of the gastrocnemius muscle. If the vessel takes an anomalous route medial to the tibial head of the muscle or if abnormal fascial slips are present, the popliteal artery may be subject to compression.[44] When compression causes claudication or thrombosis, the syndrome is termed *popliteal entrapment.* Those typically affected are active men of heavy build between 20 and 40 years of age.

Classical angiographic findings are medial deviation of the popliteal artery and stenosis. Unfortunately, no narrowing or abnormal course may be evident in many with the clinical sydrome.[45] A combination of passive dorsiflexion of the foot with active plantar flexion against resistance elicits marked narrowing or occlusion. Poststenotic dilatation, mural irregularity, or aneurysm may also be observed, and the condition is very often bilateral. Although false-positive noninvasive studies have been reported, duplex sonography, CT scan, and MRI (including magnetic resonance angiography) may play an increasing role in evaluation.[44]

Cystic Adventitial Disease

Another cause of claudication, predominantly in young men, is cystic adventitial disease. Arterial compromise of the popliteal artery results from compression by a unicameral or multilocular cyst of the vessel wall. The cause of the cyst is unclear, but microtrauma or congenital mucous cell rests may be responsible. Symptoms may be sudden in onset, and confusion with popliteal entrapment syndrome is not unusual.[46] Ultrasonography and CT scan have been of value in making the diagnosis.[47,48] Angiography demonstrates a smooth, scalloped, or hourglass-shaped narrowing of the popliteal artery without poststenotic dilatation.

Tumors and Arteriovenous Malformations

Osseous and soft tissue tumors are diagnosed by plain radiography, scintigraphy, CT scan, ultrasonography, or MRI. Angiography is reserved for preoperative evaluation, defining tumor vascularity and feeding vessels. In selected cases treatment may call for local arterial infusion of chemotherapeutic agents or embolization (see Chapter 12 entitled Embolotherapy).

Congenital arteriovenous (AV) malformations of the pelvis and extremities can cause bleeding, ulceration, and disfigurement. They may behave in a quite malignant fashion, requiring extensive surgery or amputation for control. Unfortunately, many recur after treatment. As in malignant tumors, arteriography serves to define the vascular anatomy prior to surgery, or it may be used to palliate by injection of particulate emboli or sclerosing agents. Chronic AV fistulae may develop multiple feeding arteries and draining veins, simulating AV malformations.[49] Evaluation must include rapid serial-film angiography with superselective injection. The distinction of AV fistula from a vascular malformation is important because embolic occlusion of the AV communication in a fistula is definitive therapy and the lesion should not recur.

TRAUMA

When a patient has sustained major trauma and an enlarging extremity hematoma, hypotension, absent or diminshed pulse, or neurologic deficit is present, emergency angiography is usually indicated to define arterial disruption or occlusion, although color-flow duplex sonography may allow noninvasive diagnosis of some injuries. Positive angiographic findings include compression, thrombosis, spasm, extravasation, pseudoaneurysm, intimal injury, and arteriovenous fistula. Digital subtraction angiography, despite its lower spatial resolution, can be as accurate for a diagnosis as conventional film angiography.[50] Scout films are indispensable and each site of suspected injury must be examined in at least two projections. Entry and exit sites of bullets or other projectiles should be indicated by radiopaque markers. Properly performed angiography has 92% to 98% accuracy in extremity trauma.[51,52]

Vessel narrowing may represent spasm or external compression from a compartment syndrome. Radiolucent angiographic strips in a longitudinal orientation within a vessel often represent flow or layering phenomena and must not be mistaken for intimal flaps. Filling defects must be constant and visible on more than one projection for the diagnosis of intimal injury to be made. Flaps typically appear as thin, transverse lines or globules attached to the vessel wall in at least one view.[53] When arterial occlusion is found, its precise cause cannot reliably be determined by angiography.

Except for a few specific forms of trauma (such as high-power gunshot wound), lack of suggestive physical findings is highly predictive of normal angiography.[54] If a patient does not have absent or diminished pulse, neurologic deficit, bruit, murmur, or signs of active bleeding, and angiography is requested merely because of the proximity of penetrating trauma to a major vessel, the chance of uncovering a significant abnormality is less than 5% in most reports.[54–57] If an asymptomatic intimal flap, small pseudoaneurysm, or AV fistula *is* found, it can be treated conservatively with little risk to the patient.[58,59] Even those surgeons advocating continued application of arteriography for "proximity" indications have found that delay of angiography of up to 24 hours has not led to any complications in such patients.[60]

Routine arteriography after knee trauma has been recommended in the past, particularly for those with dislocation or associated femoral fractures, because of the high morbidity of traumatic popliteal artery occlusion.[61,62] Recently, Treiman and colleagues described their experience in treating 220 patients with knee dislocations: 19% of patients with anterior and 31% with posterior dislocations had popliteal artery injury, but *all* of the injuries needing surgical intervention were evident by diminished or absent distal pulses.[63] As long as patients with knee dislocation and intact distal pulses can be carefully observed for at least 48 hours, routine arteriography does not appear to be necessary.[63,64] Duplex sonography may allow rapid assessment of equivocal findings in cases of dislocation or other extremity injuries, but its accuracy remains to be defined.

NONINVASIVE STUDIES

Nonangiographic examinations are valuable in screening patients for vascular disease and selecting who might benefit by arteriography. Segmental Doppler blood pressure measurements, which are easy to perform and generate an ankle-brachial pressure index, are extremely useful in the detection of significant arterial obstruction. However, noninvasive imaging examinations are being actively developed in the hope of increasing sensitivity and perhaps someday replacing catheter angiography. At present, velocity ratios determined by duplex ultrasonography are detecting graft and other stenoses before they are suggested by symptoms or segmental pressure changes.[33]

Various strategies are being employed to develop magnetic resonance angiography, and many obstacles have been overcome.[13,23,65] Nevertheless, limitations imposed by ferromagnetic vascular clips, imaging times, in-plane flow, and other problems remain. Spiral CT angiography allows noninvasive examination of vascular anatomy but is constrained by the need to inject larger volumes of iodinated contrast material, the limited extent of the vascular anatomy that may be examined at one time, spatial resolution, and image processing requirements.[22] Catheter aortography and lower extremity arteriography are likely to diminish in importance in the coming years, but they are certain to maintain a role in the primary diagnosis of vascular disease.

REFERENCES

1. Genton E, Clagett GP, Salzman EW: Antithrombotic therapy in peripheral vascular disease. *Chest* 1986; 89:75–81.
2. Hessel SJ, Adams DF: Complications of angiography. *Radiology* 1981; 138:273–281.

3. Wade GL, Smith DC, Mohr LL: Follow-up of 50 consecutive angiograms obtained utilizing puncture of prosthetic vascular grafts. *Radiology* 1983; 146:663–664.
4. Veterans Administration Cooperative Study Group 141: Comparative evaluation of prosthetic, reversed, and in situ vein bypass grafts in distal popliteal and tibial-peroneal revascularization. *Arch Surg* 1988; 123:434–438.
5. Taylor LM, Jr, Hamre D, Dalman RL, Porter JM: Limb salvage vs amputation for critical ischemia: The role of vascular surgery. *Arch Surg* 1991; 126:1251–1258.
6. Karacagil S, Almgren B, Bowald S, Eriksson I: A new method of angiographic runoff evaluation in femorodistal reconstructions: Significant correlation with early graft patency. *Arch Surg* 1990; 125:1055–1058.
7. Gavant ML: Digital subtraction angiography of the foot in atherosclerotic occlusive disease. *South Med J* 1989; 82:328–334.
8. Hol PK, Heldaas J, Skjennald A: Demonstration of pedal arterial arcades in occlusive arteriosclerotic disease. *Acta Radiol* 1989; 30:61–63.
9. Kahn PC, Boyer DN, Moran JM, Callow AD: Reactive hyperemia in lower extremity arteriography: An evaluation. *Radiology* 1968; 90:975–980.
10. Zagoria RJ, D'Souza VJ, Sharling ES: Prosthetic arterial graft occlusion: A complication of tourniquet use during arteriography. *Radiology* 1988; 167:121–122.
11. Kozak BE, Bedell JE, Rösch J: Small vessel leg angiography for distal vessel bypass grafts. *J Vasc Surg* 1988; 8:711–715.
12. Cohen MI, Vogelzang RL: A comparison of techniques for improved visualization of the arteries of the distal lower extremity. *Am J Roentgenol* 1986; 147:1021–1024.
13. Owen RS, Carpenter JP, Baum RA, et al: Magnetic resonance imaging of angiographically occult runoff vessels in peripheral arterial occlusive disease. *N Engl J Med* 1992; 326:1577–1581.
14. Jurriaans E, Wells IP: Bolus chasing: A new technique in peripheral arteriography. *Clin Radiol* 1993; 48:182–185.
15. Sethi GK, Scott SM, Takaro T: Multiple plane angiography for more precise evaluation of aortoiliac disease. *Surgery* 1975; 78:154–159.
16. Mandell VS, Jaques PF, Delany DJ, Oberheu V: Persistent sciatic artery: Clinical, embryologic, and angiographic features. *Am J Roentgenol* 1985; 144:245–249.
17. Rosenbloom MS, Flanigan DP, Schuler JJ, et al: Risk factors affecting the natural history of intermittent claudication. *Arch Surg* 1988; 123:867–870.
18. Holmes DR, Jr, Burbank MK, Fulton RE, Bernatz PE: Arteriosclerosis obliterans in young women. *Am J Med* 1979; 66:997–1000.
19. Katz S, Andros G, Kohl R, et al: Arterial emboli of venous origin. *Surg Gynecol Obstet* 1992; 174:17–21.
20. Trede M, Storz LW, Petermann C, Schiele U: Pitfalls and progress in the management of abdominal aortic aneurysms. *World J Surg* 1988; 12:810–817.
21. Cho SI, Johnson WC, Bush HL, Jr, et al: Lethal complications associated with nonrestrictive treatment of abdominal aortic aneurysms. *Arch Surg* 1982; 117:1214–1217.

22. Dillon EH, Vanleeuwen MS, Fernandez MA, Mali WPTM: Spiral CT angiography. *Am J Roentgenol* 1993; 160:1273–1278.
23. Mistretta CA: Relative characteristics of MR angiography and competing vascular imaging modalities. *J Magn Reson Imaging* 1993; 3:685–698.
24. Rösch J, Keller FS, Porter JM, Baur GM: Value of angiography in the management of abdominal aortic aneurysm. *Cardiovasc Radiol* 1978; 1:83–94.
25. Harris JA, Bis KG, Glover JL, et al: Penetrating atherosclerotic ulcers of the aorta. *J Vasc Surg* 1994; 19:90–99.
26. Gmelin E, Burmester E, Valesky A, Weiss H-D: Das sogenannte "inflammatorische aneurysma" der bauchaorta. *Rofo* 1984; 141:56–60.
27. Gonda RL, Jr, Gutierrez OH, Azodo MVU: Mycotic aneurysms of the aorta: Radiologic features. *Radiology* 1988; 168:343–346.
28. Richardson JW, Greenfield LJ: Natural history and management of iliac aneurysms. *J Vasc Surg* 1988; 8:165–171.
29. Carpenter JP, Barker CF, Roberts B, et al: Popliteal artery aneurysms: Current management and outcome. *J Vasc Surg* 1994; 19:65–73.
30. Grigg MJ, Nicolaides AN, Wolfe JHN: Detection and grading of femorodistal vein graft stenoses: Duplex velocity measurements compared with angiography. *J Vasc Surg* 1988; 8:661–666.
31. Teeuwen C, Eikelboom BC, Ludwig JW: Clinically unsuspected complications of arterial surgery shown by post-operative digital subtraction angiography. *Br J Radiol* 1989; 62:13–19.
32. Beidle TR, Brom-Ferral R, Letourneau JG: Surveillance of infrainguinal vein grafts with duplex sonography. *Am J Roentgenol* 1994; 162:443–448.
33. Polak JF: Arterial sonography: Efficacy for the diagnosis of arterial disease of the lower extremity. *Am J Roentgenol* 1993; 161:235–243.
34. Berkowitz HD, Fox AD, Deaton DH: Reversed vein graft stenosis: Early diagnosis and management. *J Vasc Surg* 1992; 15:130–142.
35. Carney WI, Jr, Balko A, Barrett MS: In situ femoropopliteal and infrapoplitcal bypass: Two-year experience. *Arch Surg* 1985; 120:812–816.
36. Gad A: Aortoduodenal fistula revisited. *Scand J Gastroenterol* 1989; 24:97–100.
37. Sprayregen S, Veith FJ, Bakal CW: Catheterization and angioplasty of the nonopacified peripheral autogenous vein bypass graft. *Arch Surg* 1988; 123:1009–1012.
38. Waneck R, Jantsch H, Lechner G, et al: Dynamic angiography in below-knee bypass grafts. *Vasc Surg* 1988; 23:95–101.
39. Hagen B, Lohse S: Clinical and radiologic aspects of Buerger's disease. *Cardiovasc Intervent Radiol* 1984; 7:283–293.
40. Ohta T, Shionoya S: Fate of the ischaemic limb in Buerger's disease. *Br J Surg* 1988; 75:259–262.
41. Bagby RJ, Cooper RD: Angiography in ergotism: Report of two cases and a review of the literature. *Am J Roentgenol* 1972; 116:179–186.
42. Sano K, Aiba T, Saito I: Angiography in pulseless disease. *Radiology* 1970; 94:69–74.
43. Lüscher TF, Lie JT, Stanson AW, et al: Arterial fibromuscular dysplasia. *Mayo Clin Proc* 1987; 62:931–952.

44. Murray A, Halliday M, Croft RJ: Popliteal artery entrapment syndrome. *Br J Surg* 1991; 78:1414–1419.
45. Greenwood LH, Yrizarry JM, Hallet JW, Jr: Popliteal artery entrapment: Importance of the stress runoff for diagnosis. *Cardiovasc Intervent Radiol* 1986; 9:93–99.
46. Jasinski RW, Masselink BA, Partridge RW, et al: Adventitial cystic disease of the popliteal artery. *Radiology* 1987; 163:153–155.
47. Jantsch J, Lechner G, Kretschmer G: Sonographische diagnose einer zystis-chen adventitia-degeneration (ZAD). *Rofo* 1985; 143:600–601.
48. Wilbur AC, Woelfel GF, Meyer JP, et al: Adventitial cystic disease of the popliteal artery. *Radiology* 1985; 155:63–64.
49. Lawdahl RB, Routh WD, Vitek JJ, et al: Chronic arteriovenous fistulas mas-querading as arteriovenous malformations: Diagnostic considerations and therapeutic implications. *Radiology* 1989; 170:1011–1015.
50. Sibbitt RR, Palmaz JC, Garcia F, Reuter SR: Trauma of the extremities: Prospective comparison of digital and conventional angiography. *Radiology* 1986; 160:179–182.
51. Rose SC, Moore EE: Emergency trauma angiography: Accuracy, safety, and pitfalls. *Am J Roentgenol* 1987; 148:1243–1246.
52. Snyder WH, Thal ER, Bridges RA, et al: The validity of normal arteriography in penetrating trauma. *Arch Surg* 1978; 113:424–428.
53. Rose SC, Moore EE: Angiography in patients with arterial trauma: Correlation between angiographic abnormalities, operative findings, and clinical outcome. *Am J Roentgenol* 1987; 149:613–619.
54. Frykberg ER, Crump JM, Vines FS, et al: A reassessment of the role of arteri-ography in penetrating proximity trauma: A prospective study. *J Trauma* 1989; 29:1041–1050.
55. Lipchik EO, Kaebnick HW, Beres JJ, Towne JB: The role of arteriography in acute penetrating trauma to the extremities. *Cardiovasc Intervent Radiol* 1987; 10:202–204.
56. McDonald EJ, Jr, Goodman PC, Winestock DP: The clinical indications for arteriography in trauma to the extremity. *Radiology* 1975; 116:45–47.
57. Hartling RP, McGahan JP, Blaisdell EW, Lindfors KK: Stab wounds to the extremities: Indications for angiography. *Radiology* 1987; 162:465–467.
58. Frykberg ER, Vines FS, Alexander RH: The natural history of clinically occult arterial injuries: A prospective evaluation. *J Trauma* 1989; 29:577–583.
59. Stain SC, Yellin AE, Weaver FA, Pentecost MJ: Selective management of nonocclusive arterial injuries. *Arch Surg* 1989; 124:1136–1141.
60. King TA, Perse JA, Marmen C, Darvin HI: Utility of arteriography in pene-trating extremity injuries. *Am J Surg* 1991; 162:163–165.
61. Wagner WH, Calkins ER, Weaver FA, et al: Blunt popliteal artery trauma: One hundred consecutive injuries. *J Vasc Surg* 1988; 7:736–748.
62. Kaufman SL, Martin LG: Arterial injuries associated with complete disloca-tion of the knee. *Radiology* 1992; 184:153–155.
63. Treiman GS, Yellin AE, Weaver FA, et al: Examination of the patient with a knee dislocation: The case for selective arteriography. *Arch Surg* 1992; 127:1056–1063.

64. Dennis JW, Jagger C, Butcher JL, et al: Reassessing the role of arteriograms in the management of posterior knee dislocations. *J Trauma* 1993; 35:692–697.
65. Swan JS, Grist TM, Weber DM, et al: MR angiography of the pelvis with variable velocity encoding and a phased-array coil. *Radiology* 1994; 190:363–369.

3

Renal Angiography

KEY CONCEPTS

1. Arteriography is performed in prospective renal donors to define arterial supply, which is subject to variation, and to detect unsuspected disease.
2. Angiography in renal tumor is used primarily to demonstrate tumor vascularity, arterial supply, and the extent of any venous invasion.
3. Renal adenoma or oncocytoma can be suggested by the absence of malignant features on the angiogram, but a positive diagnosis requires surgical resection.
4. Poststenotic dilatation, collateral vessels, and a pressure gradient greater than 20 mm Hg imply a significant renal artery stenosis.
5. Lateralized selective renal vein renin elevation helps predict response of hypertension to revascularization, but lack of lateralization does not mean a patient will not benefit from surgery or percutaneous angioplasty.

INDICATIONS

Angiography was a valuable diagnostic tool in the study of renal abnormalities in the 1960s, but even at that time its limitations were being recognized.[1] Today arteriography remains an essential part of the evaluation of those with suspected renovascular hypertension, renal artery stenosis, and acute arterial occlusion. This holds true for renal transplants as well. Angiography also still plays a useful role for many patients with renal neoplasms, not so much to make a diagnosis as to define arterial anatomy and to assess the vascularity of the tumor prior to surgery or palliative embolization. Tumor extension into renal vein or inferior vena cava (IVC) may require invasive studies for confirmation and precise delineation of involvement, but in most cases cavography can be replaced by sonography or magnetic resonance imaging studies.[2]

Depiction of vascular anatomy is also the major reason for study of prospective renal donors, and magnetic resonance angiography has not yet reached a level of diagnostic accuracy sufficient to replace catheter arteriography before donor nephrectomy.[3] Other indications for renal angiography include hematuria of unresolved cause, trauma, renal arteriovenous malformation, arteriovenous fistula, and aneurysm. Rarely, a request may be made for examination of a patient with suspected polyarteritis nodosa or other systemic vasculitis. In general, arteriography has no place in the evaluation of diffuse renal parenchymal disease.

ANATOMIC CONSIDERATIONS
AND RENAL DONOR ANGIOGRAPHY

Each kidney is usually supplied by a single vessel arising from the abdominal aorta caudal to the superior mesenteric artery origin, near the level of the L1-2 interspace. However, in a large number of people multiple renal arteries supply one or both kidneys, sometimes arising as caudally as the iliac arteries. The incidence of multiple vessels varies between 33% and 44%.[4,5] The renal artery normally provides branches to the adrenal gland and upper ureter. There is often a major anteroposterior bifurcation before further ramifications form the segmental, interlobar, arcuate, and interlobular arteries.

Although the renal arterial circulation is often considered in isolation from surrounding organs, communications with the aorta and with intercostal, lumbar, hepatic, and inferior mesenteric arteries do occur normally.[6] They are important for providing collateral flow in cases of renal artery obstruction. These communications should also be kept in mind in the arteriographic staging of renal cell carcinoma and when therapeutic embolization is pursued.

Because of the proximity of the right kidney to the IVC, the right renal vein is short. Two to four right renal veins may be present in up to 15% of the population.[7] A single preaortic vein usually drains the left kidney, but a circumaortic venous ring is seen in 7%, and an isolated retroaortic vein, characteristically lower in position than L1 or L2 (the normal level of renal veins), can be found in 2% of patients.[7] Rich retroperitoneal communications exist on the venous side of the renal circulation, explaining why some patients with chronic renal vein thrombosis are asymptomatic.[8]

In renal transplantation the left kidney is usually selected from the donor because of the greater length of its vein. Any arterial ureteral branches or bifurcations within 1 cm of the aorta pose technical problems, and such kidneys, as well as those with multiple arteries, are less desirable for transplantation. After intravenous urography and ultrasound are used to screen out those donors with an obvious renal abnormality, arteriography is performed to define the blood supply to each kidney, as well as to uncover the presence of atherosclerosis, fibromuscular disease, infarct, or unsuspected tumor prior to surgery. In the series studied by Walker and colleagues, arteriography led to the choice of the right kidney in 24% of prospective donors.[4]

Renal donors are best examined by aortography in the anteroposterior projection. Intravenous digital subtraction angiography (DSA) has little advantage over outpatient arteriography with small-bore catheters and is subject to greater diagnostic error. Intraarterial DSA can allow accurate identification of multiple renal vessels;[9] nevertheless, the superior spatial resolution provided by conventional film studies is preferred in order to exclude lesions of fibromuscular dysplasia and other subtle abnormalities. However, DSA can be used as a supplement to film arteriography by allowing oblique views to be obtained and assessed rapidly, if there are any questionable abnormalities.

When assessing the renal arteries by aortic injection, the sideholes of the pigtail catheter must be placed below the origin of the superior mesenteric artery, and the injection rate should not exceed 20 ml/second. Otherwise, opacification of celiac and mesenteric branches may confuse interpretation. When doubts about renal vascular anatomy cannot be resolved by aortography, selective injections are indicated.

TUMORS

Renal Cell Carcinoma

Any solid renal mass in an adult without another known primary tumor must be considered renal cell carcinoma until proven otherwise. Percutaneous needle biopsy is not particularly useful in this situation, and it is not obtained in potentially resectable tumors.[10] Computed tomography (CT) is helpful in demonstrating fat in benign angiomyolipomas, but other neoplasms have nonspecific findings on cross-sectional imaging. Cortical nodules (enlarged columns of Bertin) show normal excretory function on radionuclide scans. As noted earlier, angiography is no longer used primarily for diagnosis but for operative planning.

Renal cell carcinoma is a major cause of death in people with von Hippel-Lindau disease, an autosomal dominant hereditary disease predisposing one to multiple benign and malignant tumors of various organs. Aggressive use of arteriography to diagnose renal malignancies has been promoted in the past, but Miller and associates found that only 35% of lesions resected could be demonstrated, and tumors as large as 2.5 cm escaped detection.[11] Even in such patients, arteriography is best reserved for defining vascular anatomy before surgery.

Vascularity

Most renal cell carcinomas are hypervascular, with bizarre enlarged tumor vessels and arteriovenous shunting typically present. However, about 10% of these tumors are hypovascular or avascular, and the diagnosis of malignancy is not made by angiographic criteria alone. The common dilemma of the past—renal carcinoma versus cyst—has been essentially resolved by sonography. Years ago Emmett and colleagues found only one case of malignancy intimately associated with a simple renal cyst among hundreds that had been subjected to surgical exploration, and in that case cyst aspiration would have been diagnostic (see Chapter 21 entitled Genitourinary Interventions).[12] Tumors with markedly increased vascularity may be treated by preoperative embolization to decrease blood loss, but routine embolization of carcinomas undergoing resection has generally fallen from favor (see Chapter 12 entitled Embolotherapy).

Venous Invasion

Traditionally, preoperative angiograms have included study of the IVC because renal cell carcinoma has a definite tendency to invade the renal veins, and caval extension may complicate up to 9% of those submitting to surgery.[13] Because the right renal vein is shorter, right-sided tumors are more likely to involve the IVC. At times, arterial injection shows neovascularity within the renal vein or IVC. Caval tumor thrombus does not adversely influence prognosis if nodal metastases are absent, but it does change the surgical approach.[14,15] Tumor may grow up the vena cava into the right side of the heart, and defining the cranial extent of any venous involvement is mandatory for planning resection because thoracotomy may be needed. It is noteworthy that most patients with tumor invasion of the cava do not have symptoms of IVC obstruction.

In the past, vena cavography with iodinated contrast medium has been the procedure of choice for delimiting venous extension of tumor, with accuracy of up to 95%.[16] Even so, misinterpretation of nonopacified venous inflow and technical problems have produced false-positive studies.[17] Similar streaming artifacts can cause problems in interpreting CT examinations. At present, intravascular tumors extending toward or above the diaphragm can be rapidly and noninvasively assessed by ultrasound. Magnetic resonance techniques have also shown high accuracy for determining the upper extent of tumor thrombus.[2]

Tumor Staging

Clinical staging of renal cell carcinoma as described by Robson is as follows: stage I, neoplasm confined within renal capsule; stage II, extracapsular extension without penetration of the perinephric fascia; stage IIIA, venous invasion; stage IIIB, involvement of regional lymph nodes; stage IIIC, venous and lymph node involvement; stage IVA, invasion of an adjacent organ; and stage IVB, distant metastases.[10] Other than for confirming the presence and defining the extent of venous invasion, angiography is not as good as CT in staging. Parasitic blood supply from retroperitoneal and other arteries does not imply extracapsular extension, for it is seen in many tumors confirmed histologically to be entirely intracapsular.[6]

Angiographic Approach

Aortography is followed by selective renal artery catheterization. A relatively large volume of contrast medium can be injected into the kidney to be removed. A total of 25 to 30 ml often allows the renal vein to be visualized, especially when DSA is employed. If there is any hint of abnormality in the contralateral kidney, a selective arteriogram should be obtained. Synchronous renal cell carcinomas are not rare, particularly in patients with von Hippel-Lindau disease.

Injection of epinephrine (10 to 25 µg) directly into the renal artery has been used to accentuate neovascularity within tumors in the past.[18] Such enhancement is felt to represent a diminished vasoconstrictive response of abnormal arteries in comparison to healthy intrarenal vessels. Even when arteriography had greater diagnostic importance, the value of this maneuver was questioned.[19] Intraarterial epinephrine has also been used to temporarily diminish renal blood flow for selective renal venography. Venous encasement and occlusion are commonly present in tumors with no demonstrable neovascularity.[20] Even so, renal venography is now rarely required for diagnosis.

Other Malignancies

Urothelial tumors and most neoplasms metastatic to the kidneys are hypovascular. Although vascular encasement from transitional cell carcinoma is occasionally seen, angiography does not play a significant role in the evaluation of these tumors. Lymphoma often involves the kidney but usually when it is widespread elsewhere. Lymphomas are likely to be multinodular and can diffusely infiltrate. Presentation of a single renal mass is the exception, and angiography shows no specific features, only stretching of vessels and little, if any, neovascularity.[21]

Benign Masses
Renal Adenomas/Oncocytomas
Adenomas, which are usually small and asymptomatic, are fairly common benign tumors of the kidney. Renal oncocytomas are adenomas arising from the proximal tubular epithelium.[22] They can grow quite large, but necrosis and hemorrhage are unusual. Flank pain may be the presenting symptom, but most lesions are found incidentally. On arteriography there may be peripheral hypervascularity, but the majority of adenomas are hypovascular.[22-24] Parenchymal enhancement tends to be homogeneous and approximates that of adjacent normal kidney. A wheel-spoke arterial pattern has been described as characteristic of oncocytoma, but it is seen in fewer than one third of lesions and does not exclude the diagnosis of renal cell carcinoma when it is present.[22] Features that favor oncocytoma include a sharply circumscribed homogeneous lesion and the absence of findings typical for renal cell carcinoma: bizarre tumor vessels, arteriovenous shunting, venous invasion, and vascular encasement. The diagnosis of benign lesion can be suggested, but malignancy must be assumed until tissue is examined histologically. The use of needle biopsy is controversial, and complete resection is standard therapy.[24] When adenoma or oncocytoma is suspected, surgery can be limited to partial nephrectomy.

Other Nonmalignant Masses
Angiomyolipomas can grow large and bleed. Nowadays, smaller asymptomatic lesions are being detected by ultrasonography and CT scan. They occur much more frequently in women. Although small, berrylike aneurysms are sometimes present, most lesions have nonspecific arteriographic findings.[25] Fortunately, the characteristic fat content in almost all angiomyolipomas can be demonstrated by CT scan.

By their clinical presentation, abscesses and inflammatory masses are not a differential diagnostic problem. Needle aspiration and catheter drainage can confirm the presence of abscess. In the past, the peripheral neovascularity common to renal carbuncles could be confused with that of carcinoma.

Renal cortical nodules represent ectopic cortical hyperplasia or persistent renal lobulation. Cortical nodules tend to occur at the junction of the upper and middle thirds of the kidney and may be associated with partial or complete duplication of the renal collecting system.[26] If adjacent scarring is present from a previous infarct, a cortical nodule can appear quite exophytic.[27] Angiography shows a normal or dense homogeneous blush with no abnormal feeding vessels. Almost all cortical nodules can now be diagnosed by noninvasive means.

ANGIOGRAPHY IN HYPERTENSION

Nearly one quarter of the U. S. population is estimated to be hypertensive, and perhaps 250,000 have renovascular problems causing hypertension.[28] Finding this latter set of patients is important, for renovascular hypertension is potentially curable by percutaneous angioplasty or surgery. The major problem is to determine which patients should be subjected to arteriography. Renovascular hypertension must be suspected in hypertensive individuals under 30 years of age, those with onset of hypertension after 50 years of age, patients with deteriorating renal function and improved blood pressure after administration of angiotensin converting enzyme (ACE) inhibitors, and anyone with rapid deterioration and poor control of blood pressure. Even so, physical examination, history, and screening tests such as intravenous urography and plasma renin activity lack sensitivity and accuracy.[29]

Radionuclide scans following administration of ACE inhibitors show great promise as a screening measure for selected patients at high risk for renovascular disease.[30] Other new screening tests that rely on anatomic rather than functional imaging include color-flow duplex ultrasound, spiral CT angiography, and magnetic resonance angiography.[31–33] Technical limitations are yet to be overcome, however, and the role of each of these modalities remains to be established in practice.

Atherosclerosis versus Fibromuscular Disease

Most renovascular hypertension results from atherosclerosis, but fibromuscular dysplasia (FMD) is a common cause among younger patients. Atherosclerotic stenoses are likely to become worse and carry the risk of producing arterial occlusion and renal insufficiency.[28] Risk of renal functional impairment is lower in FMD. Other conditions that can produce hypertension by renal artery narrowing include Takayasu's arteritis and neurofibromatosis.

Atherosclerotic lesions are more likely to affect patients older than 60 years of age. They may be concentric or eccentric and smooth or irregular, and they are often bilateral. Stenosis is most common in the proximal 2 cm of a renal artery, and a lesion within 1 cm of the aorta (particularly if aortic plaques are present) can be considered an ostial lesion for purposes of balloon angioplasty. Percutaneous transluminal angioplasty is less effective in treating ostial lesions. In performing arteriography in patients with atherosclerosis, great care should be taken to be sure that the origin of each

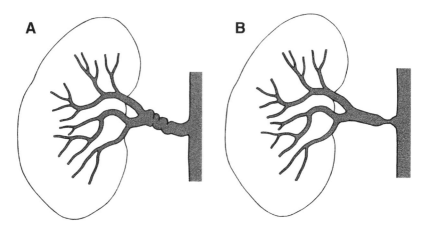

Fig. 3-1 (**A**) Typical appearance of renal artery stenosis from fibromuscular dysplasia and (**B**) atherosclerosis.

renal artery is profiled. Oblique views must be routinely obtained to avoid missing an ostial stenosis.

Fibromuscular dysplasia is responsible for 20% to 50% of renovascular hypertension, and it is mainly a disease of young white women.[34] In comparison with atherosclerotic stenoses, the lesions of FMD tend to be more peripheral, and they may affect branch arteries. Balloon angioplasty is particularly well suited for the treatment of these patients.

There are a number of histologic varieties of FMD, and some have characteristic angiographic findings. The majority of patients with FMD have medial fibroplasia with mural aneurysms, a lesion producing the classic "string of beads" appearance (Fig. 3–1). It is to be noted that aneurysms of FMD rarely rupture. Perimedial fibroplasia (15% to 25% of all FMD) has a similar appearance, but it usually lacks true aneurysms.[35] The rarer varieties of FMD—intimal fibroplasia and periarterial fibroplasia—can produce smooth stenoses or webs. Medial dissection, a complication of fibromuscular dysplasia, affects 5% to 10% of patients.[35] Although many people may have asymptomatic FMD, Cragg and associates found that 26% of patients whose renal lesions were found incidentally did develop hypertension within 5 years.[36]

Prediction of Response to Correction of Stenosis

When a stenotic lesion (70% or greater luminal narrowing) is discovered, its relationship to hypertension is not always clear, particularly in those with atherosclerosis. Many stenoses are caused by exacerbation of atherosclerosis in patients with essential hypertension. If renal function is marginal, treatment of significant occlusive disease can be argued, even when improvement in blood pressure is unlikely. Even in the absence of gross renal dysfunction, the combined use of ACE inhibitors and diuretics predisposes stenotic renal arteries to occlude.[37] Treatment of renal artery stenosis may be justified in patients needing such a medical regimen. In other patients the risks of nonmedical management must be justified by expected correction of hypertension. It is for this reason that selective renal vein renin sampling has been developed.

High blood pressure from ischemia results from excessive renin secretion by the kidney affected. Renin stimulates the production of angiotensin II and aldosterone, promoting sodium and fluid retention. Normally, each kidney adds about 24% to the renal artery renin, but excessive production by one kidney induces a feedback suppression of renin production by the opposite kidney.[7] A ratio of 1.5:1 or more of renin levels obtained from selective renal venous blood might be expected in this situation. Problems arise if both kidneys are affected by vascular disease. Lateralization of renins is predictive of response of hypertension to revascularization in 70% to 95% of patients, but 20% to 50% of patients in whom lateralization does *not* occur also improve.[7,28]

The presence of enlarged retroperitoneal, ureteral, and capsular arteries correlates well with ischemia.[38,39] Such collateral vessels are a good sign that intervention will be beneficial. Unfortunately, collateral arteries are demonstrated in only a portion of patients with renovascular hypertension. Poststenotic dilatation or measurement of a gradient of at least 20 mm Hg across the lesion can also be taken as indicative of significant narrowing.

Selective Venous Sampling for Renin

Selective samples are obtained from a catheter introduced from the femoral vein. It is best to have one or two sideholes placed near the tip of the catheter; otherwise, problems are encountered with "sidewalling" during aspiration. Cobra or Simmons catheters can be used, as can a multipurpose angled catheter. A deflecting guidewire is necessary to re-form the curve of the Simmons catheter at the junction of the iliac veins. A deflecting wire is also usually needed for selecting the renal veins with a multipurpose catheter.

Contrast material is injected before each set of samples is obtained in order to check the position of the catheter tip. After 1 to 2 ml is withdrawn to clear the catheter of flush solution or contrast medium, two samples of 7 ml each are drawn at each sampling position. Appropriate collection tubes are filled and kept on ice until the samples reach the laboratory. Each renal vein is sampled, in addition to mixed venous blood from the IVC and aortic blood (if an arterial catheter is in place for renal arteriography). If multiple veins drain one kidney, each should be sampled separately. If a branch renal artery stenosis is found, superselective sampling of the renal vein is in order.

Various maneuvers have been recommended to accentuate differences in renin secretion; among these are premedication with captopril, salt depletion, controlled hypotension, or upright posture (maintained at least 20 minutes before sampling).[7] Selective renal arteriography has not been shown to affect renin levels substantially, so samples can be taken immediately after arterial study. Beckman and Abrams recommend stimulatory maneuvers only if baseline supine sampling gives normal or borderline values.[7]

Angiography and Pheochromocytoma

Another potentially correctable cause of hypertension is pheochromocytoma, found in fewer than 1% of hypertensive persons.[40] About 10% are part of the constellation of tumors called *multiple endocrine neoplasia, type II,* a condition inherited as a dominant trait. The majority of tumors are benign, but the incidence of malignancy varies from 5% to 33%.[40] All but 10% arise in the adrenal medulla. Most extraadrenal pheochromocytomas (paragangliomas) are found in the abdomen.

Angiography is not normally indicated when CT shows an adrenal mass and when urinary catecholamine values are consistent with the diagnosis. A new radionuclide study utilizing metaiodobenzylguanidine (MIBG) may even be better than CT scanning for tumor localization.[40] Angiography has an accuracy of 80% to 90%, usually showing a hypervascular mass, but it should be reserved for cases in which noninvasive examinations are equivocal. Patients must be premedicated with α- and β-adrenergic blockers (phenoxybenzamine, 10 to 40 mg twice daily, and propranolol, 10 mg three times daily) to prevent a possible hypertensive crisis. Blood pressure must be carefully monitored during the procedure, and an acute hypertensive episode can be treated with intravenous phentolamine.

TRANSPLANTS

Problems with renal transplantation persist despite improvements in patient care. Suspected rejection can be accurately assessed by radionuclide perfusion and excretion studies, but arteriography is recommended if a primary vascular problem is under consideration.[41] Anastomotic or nonanastomotic stenosis, occlusion, infarct, and arteriovenous fistula are best demonstrated by catheter studies, and intraarterial DSA can minimize the amount of contrast medium needed. Biplane film arteriography is an alternative, with the lateral view often providing critical information. One should be aware of the type of anastomosis present (end to end to internal iliac artery or end to side to external iliac) in order to tailor the study and provide for any necessary catheter intervention (see Chapter 10 entitled Percutaneous Angioplasty, Recanalization, and Vascular Stents).

Angiographic results can be normal in cases of acute tubular necrosis, but study using contrast material is unnecessary and detrimental for such patients. Hyperacute rejection may be difficult to distinguish from acute arterial thrombosis by radionuclide studies, and transplant arteriography is diagnostic.[42] Arterial transit time of less than 2 seconds is normal, but delayed contrast clearance, lack of small artery opacification ("pruned-tree" appearance of the intrarenal vessels), and absence of nephrogram are diagnostic of rejection. Findings of chronic rejection include small vessel irregularity, cortical infarcts, and small artery aneurysms.

RENAL ARTERY ANEURYSM

The incidence of renal artery aneurysm found at autopsy is 0.3% to 0.7%.[43] Despite this, renal artery aneurysms rarely cause clinical problems, and many are found incidentally because of calcification seen on plain abdominal films or on angiograms performed for other reasons. Aneurysms typically involve the main renal artery or a first-order branch. They occur with equal frequency in men and women, and mean age of presentation is 60 years. Tham and associates described 69 patients with aneurysms not treated surgically, and found no case of rupture in a mean 4-year follow-up.[43] They believe the risk of rupture has been exaggerated, and asymptomatic lesions can be treated conservatively, even if they are larger than 2 cm in diameter. Aneurysms should be resected if they are associated with hematuria (all other potential causes being excluded), flank pain, or hypertension. Primary repair has produced excellent relief of hypertension in selected patients.[44] A renal aneurysm of any size should be repaired in a woman planning to have children, for risk of aneurysm rupture during pregnancy is substantial.[44,45]

MISCELLANEOUS CONDITIONS

Vasculitis

Polyarteritis nodosa is a systemic vasculitis that has been associated with small artery aneurysms in multiple viscera, particularly in the kidney. The disease is characterized by fibrinoid medial necrosis of medium-sized and small arteries. Although aneurysms are virtually pathognomonic, only a minority of patients with polyarteritis nodosa have aneurysms, and angiography is not justified as a screening measure.[46] It should be noted that aneurysms may regress with clinical improvement of the patient.

When present, microaneurysms must be distinguished from mycotic lesions. Identical aneurysms can be found in hypersensitivity or drug-induced angiitis.[47] Other findings of vasculitis include irregularity, stenosis, and occlusion of intrarenal branches, and nephrograms may have a spotted or striated pattern.[48,49]

Renal Trauma

The effects of renal trauma can usually be determined by excretory urography, radionuclide scan, or CT scan. Renal infarcts, tears, and contusions can all be accurately detected with CT scan, but arterial injury is easily missed.[50] If a patient deteriorates clinically and arterial injury is suspected, renal arteriography should be performed to detect arterial laceration, intimal flap, arteriovenous fistula, or occlusion. Delayed massive hematuria after penetrating renal injury is not rare (incidence of 13% to 19%); in such a situation, renal arteriography is not only diagnostic but also very often therapeutic through the delivery of occluding coils or other emboli.[51]

Hematuria of Unresolved Origin

Angiography is not usually helpful in cases of nontraumatic unilateral hematuria that cannot be diagnosed by other means. Mitty and Goldman reviewed 48 patients with documented unilateral gross hematuria and found only six angiographic abnormalities, including emboli and vascular malformations.[52] Forniceal and suburethelial veins are thin-walled and may be a source of bleeding, but they cannot be demonstrated reliably by angiography. Compression of the left renal vein between aorta and superior mesenteric artery (the "nutcracker" phenomenon) has been implicated in some cases of hematuria. Nishimura and associates found a significant elevation in left renal vein pressure in patients with left renal bleeding versus controls, and they define a left renal vein–IVC pressure gradient of 3 mm Hg or more as abnormal.[53] The filling of ureteral or capsular veins on arterial or venous injection may alert one to the diagnosis.

Renal Venography and Renal Vein Thrombosis

Renal venography has lost much of its past importance, especially in the diagnosis of malignant neoplasms. Today it is most often performed prior to placement of splenorenal shunts or to make the diagnosis of renal vein thrombosis. The main renal vein is usually well demonstrated by selective catheterization with a multi-sidehole catheter and injection of contrast medium at 15 ml/second for 2 seconds. Rapid filming or high DSA frame rate (2 to 3 frames per second) gives best results. Demonstration of intrarenal branches requires a similar injection of contrast material immediately after the administration of epinephrine (10 µg) directly into the renal artery.[7]

Acute renal vein thrombosis results in a tense, swollen kidney, but occlusion of more gradual onset, or chronic occlusion, may produce few symptoms. Most cases of renal vein thrombosis in adults are the result of trauma or an underlying disease, such as pancreatitis, retroperitoneal fibrosis, tumor, or diffuse parenchymal disease (e.g., glomerulonephritis).[8] It appears that nephrotic syndrome predisposes one to renal vein thrombosis, not vice versa. Renal vein thrombosis is often overlooked in the absence of nephrotic syndrome or anuria, but it should be included in the differential diagnosis of sudden deterioration in renal function in renal transplant patients or those with known renal disease.[54] Standard treatment is systemic anticoagulation, but local thrombolytic infusion has been reported.[55]

REFERENCES

1. Chait A: Current status of renal angiography. *Urol Clin North Am* 1985; 12:687–698.
2. Roubidoux MA, Dunnick NR, Sostman HD, Leder RA: Renal carcinoma: Detection of venous extension with gradient-echo MR imaging. *Radiology* 1992; 182:269–272.
3. Debatin JF, Sostman HD, Knelson M, et al: Renal magnetic resonance angiography in the preoperative detection of supernumerary renal arteries in potential kidney donors. *Invest Radiol* 1993; 28:882–889.
4. Walker TG, Geller SC, Delmonico FL, et al: Donor renal angiography: Its influence on the decision to use the right or left kidney. *Am J Roentgenol* 1988; 151:1149–1151.
5. Spring DB, Salvatierra O, Jr, Palubinskas AJ, et al: Results and significance of angiography in potential kidney donors. *Radiology* 1979; 133:45–47.
6. Wilkins RA, Sandin B, Price A, Twomey B: Extrarenal arterial connections of the normal renal artery. *Cardiovasc Intervent Radiol* 1986; 9:119–122.
7. Beckman CF, Abrams HL: Renal venography: Anatomy, technique, applications, analysis of 132 venograms, and a review of the literature. *Cardiovasc Intervent Radiol* 1980; 3:45–70.
8. Keating MA, Althausen AF: The clinical spectrum of renal vein thrombosis. *J Urol* 1985; 133:938–945.
9. Petty W, Spigos DG, Abejo R, et al: Arterial digital angiography in the evaluation of potential renal donors. *Invest Radiol* 1986; 21:122–124.
10. Levine E: Renal cell carcinoma: Radiological diagnosis and staging. *Semin Roentgenol* 1987; 22:248–259.
11. Miller DL, Choyke PL, Walther MM, et al: Von Hippel–Lindau disease: Inadequacy of angiography for identification of renal cancers. *Radiology* 1991; 179:833–836.
12. Emmett JL, Levine SR, Woolner LB: Coexistence of renal cyst and tumour: Incidence in 1007 cases. *Br J Urol* 1963; 35:403–410.
13. Kadir S, Coulam CM: Intracaval extension of renal cell carcinoma. *Cardiovasc Intervent Radiol* 1980; 3:180–183.
14. Selli C, Barbanti G, Barbagli G, et al: Caval extension of renal cell carcinoma: Results of surgical treatment. *Urology* 1987; 30:448–452.
15. Henriksson C, Aldenborg F, Haljamäe H, et al: Renal cell carcinoma with vena cava extension: Diagnosis and surgical features of 41 cases. *Scand J Urol Nephrol* 1987; 21:291–296.
16. Hatcher PA, Paulson DF, Anderson EE: Accuracy in staging of renal cell carcinoma involving vena cava. *Urology* 1992; 39:27–30.

17. Selby JB, Pryor JL, Tegtmeyer CJ, Gillenwater JY: Inferior vena caval invasion by renal cell carcinoma: False positive diagnosis by venacavography. *J Urol* 1990; 143:464–467.
18. Abrams HL: The response of neoplastic renal vessels to epinephrine in man. *Radiology* 1964; 82:217–223.
19. Meaney TF: Errors in angiographic diagnosis of renal masses. *Radiology* 1969; 93:361–366.
20. Smith JC, Jr, Rösch J, Athanasoulis CA, et al: Renal venography in the evaluation of poorly vascularized neoplasms of the kidney. *Am J Roentgenol* 1975; 123:552–556.
21. Seltzer RA, Wendlund DE: Renal lymphoma: Arteriographic studies. *Am J Roentgenol* 1967; 101:692–695.
22. Ambos MA, Bosniak MA, Valensi QJ, et al: Angiographic patterns in renal oncocytomas. *Radiology* 1978; 129:615–622.
23. Holt RG, Neiman HL, Korsower JM, Newhouse J: Angiographic features of benign renal adenoma. *Urology* 1975; 6:764–767.
24. Drüber C, Schweden F, Klose K-J, et al: Das onkozytom der niere. *Rofo* 1988; 148:227–233.
25. Bret PM, Bretagnolle M, Gaillard D, et al: Small, asymptomatic angiomyolipomas of the kidneys. *Radiology* 1985; 154:7–10.
26. Popky GL, Bogash M, Pollack H, Longacre AM: Focal cortical hyperplasia. *J Urol* 1969; 102:657–660.
27. King MC, Friedenberg RM, Tena LB: Normal renal parenchyma simulating tumor. *Radiology* 1968; 91:217–222.
28. Working Group on Renovascular Hypertension: Detection, evaluation, and treatment of renovascular hypertension. *Arch Intern Med* 1987; 147:820–829.
29. Greminger P, Schneider E, Siegenthaler W, Vetter W: Renovaskuläre hypertonie. *Internist (Berl)*1988; 29:246–251.
30. Sfakianakis GN, Bourgoignie JJ, Georgiou M, Guerra JJ: Diagnosis of renovascular hypertension with ACE inhibition scintigraphy. *Radiol Clin North Am* 1993; 31:831–848.
31. Davidson RA, Wilcox CS: Newer tests for the diagnosis of renovascular disease. *JAMA* 1992; 268:3353–3358.
32. Galanski M, Prokop M, Chavan A, Schaefer CM, Jandeleit K, Nischelsky JE: Renal arterial stenoses: Spiral CT angiography. *Radiology* 1993; 189: 185–192.
33. Grist TM, Kennell TW, Sproat IA, et al: Prospective evaluation of renal MR angiography: Comparison with conventional angiography in 35 patients. Presented at the *79th Meeting of the Radiological Society of North America*, 30 November, 1993, Chicago, Ill.
34. Lüscher TF, Lie JT, Stanson AW, et al: Arterial fibromuscular dysplasia. *Mayo Clin Proc* 1987; 62:931–952.
35. Harrison EG, Jr, McCormack LJ: Pathologic classification of renal arterial disease in renovascular hypertension. *Mayo Clin Proc* 1971; 46:161–167.
36. Cragg AH, Smith TP, Thompson BH, et al: Incidental fibromuscular dysplasia in potential renal donors: Long-term clinical follow-up. *Radiology* 1989; 172:145–147.

37. Postma CT, Hoefnagels WHL, Barentsz JO, et al: Occlusion of unilateral stenosed renal arteries: Relation to medical treatment. *J Hum Hypertens* 1989; 3:185–190.
38. Abrams HL, Cornell SH: Patterns of collateral flow in renal ischemia. *Radiology* 1965; 84:1001–1012.
39. Meyers MA, Friedenberg RM, King MC: The significance of the renal capsular arteries. *Br J Radiol* 1967; 40:949–956.
40. Samaan NA, Hickey RC, Shutts PE: Diagnosis, localization, and management of pheochromocytoma: Pitfalls and follow-up in 41 patients. *Cancer* 1988; 62:2451–2460.
41. Prager P, Clorius JH, Dreikorn K: Beitrag der digitalen subtraktionsangiographie zur diagnostik von abstoßungsreaktionen nach nierentransplantation. *Rofo* 1985; 143:426–431.
42. Hamway S, Novick A, Braun WE, et al: Impaired renal allograft function: A comparative study with angiography and histopathology. *J Urol* 1979; 122:292–297.
43. Tham G, Ekelund L, Herrlin K, et al: Renal artery aneurysms: Natural history and prognosis. *Ann Surg* 1983; 197:348–352.
44. Bulbul MA, Farrow GA: Renal artery aneurysms. *Urology* 1992; 40:124–126.
45. Cohen JR, Shamash FS: Ruptured renal artery aneurysms during pregnancy. *J Vasc Surg* 1987; 6:51–59.
46. Sellar RJ, Mackay IG, Buist TAS: The incidence of micro-aneurysms in polyarteritis nodosa. *Cardiovasc Intervent Radiol* 1986; 9:123–126.
47. Fisher RG: Renal artery aneurysms in polyarteritis nodosa: A multiepisodic phenomenon. *Am J Roentgenol* 1981; 136:983–985.
48. Vázquez JJ, San Martin P, Barbado FJ, et al: Angiographic findings in systemic necrotizing vasculitis. *Angiology* 1981; 32:773–779.
49. Warren BH, Rösch J: Angiography in the diagnosis of renal scleroderma. *Radiologia Clin* 1977; 46:194–202.
50. Lang EK, Sullivan J, Frentz G: Renal trauma: Radiological studies. *Radiology* 1985; 154:1–6.
51. Heyns CF, van Vollenhoven P: Increasing role of angiography and segmental artery embolization in the management of renal stab wounds. *J Urol* 1992; 147:1231–1234.
52. Mitty HA, Goldman H: Angiography in unilateral renal bleeding with a negative urogram. *Am J Roentgenol* 1974; 121:508–517.
53. Nishimura Y, Fushiki M, Yoshida M, et al: Left renal vein hypertension in patients with left renal bleeding of unknown origin. *Radiology* 1986; 160:663–667.
54. Clark RA, Wyatt GM, Colley DP: Renal vein thrombosis: An underdiagnosed complication of multiple renal abnormalities. *Radiology* 1979; 132:43–50.
55. Robinson JM, Cockrell CH, Tisnado J, et al: Selective low-dose streptokinase infusion in the treatment of acute transplant renal vein thrombosis. *Cardiovasc Intervent Radiol* 1986; 9:86–89.

4

Hepatic Angiography

KEY CONCEPTS

1. Hepatic arterial anatomy is variable; partial supply from superior mesenteric and left gastric arteries is common.
2. Normal liver is perfused by the hepatic artery and portal vein; malignant tumors are supplied by the hepatic artery only.
3. Hepatocellular carcinoma is associated with hepatitis and cirrhosis. It has a propensity for venous invasion.
4. Computed tomographic arteriography, computed tomographic portography, and arterial injection of lymphographic oily contrast agents can improve tumor detection. Spiral computed tomography optimizes results.
5. Knowledge of hepatic segmental anatomy is required to interpret studies guiding surgical resection of metastases.
6. Hepatic venous obstruction causes Budd-Chiari syndrome.

INDICATIONS

With the development of noninvasive diagnostic imaging techniques, the role of hepatic angiography has narrowed and become more strictly defined. One of the chief uses of arteriography remains in the evaluation of hepatic neoplasms when radionuclide scan, computed tomographic scan, ultrasonography (US), magnetic resonance imaging (MRI), or needle biopsy fail to produce a satisfactory diagnosis. Such may be the case if a large regenerating nodule needs to be differentiated from possible hepatocellular carcinoma. Similarly, a tumor not clearly malignant on histologic sampling may have unequivocally malignant features (vascular encasement, portal occlusion) on angiography. Rarely cavernous hemangioma may have an atypical appearance on computed tomography (CT), ultrasonography, and other noninvasive imaging but can be confidently diagnosed arteriographically.

Often the nature of a hepatic malignancy is known, but the precise location, number of satellite nodules or metastases, and presence of vascular invasion must be defined before surgical resection for cure can be pursued. Arteriography remains a prime diagnostic tool in this situation. If a tumor is unresectable, one may still choose to treat by transcatheter embolization or selective arterial infusion of chemotherapeutic agents.

Other current indications include preoperative evaluation for portal hypertension (see Chapter 5 entitled Portal Venography, Portal Hypertension, and TIPS), liver transplantation, vascular malformations, trauma, and Budd-Chiari syndrome.

ANATOMY

The anatomy of the liver differs from that of the other viscera by its dual blood supply: arterial and portal venous. Within the liver the branches parallel one another and terminate in the ascinus, the organ's basic functional unit. Blood flows through the hepatic sinusoids into the venules at the periphery of each ascinus. These small vessels drain into the three major hepatic veins (right, middle, and left), which enter the inferior vena cava (IVC) and define surgical lines of cleavage.

The morphologic division between right and left lobes corresponds to a line drawn between the gallbladder and IVC, not to any surface features. The right lobe is composed of anterior and posterior segments, each with superior and inferior subsegments. The left lobe contains medial and lateral segments (medial segment representing the quadrate lobe of older terminology). The caudate lobe, lying posterior to the porta hepatis and medial segment of the left lobe, anterior to the IVC, and connected laterally to the right lobe, receives arterial and portal branches from both the major lobar divisions; it drains by small veins directly into the IVC.

A modification of the Couinaud anatomic nomenclature is widely accepted internationally and may become standard in the United States. By this concept, the right and left hepatic lobes are each divided as described in the previous paragraph, and each of these four segments is divided into superior and inferior subsegments by a transverse line drawn through the right and left portal branches (Fig. 4-1).[1] These subsegments are identified by the following numbers:

      I—caudate lobe
      II—left lateral superior subsegment
      III—left lateral inferior subsegment
      IV—left medial subsegment
      V—right anterior inferior subsegment
      VI—right posterior inferior subsegment
    VII—right posterior superior subsegment
  VIII—right anterior superior subsegment

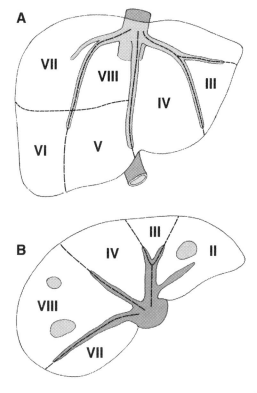

Fig. 4-1 **A,** Anterior view of the liver with segments identified by the modified Couinaud numbering system. **B,** Transverse section through the liver at the confluence of hepatic veins and inferior vena cava. Lesions present in segments II and VIII.

This system can be used to clearly communicate the distribution of hepatic neoplasms before any planned surgical resection.

The arterial supply of the liver is quite variable (Fig. 4-2), and 10 anatomic categories have been described by Michels.[2] He found that only 55% of the cadavers studied had complete arterial supply through a common hepatic artery arising from the celiac axis. A branch of the superior mesenteric artery (SMA) provided either a complete blood supply (replaced right hepatic artery) or incomplete supply (accessory right hepatic artery) to the right lobe in 17%. Replaced or accessory left hepatic arteries arose from the left gastric artery in 25%. Rarely, one may find the hepatic artery originating entirely from the SMA or left gastric artery. The middle hepatic (artery to the medial segment of the left lobe) is as likely to come from the right hepatic artery as from the left. These variations obviously have relevance for planning surgical resection or transplantation and for performing therapeutic emboliza-

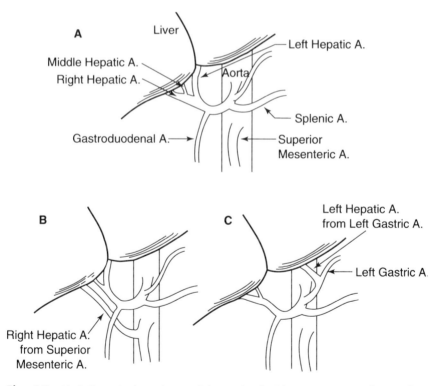

Fig. 4-2 Variations in hepatic arterial supply. **A,** Most common celiac and hepatic arterial anatomy; **B,** right hepatic artery "replaced" to superior mesenteric artery; **C,** left hepatic artery arising from the left gastric artery.

tion or chemoinfusion. One must be prepared to perform SMA and left gastric injections for complete arteriographic study of the liver.

TECHNICAL ASPECTS

Aortography is not ordinarily necessary prior to selective catheterization, but if celiac occlusion is suspected and the celiac artery cannot be entered, a lateral aortogram (by digital subtraction or conventional film studies) may be helpful.

Catheters most often used in hepatic arterial studies from the femoral approach are those with downward or reverse curves such as Cobra, sidewinder, or MK-2 shapes. If the celiac artery takes a right-angle or cephalad course, an H1H catheter can be employed successfully at times. Depending on the anatomy, preformed catheters may not enter the celiac or hepatic artery, and it may be necessary to custom form a tip configuration by steam. Rarely, a narrow or acutely angled celiac artery can be engaged only from an axillary or brachial artery approach. An upper extremity approach may also allow much more selective placement of the catheter if embolization is indicated.

The smaller, high-torque catheters now available tend to pass farther peripherally for superselective injections. If distal placement is desired, torque-control guidewires and coaxial catheter systems may be tried. One should be aware of the potential for arterial spasm during manipulations. A sidehole near the catheter tip prevents problems with "sidewalling" during aspiration and also decreases the jet effect from the tip during power injections. For embolization, however, only endhole catheters are used in order to ensure that no injected particles remain lodged within the catheter.

Conventional Hepatic Arteriography

In conventional hepatic arteriography, flow within the vessel selected should be approximated by the injection rate (generally between 6 and 10 ml/second). A test injection with fluoroscopic observation can give an idea of the flow that is present, as well as the stability of catheter position. Sensitivity of arteriography is much improved if the common or proper hepatic artery is selected, rather than just the celiac axis.[3] Between 30 and 40 ml of contrast medium is injected. Filming should be rapid (one or two films per second) during the first few seconds and then may be slowed to cover a total of 25 to 30 seconds in order to include both parenchymal and venous phases. Digital subtraction angiography (DSA) improves tissue contrast during the parenchymal phase and is useful if the patient is able to suspend respiration for 30 to 40 seconds.

Computed Tomography-Angiography

Computed tomography-angiography shows increased sensitivity for detection of neoplasm. It immediately follows standard angiography, and it is advisable to limit the amount of contrast medium injected during the preliminary study. To this end, DSA may minimize the contrast medium dose needed to define the arterial supply to the liver. Limiting the dose injected for arteriography provides for maximal contrast of lesion to normal liver during the CT portion of the examination. Computed tomography-angiography may be performed in one of two ways.

In CT-arteriography, the hepatic artery is injected with 8 to 12 ml of 30% contrast per CT slice.[4] This technique is no longer commonly used, but the introduction of spiral CT may lead to renewed application with a modified protocol. Spiral CT allows much more rapid scan acquisition and many more images to be reconstructed than conventional CT. For spiral CT-arteriography 25 ml of diluted contrast medium may be injected at 1 ml/second with scanning commencing 1 second after the onset of injection.[5] The entire liver can be examined before the injection has ended. In CT-arteriography most lesions appear hypervascular, unlike CT-portography, in which they appear hypovascular in comparison to surrounding normal liver. Variations in hepatic arterial supply pose problems for CT-arteriography, for injection of a single vessel produces enhancement of only part of the liver if accessory or replaced hepatic arteries are present.

With CT-portography the catheter is placed in the SMA beyond any branches that might supply the liver. Scanning begins 10 to 20 seconds after the onset of injection of contrast medium (300 mg iodine/ml); a total volume of 100 to 150 ml is injected at 2 to 3 ml/second.[6,7] If a spiral CT scanner is available, 50 to 150 ml of iodinated contrast medium are injected at a similar rate with an imaging delay of 30 to 40 seconds.[5,8] Beam collimation of 8 mm and a table motion of 8 mm/second allow most livers to be covered in the course of a single breath-hold.

A novel variation of CT-portography described by Sawada and colleagues involves percutaneous splenic puncture with a specially designed 23-gauge needle.[9] The needle contains two sideholes and an adjustable stopper for limiting depth of insertion; it allows injection of dilute contrast medium at the rate of 0.5 to 1 ml/second. They found that acceptable diagnostic studies could be obtained in most patients, who could be discharged after a short period of postprocedural observation. One early report of MR-portography (with injection of a gadolinium-containing contrast agent into the SMA) indicates that it has no advantage over CT-portography in the detection of metastases.[10]

No matter what specific technique is used, CT-portographic studies must be read with care. False-positive interpretations can arise from detection of benign lesions (such as hemangiomas or cysts), as well as from unappreciated injection of small bubbles or incomplete mixing of contrast medium with unopacified splenic venous blood, causing decreased enhancement of portions of the liver.[11] The presence of a straight-bordered, nonopacified, wedge-shaped peripheral segment of parenchyma is often a benign finding (although it may also represent a central tumor obstructing more peripheral portal venous flow). Hepatic veins scanned too early after contrast medium injection must not be misconstrued as metastases. Another possible source of error is the medial segment of the left lobe adjacent to the porta hepatis, which, by a variant blood supply, may be hypodense with respect to the rest of the liver.[11] Subcapsular areas of hypoperfusion are sometimes seen in the absence of disease. With each of these potential problems, repeat delayed scans should show disappearance of any benign defect.

Where available, a spiral scanner should be used for CT-arteriography or CT-portography for a number of reasons. Rapid scanning during a compact contrast medium bolus permits maximum differentiation of lesion from normal liver. Complete coverage of the liver during a single breath-hold minimizes artifacts and permits multiplanar reconstruction. Overlapping reconstruction (at 2-mm to 4-mm intervals) makes the centering of nearly any small lesion within a slice more likely, decreasing partial-volume effects. These combined advantages can lead to 94% to 96% sensitivities for tumor.[5]

Oil-based iodinated contrast agents such as Lipiodol (iodized oil) or Ethiodol (ethiodized oil) have a propensity to accumulate in primary hepatic tumors. This effect has been exploited for diagnosis, but some would dispute its utility.[12] These oily contrast agents can be injected into the hepatic artery (2 to 20 ml, with or without chemotherapeutic agents in emulsion) and followed by plain radiography or CT scanning.[13]

Portal Venography
The portal venous system may be opacified by various techniques (see Chapter 5 entitled Portal Venography, Portal Hypertension, and TIPS), the most widely used being arterial portography. The splenic artery or SMA is injected with a large volume of contrast medium (50 to 60 ml) and filming carried out to 30 seconds. If opacification of the portal vein is inadequate, SMA injection may be repeated after tolazoline (40 mg) is administered into the artery.

Hepatic Venography
Hepatic venography is performed with an endhole or occlusion balloon catheter. If introduced from the femoral vein, the catheter is guided into a major hepatic vein by means of a tip-deflecting guidewire. Small volumes of contrast medium are injected by hand to gauge the size of the vein as well as the flow rate. A free hepatic venogram is obtained by injection with

unobstructed flow around the catheter. Wedge hepatic venogram requires either occlusion balloon inflation or such peripheral tip placement that the catheter itself effects occlusion. In a wedge injection, no more than several milliliters of contrast medium should be injected by hand. Digital imaging allows very dilute contrast material to be used, lessening the chance of hepatic infarction resulting in the area of parenchymal stain. Pressure measurements are routinely obtained during hepatic vein catheterization (see Chapter 5).

MASS LESIONS

The diagnostic accuracy of angiography in the liver has been variously reported between 74% and 96%.[14] The presence of cirrhosis or obstructive jaundice can make diagnostic interpretation considerably more difficult, particularly for small focal lesions. Many tumors can have a nonspecific angiographic appearance, and needle or open biopsy may be necessary to establish a diagnosis. Nevertheless, certain lesions may have a characteristic enough appearance to make angiography worthwhile.

Benign Tumors
Cavernous Hemangiomas
Cavernous hemangiomas are encountered very frequently in CT, US, and radionuclide examinations. An incidence of up to 7% has been noted in autopsy studies; metastases are the only mass lesions seen more commonly in the liver.[15] Cavernous hemangiomas are almost always incidental findings and not the reason for the imaging procedure. Very rarely a large lesion may cause symptoms by mass, bleeding, or arteriovenous (AV) shunting. Cavernous hemangioma occurs more commonly in women, and multiple lesions may be detected in 10% of cases. Appearance on dynamic contrast material–enhanced CT is quite characteristic: initially hypodense, then showing peripheral areas of focal enhancement followed by diffuse hyperdensity at 2 minutes, and finally isodense on delayed scans. Red cell radionuclide scanning can also be used to make a reliable diagnosis. Hemangiomas produce intense signal on T_2-weighted MR images, and MR may become recognized as the most accurate imaging study available.[16,17] For the rare cavernous hemangioma that does not exhibit conventional features, aspiration needle biopsy may be safely performed as long as thin needles (no larger than 20 gauge) are employed. One should alert the examining pathologist to the suspected diagnosis, so that endothelial elements can be specifically sought in the biopsy sample.[18]

If a cavernous hemangioma is studied by arteriography, the following are pathognomonic as a constellation of findings:
1. Normal-sized feeding artery

2. Absence of neovascularity or AV shunting
3. Early peripheral ring or C-shaped accumulation of contrast material
4. Persistent "cotton-wool" pooling of contrast material to at least 20 seconds

Focal Nodular Hyperplasia

Focal nodular hyperplasia is not a neoplasm, but rather a hamartomatous lesion containing hepatocytes, Kupffer cells, and biliary elements. It is generally found in young women, is asymptomatic, and may be associated with the use of oral contraceptives, although the association is not very strong.[19] There have been no reliable reports of malignant degeneration, and severe complications arise only exceptionally (bleeding in less than 3%), so that routine surgical intervention is not indicated.[19] Multiple foci are found in 13% to 45%, and because of the presence of reticuloendothelial cells, there is significant uptake of radionuclide within the tumor in roughly half of cases examined.[19–21] An enhancing central scar is sometimes seen on CT scans or on early gradient-echo MR images after injection of gadolinium-containing contrast agents, but findings are often nonspecific.[8,16] If the lesion is "cold" by scintigraphy and other imaging techniques are not helpful, angiography may be the next step in evaluation. Characteristic angiographic findings of focal nodular hyperplasia include:

1. Hypervascular lesion with very tortuous vessels, but without frankly malignant neovascularity
2. Dense capillary stain of a sharply marginated mass
3. Septations visible within the capillary stain (in about one third), radiating from a small fibrous core (wheel-spoke pattern)

Previous reports of a central feeding vessel as typical of focal nodular hyperplasia have not proved useful in the differentiation of this entity from hepatic adenoma in most cases.[19–21] Although the features listed are quite specific of the category as a whole, two thirds of "cold" hypervascular lesions still require biopsy to differentiate focal nodular hyperplasia from hepatic adenoma.[20]

Hepatic Adenoma

Hepatic adenoma is a true neoplasm of clinical importance in that it is often complicated by necrosis and may present with catastrophic bleeding. In addition, there appears to be a small potential for malignant degeneration.[20] For these reasons, adenomas are not ordinarily treated conservatively. The great majority arise in younger women, and there is a strong association with the use of oral contraceptives or anabolic steroids. Because of hemorrhage and necrosis, most adenomas are symptomatic when discovered, and the CT and US appearances are quite heterogeneous and nonspecific. Present MR techniques have not been able to distinguish these tumors from hepatocellular carcinomas.[16] Hepatic adenomas do not usually contain Kupffer cells and do not accumulate tagged sulfur colloid. On angiography, they manifest the following:

1. Well-circumscribed mass somewhat larger (8 to 15 cm) than typical focal nodular hyperplasia
2. Hypovascular in about 50%
3. Blush rather homogeneous (somewhat less intense than in focal nodular hyperplasia) but for hypovascular areas corresponding to hemorrhage or necrosis

Needle biopsy is of limited value because hepatocellular carcinomas may contain areas of well-differentiated cells. If such tissue is sampled by needle, a malignant tumor may be misdiagnosed as a benign adenoma. Therefore, a confident diagnosis of adenoma usually requires open biopsy and resection.

Malignant Tumors

An important point about both primary and secondary malignant tumors in the liver is that they almost uniformly obtain blood supply from the arterial circulation only, not from portal vessels. This point has practical implications for both diagnostic studies and therapeutic catheter interventions. The reason that selective hepatic arterial injection of contrast medium is better than celiac injection is that in the former, contrast between a neoplastic focus and normal liver is enhanced because of unopacified portal blood "washing out" normal parenchyma in the face of persistent capillary stain in the tumor.[3] At times, a treated lesion persists on US or CT despite the fact that no viable tissue is present. Lack of capillary stain on a posttreatment angiogram appears reliable in confirming a positive response.[3]

Hepatocellular Carcinoma

Hepatocellular carcinoma is the most frequent primary tumor of the liver. In the majority of patients it arises within a previously diseased and cirrhotic liver, and there is a strong propensity for those with a history of hepatitis B to develop this tumor. Hepatocellular carcinoma is one of the most common neoplasms in Asia. It is a highly malignant lesion, and the 5-year survival of those not undergoing tumor resection is 0%.[22] At present, surgery provides the only hope of cure, with 21% to 30% 5-year survival after resection.[22,23] At the time of tumor discovery, many patients already have satellite nodules or metastases, and these findings (or vascular invasion) may preclude surgical therapy. Spiral CT and MRI can demonstrate vascular invasion reliably, and they are first-line imaging studies for diagnosis and staging.[8,16]

Hepatic angiography is quite sensitive in the detection of hepatocellular carcinomas larger than 2 cm diameter, with 93% of such tumors identified by conventional selective arteriography.[24] False-negative studies occur in smaller lesions or in diffuse infiltrating tumors. The latter tend to be hypovascular, lack mass effect, and are very difficult to recognize angiographically, but they comprise only 5% to 7% of all hepatocellular carcinomas.[25]

Angiographic features that may be found in hepatocellular carcinoma include:

1. Mass effect and hypervascularity
2. Irregular tumor vessels
3. Nodular or irregular tumor stain
4. Arteriovenous shunting
5. "Threads and streaks" sign of tumor thrombus in portal or hepatic veins
6. Portal vein occlusion

Portal hypertension, new or abruptly worsening, may be the first clinical sign of malignancy. Massive AV shunting can produce portal hypertension, as can tumor obstructing portal flow. The portal vein does not normally opacify with selective hepatic artery injection. The "threads and streaks" sign described in portal vein invasion represents the vascularity of the tumor thrombus itself.[26] Segmental staining after an arterial injection is an indirect sign of tumor with focal portal obstruction.[27]

Hepatocellular carcinoma may be confused angiographically with hypervascular metastases from another primary tumor. False-positive studies can also result in those with macronodular cirrhosis.[28] The lack of sensitivity of angiography in detection of lesions smaller than 2 cm, as well as the invasive nature of the study, does not permit it to be used as an aggressive screening measure for those at high risk for hepatocellular carcinoma. The best available screens at present appear to be serum α-fetoprotein determination and US scanning.

When angiography is performed, it can be enhanced by selective intraarterial injection of a lymphographic oily contrast agent (Lipiodol or Ethiodol). Injection of 2 to 5 ml of the agent results in its accumulation and persistence in hepatic tumors, particularly in hepatocellular carcinoma, whereas normal liver parenchyma is clear of the contrast material within 1 month.[29,30] With performance of CT at intervals after oily contrast injection, more tumor nodules can be recognized than with angiography alone.[30,31] As already noted, however, not everyone has found oily contrast agents to be useful for diagnosis.[12] What may be of greater benefit for preoperative staging is CT-portography, which in one multiinstitutional review was 87% accurate in determining extent of tumor.[7]

Fibrolamellar Hepatocellular Carcinoma
Fibrolamellar hepatocellular carcinoma is a distinct clinical variant of primary liver cancer that occurs in a much younger group of patients (mean

age at presentation is 20 years) and has a distinctly better prognosis.[23] These tumors tend to be quite large, and they often contain calcification visible on plain radiographs. On angiograms they usually appear hypervascular, but the presence of fibrous septae or areas of necrosis can make their differentiation from focal nodular hyperplasia or hepatic adenoma difficult. Detection of satellite nodules may be helpful, but in most cases surgery is needed to establish the diagnosis.[23] Pleomorphism of tissue within the tumor makes diagnosis by needle biopsy unlikely.

Cholangiocarcinoma

Cholangiocarcinoma is the only liver tumor that commonly causes vascular encasement and arterial occlusion. The tumor tends to be hypovascular and infiltrating, and obstructive jaundice is the typical clinical presentation.[32] With availability of US, CT, MRI, percutaneous biliary drainage, and percutaneous biopsy, angiography is rarely needed for diagnosis or determining the extent of disease.

Hepatic Angiosarcoma

This is an aggressive malignancy associated with occupational exposure to vinyl chloride. True tumor vessels may be difficult to identify.[33] Hepatic angiosarcomas tend to have hypervascular rims and hypovascular centers, features that are far from specific. These lesions are associated with cirrhosis and periportal fibrosis.

Metastases

Vascularity of hepatic metastases is related to that of the tumor of origin. Most are hypervascular and manifest a capillary stain. Metastases do not characteristically produce AV shunting or portal vein occlusion, but these features are sometimes encountered.[34] Angiography today is generally reserved for those in whom surgical resection is contemplated. The role of film angiography and DSA is to determine vascular anatomy; the extent of disease is best determined by CT-portography, preferably with a spiral CT scanner.

Resection of solitary (or a limited number of) hepatic metastases has been associated with prolonged survival, particularly for metastases of colorectal primaries, although some surgeons remain skeptical.[35] Even if the value of resection is conceded, the expense and morbidity of surgery do not allow exploration of every patient found to have a liver metastasis without evidence of disease elsewhere. Although intraoperative ultrasound is very sensitive for identifying metastases, it requires a wide operative exposure.[36] Reliable nonoperative means of screening out those who would not benefit from surgery are desirable. To this point, CT-portography has been the most effective method of detecting otherwise occult

the liver. The spaces have diameters of 2 to 6 mm, can be distributed focally or diffusely, and lack an endothelial lining or communication with venules.[49,50] The spaces fill with contrast material on the late arterial phase and persist through the venous phase of an arteriogram. When focal, a sharply defined collection can appear similar to a hypervascular nodule. There is some risk for intrahepatic hemorrhage.

Peliosis hepatis must be distinguished from periportal sinusoidal dilatation, a condition described only in conjunction with pregnancy or use of oral contraceptives.[51] Angiography can demonstrate punctate areas of contrast accumulation in periportal sinusoidal dilatation, but these are not as pronounced or as well circumscribed as the collections in peliosis hepatis. The lesions are dilated sinusoids, spaces possessing an endothelial lining. There is no risk of hemorrhage, and the condition resolves after pregnancy or discontinuance of oral contraceptives.

Angiography is used in prospective liver transplant recipients for determination of arterial anatomy, IVC patency, and portal vein patency.[52] In some institutions conventional arteriography is now being replaced with magnetic resonance angiography for this purpose.[53] Transplant recipients may demonstrate arterial stenosis or thrombosis postoperatively, manifesting as ischemic cholangitis or progressive hepatic failure.[54] Diffuse intrahepatic arterial narrowing may be present in cases of graft rejection.[55] Diffuse arterioportal shunting indicates severe rejection. Arteriovenous fistulae can result from biopsies in transplant patients. Another potential cause for hepatic failure in such a setting is IVC and hepatic vein thrombosis.

BUDD-CHIARI SYNDROME

The Budd-Chiari syndrome is a clinical condition caused by obstruction of hepatic venous outflow and resulting in congestion, portal hypertension, and progressive liver failure. It has been associated with malignancy, use of oral contraceptives, paroxysmal nocturnal hemoglobinuria, polycythemia rubra vera, and other myeloproliferative disorders, but one third of patients have no evident predisposing condition.[56] Onset is usually insidious; the affected individual develops hepatomegaly, pain, ascites, and edema. Obstruction can be due to thrombosis of hepatic veins or the IVC, invasion of the vessels by tumor, or vascular webs (this latter condition seen more often in Asia). Venous obstruction may be partial or complete, and the most effective treatment for complete obstruction, when possible, is surgical placement of a portocaval shunt.[56] Transjugular intrahepatic portosystemic shunt placement (TIPS) is a less invasive option now available; we have successfully treated one such patient with TIPS at the University of Wisconsin–Madison.

If the entire liver is affected, arteriography demonstrates diffuse straightening and narrowing of intrahepatic arterial branches, slowed flow, and diminished filling of peripheral vessels.[45] The hepatogram may be prolonged and diffusely mottled. Often, despite involvement of the rest of the liver, the caudate lobe has unimpeded outflow into the IVC and shows compensatory hypertrophy.

When only portions of the liver are involved, the unaffected segments enlarge and portal blood is shunted from the affected area to the unaffected segments.[57] The affected segments may manifest crowding of arterial branches and an intense hepatogram. Retrograde portal filling is sometimes observed.

Although arteriography or noninvasive studies such as US, MRI, or dynamic CT may suggest the diagnosis, the most direct and conclusive evidence for Budd-Chiari syndrome is provided by IVC cavography and hepatic venography with pressure measurements in all vessels studied. Even when all hepatic veins are thrombosed, one can usually cannulate at least one. Contrast injection then shows the typical hepatic vein–to–hepatic vein "spiderweb" collaterals. If a hepatic vein cannot be entered, power injection of contrast material into the IVC with the patient in the Valsalva maneuver may be performed. Failure to opacify any veins by reflux then gives the presumptive diagnosis of hepatic vein occlusion.[58] Multiple veins should be catheterized, when possible, to exclude the possibility of partial Budd-Chiari syndrome.

REFERENCES

1. Soyer P: Segmental anatomy of the liver: Utility of a nomenclature accepted worldwide. *Am J Roentgenol* 1993; 161:572–573.
2. Michels NA: Newer anatomy of the liver and its variant blood supply and collateral circulation. *Am J Surg* 1966; 112:337–347.
3. Chuang VP: Hepatic tumor angiography: A subject review. *Radiology* 1983; 148:633–639.
4. Freeny PC, Marks WM: Computed tomographic arteriography of the liver. *Radiology* 1983; 148:193–197.
5. Helmberger H, Bautz W, Vogel U, Lenz M: CT-Arterioportographie in Spiraltechnik zum Nachweis von Lebermetastasen. *Rofo* 1993; 158:410–415.
6. Nelson RC, Chesmar JL, Sugarbaker PH, Bernardino ME: Hepatic tumors: Comparison of CT during arterial portography, delayed CT, and MR imaging for preoperative evaluation. *Radiology* 1989; 172:27–34.
7. Small WC, Mehard WB, Langmo LS, et al: Preoperative determination of the resectability of hepatic tumors: Efficacy of CT during arterial portography. *Am J Roentgenol* 1993; 161:319–322.
8. Bluemke DA, Urban B, Fishman EK: Spiral CT of the liver: Current applications. *Semin Ultrasound CT MRI* 1994; 15:107–121.
9. Sawada S, Nakamura K, Tanigawa N, Kobayashi M: Computed tomographic percutaneous transsplenic portography. *Acta Radiol* 1993; 34:529–531.

10. Soyer P, Laissy J-P, Sibert A, et al: Focal hepatic masses: Comparison of detection during arterial portography with MR imaging and CT. *Radiology* 1994; 190:737–740.

11. Nelson RC, Thompson GH, Chezmar JL, et al: CT during arterial portography: Diagnostic pitfalls. *RadioGraphics* 1992; 12:705–708.

12. Dawson P, Adam A, Banks L: Diagnostic iodized oil embolisation of liver tumours: The Hammersmith experience. *Eur J Radiol* 1993; 16:201–206.

13. Ohishi H, Uchida H, Yoshimure H, et al: Hepatocellular carcinoma detected by iodized oil. *Radiology* 1985; 154:25–29.

14. Gutierrez OH, Rösch J: Limitations of angiographic differential diagnosis in major hepatic processes. *Rofo* 1977; 127:1–8.

15. Brant WE, Floyd JL, Jackson DE, Gilliland JD: The radiological evaluation of hepatic cavernous hemangioma. *JAMA* 1987; 257:2471–2474.

16. Powers C, Ros PR, Stoupis C, et al: Primary liver neoplasms: MR imaging with pathologic correlation. *RadioGraphics* 1994; 14:459–482.

17. Davis WD, Ferrante WA, Tutton RH, Bowen JC: Hepatic hemangioma with normal angiograms: Three case reports. *JAMA* 1990; 263:983–986.

18. Cronan JJ, Esparza AR, Dorfman GS, et al: Cavernous hemangioma of the liver: Role of percutaneous biopsy. *Radiology* 1988; 166:135–138.

19. Rogers JV, Mack LA, Freeny PC, et al: Hepatic focal nodular hyperplasia: Angiography, CT, sonography, and scintigraphy. *Am J Roentgenol* 1981; 137:983–990.

20. Casarella WJ, Knowles DM, Wolff M, Johnson PM: Focal nodular hyperplasia and liver cell adenoma: Radiologic and pathologic differentiation. *Am J Roentgenol* 1978; 131:393–402.

21. Welch TJ, Sheedy PF, Johnson CM, et al: Radiographic characteristics of benign liver tumors: Focal nodular hyperplasia and hepatic adenoma. *RadioGraphics* 1985; 5:673–682.

22. Marks WM, Jacobs RP, Goodman PC, Lim RC, Jr: Hepatocellular carcinoma: Clinical and angiographic findings and predictability for surgical resection. *Am J Roentgenol* 1979; 132:7–11.

23. Friedman AC, Lichtenstein JE, Goodman Z, et al: Fibrolamellar hepatocellular carcinoma. *Radiology* 1985; 157:583–587.

24. Takayasu K, Shima Y, Muramatsu H, et al: Angiography of small hepatocellular carcinomas: Analysis of 105 resected tumors. *Am J Roentgenol* 1986; 147:525–529.

25. Freeny PC: Angiography of hepatic neoplasms. *Semin Roentgenol* 1983; 18:114–122.

26. Okuda K, Musha H, Yoshida T, et al: Demonstration of growing casts of hepatocellular carcinoma in the portal vein by celiac angiography: The thread and streaks sign. *Radiology* 1975; 117:303–309.

27. Matsui O, Takashima T, Kadoya M, et al: Segmental staining on hepatic arteriography as a sign of intrahepatic portal vein obstruction. *Radiology* 1984; 152:601–606.

28. Shumida M, Ohto M, Ebara M, et al: Accuracy of angiography in the diagnosis of small hepatocellular carcinoma. *Am J Roentgenol* 1986; 147:531–536.

29. Nakakuma K, Tashiro S, Hiraoka T, et al: Hepatocellular carcinoma and metastatic cancer detected by iodized oil. *Radiology* 1985; 154:15–17.

30. Yumoto Y, Jinno K, Tokuyama K, et al: Hepatocellular carcinoma detected by iodized oil. *Radiology* 1985; 154:19–24.
31. Hayashi N, Yamamoto K, Tamaki N, et al: Metastatic nodules of hepatocellular carcinoma: Detection with angiography, CT, and US. *Radiology* 1987; 165:61–63.
32. Walter JF, Bookstein JJ, Bouffard EV: Newer angiographic observations in cholangiocarcinoma. *Radiology* 1976; 118:19–23.
33. Whelan JG, Jr, Creech JL, Tamburo CH: Angiographic and radionuclide characteristics of hepatic angiosarcoma found in vinyl chloride workers. *Radiology* 1976; 118:549–557.
34. Heaston DK, Chuang VP, Wallace S, de Santos LA: Metastatic hepatic neoplasms: Angiographic features of portal vein involvement. *Am J Roentgenol* 1981; 136:897–900.
35. Silen W: Hepatic resection for metastases from colorectal carcinoma is of dubious value. *Arch Surg* 1989; 124:1021–1022.
36. Soyer P, Elias D, Zeitoun G, et al: Surgical treatment of hepatic metastases: Impact of intraoperative sonography. *Am J Roentgenol* 1993; 160:511–514.
37. Leen E, Goldberg JA, Robertson J, et al: Early detection of occult colorectal hepatic metastases using duplex colour doppler sonography. *Br J Surg* 1993; 80:1249–1251.
38. Nakamura H, Tanaka T, Hori S, et al: Transcatheter embolization of hepatocellular carcinoma: Assessment of efficacy in cases of resection following embolization. *Radiology* 1983; 147:401–405.
39. Yamada R, Sato M, Kawabata M, et al: Hepatic artery embolization in 120 patients with unresectable hepatoma. *Radiology* 1983; 148:397–401.
40. Chuang VP, Wallace S: Hepatic artery embolization in the treatment of hepatic neoplasms. *Radiology* 1981; 140:51–58.
41. Mitty HA, Warner RRP, Newman LH, et al: Control of carcinoid syndrome with hepatic artery embolization. *Radiology* 1985; 155:623–626.
42. Rabinowitz JG, Kinkabwala M, Ulreich S: Macro-regenerating nodule in the cirrhotic liver. *Am J Roentgenol* 1974; 121:401–411.
43. Freeny PC: Acute pyogenic hepatitis: Sonographic and angiographic findings. *Am J Roentgenol* 1980; 135:388–391.
44. Baltaxe HA, Fleming RJ: The angiographic appearance of hydatid disease. *Radiology* 1970; 97:599–604.
45. Rösch J, Keller FS: Angiography in diagnosis and therapy of diffuse hepatocellular disease. *Radiologe* 1980; 20:334–342.
46. Casarella WJ, Martin EC: Angiography in the management of abdominal trauma. *Semin Roentgenol* 1984; 19:321–327.
47. Gelin J, Wilms G: Angiodysplasien der leber und des gastrointestinaltraktes bei morbus Rendu-Osler-Weber. *Rofo* 1985; 143:722–724.
48. Danchin N, Thisse JV, Neimann JL, Faivre G: Osler-Weber-Rendu disease with multiple intrahepatic arteriovenous fistulas. *Am Heart J* 1983; 105:856–859.
49. Lyon J, Bookstein JJ, Cartwright CA, et al: Peliosis hepatis: Diagnosis by magnification wedged hepatic venography. *Radiology* 1984; 150:647–649.
50. Tsukamoto Y, Nakata H, Kimoto T, et al: CT and angiography of peliosis hepatitis. *Am J Roentgenol* 1984; 142:539–540.

51. Fisher MR, Neiman HL: Periportal sinusoidal dilatation associated with pregnancy. *Cardiovasc Intervent Radiol* 1984; 7:299–302.
52. Cardella JF, Amplatz K: Preoperative angiographic evaluation of prospective liver recipients. *Radiol Clin North Am* 1987; 25:299–308.
53. Finn JP, Edelman RR, Jenkins RL, et al: Liver transplantation: MR angiography with surgical validation. *Radiology* 1991; 179:265–269.
54. Ludwig J, Batts KP, MacCarty RL: Ischemic cholangitis in hepatic allografts. *Mayo Clin Proc* 1992; 67:519–526.
55. Cardella JF, Amplatz K: Postoperative angiographic and interventional radiologic evaluation of liver recipients. *Radiol Clin North Am* 1987; 25:309–321.
56. McCarthy PM, van Heerden JA, Adson MA, et al: The Budd-Chiari syndrome: Medical and surgical management of 30 patients. *Arch Surg* 1985; 120:657–662.
57. Maguire R, Doppman JL: Angiographic abnormalities in partial Budd-Chiari syndrome. *Radiology* 1977; 122:629–635.
58. Floyd JL: The radiographic gamut of Budd-Chiari syndrome. *Gastroenterology* 1981; 76:381–387.

5

Portal Venography, Portal Hypertension, and TIPS

KEY CONCEPTS

1. A major indication for portal venography is definition of anatomy and flow prior to surgical shunt placement or hepatic transplantation.
2. Arterial portography does *not* define most esophageal varices, nor does it show active variceal bleeding.
3. Portal hypertension may be caused by presinusoidal or postsinusoidal venous obstruction. Cirrhosis results in an increase in postsinusoidal resistance.
4. Esophageal, colonic, small bowel, and rectal varices represent spontaneous portosystemic shunts, and all can be the source of gastrointestinal bleeding.
5. The direction of portal venous flow reverses with severe cirrhosis.
6. Corrected hepatic vein wedge pressure provides an estimation of hepatic sinusoidal pressure.
7. Transjugular intrahepatic portosystemic shunts (TIPS) can take the place of surgical shunts in selected patients, but many need continued and repeated interventions to maintain long-term shunt patency.

INDICATIONS

Portal venography is primarily used for the evaluation of patients with portal hypertension prior to portosystemic shunt surgery or TIPS. The patency and size of portal, splenic, and mesenteric veins are assessed, as well as the direction of flow and presence of portosystemic collaterals. Arterial portography is not used to make the diagnosis of esophageal varices or variceal bleeding. Fewer than 25% of patients with endoscopically documented varices demonstrate these varices by arterial injection of contrast material.[1]

Other indications for angiography of the portal venous system include problems following placement of a portosystemic shunt, suspected mesenteric venous thrombosis, colonic or small bowel varices, and preoperative localization of functioning pancreatic islet cell tumors. Hepatic transplantation is dependent on the patency and size of the portal vein, and portography may be necessary postoperatively as well as preoperatively if complications arise.[2,3] Large portosystemic collateral vessels may jeopardize portal perfusion in patients with liver transplants; preoperative recognition and intraoperative ligation improve graft and patient survival.[4] Portography is occasionally useful for determining if hepatic, pancreatic, or other intraabdominal tumors are surgically resectable.

Developments in duplex sonography and magnetic resonance imaging (MRI) may circumscribe the future use of conventional examinations with contrast material.[5–8] Portography for portal hypertension and percutaneous interventions in the treatment of portal hypertension are addressed in this chapter. For islet cell tumor localization and mesenteric thrombosis, see Chapter 6 entitled Mesenteric Angiography.

ANATOMY

The portal venous system drains blood from the small bowel, stomach, spleen, pancreas, and colon. The confluence of the superior mesenteric vein and splenic vein at the pancreatic head forms the portal vein. The inferior mesenteric vein usually enters the splenic vein several centimeters from the origin of the portal vein.

The portal vein ramifies within the liver, defining the segmental anatomy of the organ. Blood flows within the hepatic sinusoids, mixes with hepatic arterial blood, and drains into the hepatic veins at the periphery of the acinus (the basic functional unit of the liver). An older convention defines the hepatic lobule as the tissue surrounding a hepatic vein and places portal triads (portal vein, hepatic artery, and bile duct branch) at the periphery of each lobule.

If normal portal flow is obstructed, blood may pursue various collateral pathways to rejoin the systemic circulation. Potential portosystemic

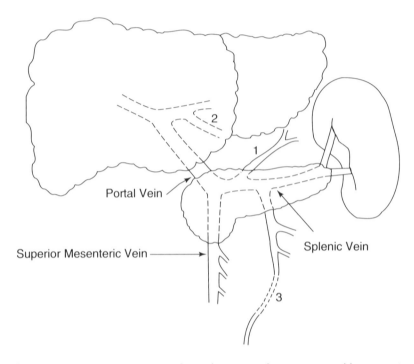

Fig. 5-1   Portosystemic venous channels commonly seen in portal hypertension: coronary vein (*1*), paraumbilical veins (*2*), inferior mesenteric/rectal veins (*3*). (Modified from Reuter SR, Redman HC, Cho KJ: *Gastrointestinal Angiography,* ed 3. 1986, Philadelphia: WB Saunders; with permission.)

communications include left portal vein to paraumbilical veins within the falciform ligament, superior rectal vein to inferior rectal vein, spontaneous splenorenal or other retroperitoneal shunts, and left gastric (coronary vein) or short gastric branches to the azygos system by way of esophageal veins (Fig. 5-1). Obstruction of main portal or splenic veins can result in the emergence of gastroepiploic, pancreatic, or biliary/gallbladder venous collaterals.[9] The propensity of gastroesophageal varices to catastrophic rupture is a prime cause of death from portal hypertension.

CAUSES OF PORTAL HYPERTENSION

The major cause of portal hypertension in the United States is Laënnec's (alcoholic) cirrhosis. The condition is characterized by bands of fibrosis throughout the liver and relatively small, homogeneous regenerating nodules. Viral hepatitis and a number of other toxic or infectious diseases may lead to postnecrotic cirrhosis, which is associated with larger regenerating nodules. Both alcoholic and postnecrotic cirrhosis produce portal venous obstruction predominantly at the *postsinusoidal* level. Other conditions causing a postsinusoidal increase in vascular resistance include Budd-Chiari syndrome (hepatic vein thrombosis) and constrictive pericarditis.

Portal hypertension may also arise from *presinusoidal* obstruction, such as tumor invasion or encasement of the portal vein, schistosomiasis, congenital hepatic fibrosis, noncirrhotic idiopathic portal hypertension (Banti's syndrome), and portal vein thrombosis. Thrombosis can result from dehydration, trauma, infection, and hypercoagulable states. Splenic vein occlusion, often consequent to pancreatitis or pancreatic malignancy, produces hypertension in a portion of the portal system. The distinction between presinusoidal and postsinusoidal blocks is important in the interpretation of studies with contrast material and in hepatic venous pressure measurements (see the section on Hemodynamic Measurements later in this chapter). Rarely, a large arteriovenous shunt produced by trauma or hepatocellular carcinoma can result in a high-output form of portal hypertension.

CLINICAL ASPECTS OF PORTAL HYPERTENSION

As mentioned, a major threat from any form of portal hypertension is exsanguination from ruptured varices. Although rectal, colonic, and other varices may develop, they do not ordinarily pose the same degree of risk that gastroesophageal varices do. Approximately 50% of patients with cirrhosis develop esophageal varices, and most of them bleed at some time.[10] Despite aggressive approaches to medical management, the prognosis of such patients has been dismal. One third may die during initial hospitalization, many rebleed within weeks of discharge, and only about one third survive 1 year.[10] Bleeding is related to the size of varices, but their size does not correlate well with portal venous pressure.[11]

Other major causes of morbidity are hepatic encephalopathy and liver failure. They are particularly problems in patients with cirrhosis as the cause of portal hypertension, and they may be precipitated by an episode of major hemorrhage. Unfortunately, encephalopathy may occur in some patients after surgical treatment with portosystemic shunt placement for decompression.

Treatment Alternatives

Propranolol, labetalol, and other medications that lower portal blood pressure have produced modest improvements in initial or recurrent bleeding rates, and they may increase survival.[12] Even so, their place in the management of portal hypertension remains controversial. Intravenous vasopressin has been used successfully to control acute hemorrhage.

In cases of active bleeding, esophageal balloon catheters, such as the Sengstaken-Blakemore tube, are effective in tamponade and are best applied in catastrophic hemorrhage. However, a high rebleeding rate after balloon deflation means that tamponade is merely a temporizing step before definitive treatment.[13]

Because of the deficiencies of more conservative treatment, various surgical portosystemic shunting procedures have been devised. A successful shunt reduces the risk of recurrent hemorrhage to 4% to 7%, and when bleeding occurs it is usually associated with thrombosis or stenosis of the shunt.[14] Emergency surgery carries a high mortality rate, and acute bleeding is best controlled by other means. Alternatives to surgery explored in the past 20 years have included percutaneous transhepatic embolization of varices, endoscopic injection sclerotherapy, and endoscopic band ligation.

Transhepatic catheter embolization of varices was investigated at various institutions, but the procedure has generally been abandoned because of a high complication rate and lack of lasting effect (see the section on Percutaneous Interventions later in this chapter). Endoscopic injection sclerotherapy has been widely applied, and it is now considered a first-line measure for preventing rebleeding.[15,16] It has the advantage of preserving hepatic perfusion, minimizing the risk of hepatic encephalopathy, and at the same time not interfering with any subsequent surgery. Nevertheless, there can be substantial morbidity from esophageal strictures, perforation, ulceration, and pneumonia, and early rebleeding (within 24 hours) can complicate 6% of sclerotherapy treatments.[17] Rebleeding within 2 years is encountered in more than one third of patients managed by endoscopic sclerotherapy.[18] Moreover, in series with randomization of patients to endoscopic sclerotherapy or surgical shunting, no survival advantage to endoscopic treatment has been demonstrated.[18,19] Endoscopic band ligation of varices may be as effective as sclerotherapy, but without as high a complication rate.[16] In any case, variceal hemorrhage after at least two separate endoscopic attempts at control during a single hospitalization is considered an indication for portosystemic shunt placement. Other considerations in choosing surgical intervention include a patient's operative risk factors and the distance from the patient's home to a hospital providing high-level emergency care.[19]

Surgical Shunts

The type of shunt created operatively depends on patient anatomy, hemodynamics, and the experience of the surgeon. Direct end-to-side and side-to-side portocaval shunts, mesocaval (i.e., superior mesenteric vein–inferior vena cava [IVC]) shunts, and splenorenal shunts have been employed. A short synthetic graft can be interposed in the placement of portocaval and mesocaval shunts. Splenorenal shunts may either be proximal (Linton) or distal (Warren). In the former, the spleen is removed. In the latter, the splenic vein is divided, and drainage from the spleen is directed into the renal vein, essentially isolating the spleen from the rest of the portal circulation.

Although the distal splenorenal shunt is technically more difficult to place, it tends to preserve antegrade (hepatopetal) flow in the portal vein. The development of hepatic encephalopathy has been correlated with loss of normal portal flow.[1] Rikkers and colleagues recently reported a series of patients with a 6-year survival rate of 53% with rebleeding in less than 17% after distal splenorenal shunt placement, outcomes substantially better than those of patients randomly assigned to endoscopic sclerotherapy.[19] For a patient to be a candidate for such a shunt, antegrade flow must be present preoperatively.

What appears to be more clinically important than flow direction are the rapidity and degree of portal vein flow reversal, for most patients with distal splenorenal shunts eventually develop hepatofugal flow.[20] Use of a flow-limiting graft in portocaval shunt surgery can accomplish the same effect with a low incidence of postoperative hepatic failure or encephalopathy (for a discussion of TIPS, see the section on Percutaneous Interventions later in this chapter).[5,21]

Patients with noncirrhotic causes of portal hypertension and good hepatic functional reserve tend to tolerate surgery (as well as variceal hemorrhage) better than those with cirrhosis. Distal splenorenal shunts have produced a mean 5.5-year survival in nonalcoholic patients, as opposed to a mean 4.3-year survival in those with alcoholic cirrhosis.[22] Also, alcoholics are more likely to die of hepatic failure than those having shunt placement for other reasons.

METHODS OF PORTOGRAPHY

Portal angiography can be performed by either direct or indirect means. The portal vein and its branches cannot be catheterized via the arterial or systemic venous circulations; consequently, direct portography requires a more invasive approach, such as hepatic or splenic puncture. For this reason, most portal studies are performed by injecting mesenteric and splenic arteries with relatively high doses of contrast medium. If portal opacification is inadequate, a direct approach can then be employed.

Arterial Portography

Arterial portography requires selective catheterization of the superior mesenteric, splenic, and hepatic arteries. Preliminary biplane aortography may demonstrate stenosis or occlusion of vessel origins, but it also increases the total amount of contrast medium used and is usually unnecessary. A

Simmons or sidewinder catheter is quite useful for selective catheterization and provides stable tip placement. Because of the large amounts of contrast medium injected, stable position is critical. If there are any doubts, a 1-second power test injection at the rate planned can be performed in order to see if the catheter "kicks out" of the selected vessel. A sidehole near the catheter tip makes dissection or inadvertent superselective injection much less likely.

Injection volumes for conventional film runs range from 50 to 80 ml for superior mesenteric artery and splenic injections. The injection rate should be matched to the normal flow of the vessel, as estimated by hand injection and fluoroscopy (usually between 6 and 10 ml/second). Filming is rapid during the arterial phase and slowed after 5 to 6 seconds. Portal opacification normally peaks 15 to 25 seconds after arterial injection, so exposures are best continued to at least 25 seconds. Portal opacification can be enhanced by administration of 50 mg of tolazoline into the artery immediately before injection of contrast material. However, tolazoline is not often needed, and it should be used with caution in patients with cardiac disease.

Digital subtraction portography has been performed successfully, and it can substantially diminish the amount of contrast agent used.[23] Patient cooperation, intravenous administration of glucagon, and minimal bowel gas are prerequisites for a satisfactory study.

Hepatic arteriography should be a part of every portal examination. The presence of tumor, arterioportal shunting, liver size, and degree of cirrhosis can be assessed. If portal flow is reversed, the portal vein may opacify only after hepatic artery injection. If selective hepatic or splenic catheterization is unsuccessful, a celiac injection may be performed.

Transhepatic Portography

The portal vein can be catheterized through a transhepatic route, utilizing a technique similar to that employed for percutaneous biliary drainage. After the lateral costophrenic angle is examined fluoroscopically to prevent puncture of low-lying lung, an 18-gauge sheath needle is directed from the midaxillary line through the right lobe toward the porta hepatis. The trocar is removed, and the sheath slowly withdrawn until blood can be aspirated. Contrast medium is then injected to confirm that a portal branch (rather than a hepatic vein or hepatic artery) has been entered. If so, a guidewire is introduced, and the sheath is advanced over it into the splenic or superior mesenteric vein. Pressure measurements are made, and contrast material injected for filming. This approach allows cannulation of the coronary vein and gastroesophageal varices with selective catheters for detailed study or possible embolization. The transhepatic approach also has been used to clear the portal vein of thrombus (by catheter thrombectomy, balloon dilatation, or venous stent placement) in selected patients immediately prior to TIPS placement.[24]

If no portal branch is entered on the first pass, the needle should not be completely removed from the liver. Instead, redirection from within the tract is advisable in order to minimize the risk of peritoneal hemorrhage or bile leakage. Entry into the extrahepatic portal vein must be avoided. At the conclusion of transhepatic portography, the tract is occluded with gelatin sponge (Gelfoam) particles or coils as the sheath is slowly withdrawn through parenchyma. Particular care should be taken to place occlusion devices near the point of entry into the liver capsule.

Transhepatic portography has the advantage of providing excellent opacification of the portal system and direct measurement of portal pressure. Disadvantages include the increased risk of bleeding, as well as possible focal trauma with thrombosis of the portal vein. Needle insertion may be quite difficult in patients with advanced cirrhosis and extensive hepatic fibrosis. Also, many such patients have impaired hemostasis, further increasing risk. Contraindications to transhepatic portography include the presence of hypervascular hepatic lesions (hepatocellular carcinoma or cavernous hemangioma) and portal vein thrombosis (with the exception of pre-TIPS therapy as noted previously).[10]

Splenoportography

This approach shares many of the advantages and disadvantages of transhepatic portography. Unlike the transhepatic approach, selective catheters cannot be safely inserted through the spleen. Splenoportography is performed with an 18-gauge sheath needle placed from a subcostal midaxillary or anterolateral approach.[25] Fluoroscopy or ultrasound can be used to guide the needle into splenic pulp along the long axis of the organ to avoid possible intervening colon. With proper placement, blood should return freely through the sheath. If there is no free return of blood, Brazzini and associates recommend a test injection with contrast material, followed by a rapid injection of 1 to 2 ml of saline to break up the pulp at the sheath tip.[25] Pressures can then be determined, and a contrast study performed with an injection of 4 to 10 ml/second. At the conclusion of splenoportography, plugs of gelatin sponge are deposited in the tract as the sheath is slowly removed. Without tract plugging, the risk of hemorrhage is substantial.

Umbilical Vein Catheterization

An alternative to transparenchymal catheterization of the portal venous system is umbilical vein cannulation.[26] A cutdown is performed in the epigastrium, and the umbilical vein remnant isolated. A sound can then be passed through the remnant until the return of blood signals that the left portal vein has been reached. An 8 Fr sheath is sutured into place, giving access to catheters for selective examination of the portal vein and its tributaries. This approach permits direct portal manometry while it minimizes the chances of peritoneal hemorrhage. A disadvantage of umbilical vein cannulation is the increased radiation dose to the radiologist from direct exposure to the beam.

HEMODYNAMIC MEASUREMENTS

An integral part of portal vein studies is the determination of portal venous pressure. This is trivial in the case of transhepatic or umbilical cannulation of the portal vein; however, if arterial portography is used, portal pressure is estimated by "corrected" hepatic vein wedge pressure.

Corrected Hepatic (Sinusoidal) Wedge Pressure

An estimation of sinusoidal pressure is obtained by subtracting a "free" hepatic venous pressure (FHVP) from that obtained with a catheter "wedged" into a hepatic vein (WHVP). The latter can be measured with an endhole catheter passed as far as possible into a hepatic vein, such that it occludes outflow through that vein. A somewhat more convenient method of obtaining the same measurement is to employ an occlusion balloon catheter. The balloon is gently inflated, and the efficacy of occlusion is checked fluoroscopically by manual injection of 1 to 2 ml of radiographic contrast medium. After the WHVP is measured, the FHVP is obtained with the balloon deflated.

Some recommend that the pressure of the IVC (rather FHVP) be subtracted from the WHVP.[27] If the diaphragm exerts a pinchcock effect on the IVC, the FHVP may more closely approximate the pressure within the right atrium rather than that of IVC and intraabdominal systemic veins. The effect of this would be to overestimate the effective portal pressure if the FHVP is used to calculate the corrected WHVP.

If a jugular venipuncture is used, selection of hepatic veins with a catheter is usually uncomplicated. When a femoral approach is used, a deflection wire is required. In this case the catheter is passed to the level of the diaphragm, and the deflecting wire advanced until its tip is 2 to 3 cm proximal to the catheter tip. (A deflecting wire should never be passed beyond the catheter tip; otherwise, injury could result.) With deflection exerted, the catheter is manipulated until its tip engages the orifice of a hepatic vein. The wire is then held in place with constant deflection as the catheter is fed off it into the vein. Deflection is gently released, and the wire is removed when satisfactory catheter position has been achieved.

A normal corrected WHVP should be less than 5 mm Hg (1 mm Hg is equivalent to 1.36 cm of water). Corrected wedge pressures reflect portal pressures in cirrhosis and other conditions producing postsinusoidal venous obstruction. However, because the degree of disease may vary from one part of a liver to another, at least two separate hepatic veins should be selected for the most accurate results.[27,28] Corrected wedge pressures are *not* elevated in cases of portal hypertension caused by presinusoidal venous obstruction.

Other Pressure Measurements and Left Renal Venography

Pressures should also be obtained from the right atrium and from the IVC below its intrahepatic portion. If a splenorenal shunt is under consideration, left renal vein pressure must be measured to exclude left renal vein hypertension, and renal venography is performed to assess size and location of the left renal vein. A circumaortic or retroaortic renal vein makes selective shunt placement more difficult.

Koolpe and Koolpe have found measurement of abdominal aortic diastolic pressure valuable because the ratio of aortic diastolic pressure to hepatic vein wedge pressure has correlated with the type and degree of cirrhosis present.[28] They also recommend that the character of the hepatic venous pressure change occurring with deflation of the occlusion balloon be observed closely (see the section on Alcoholic Cirrhosis later in this chapter).

HEPATIC VENOGRAPHY IN PORTAL HYPERTENSION

Although not a standard component of most portal studies, hepatic venography may add useful information. Injections can be made with the catheter in either a free or a wedged position. Free hepatic venography is performed with 20 ml of contrast material injected at a rate of 8 to 10 ml/second, with rapid filming. The appearance of the hepatic vein correlates well with the extent of liver disease. In combination with corrected WHVP measurements, free hepatic venography is valuable in making the diagnosis of cirrhosis in those patients presenting a high risk for biopsy.[27]

Wedge hepatic venography is performed with 4 ml of contrast material injected over 2 seconds. A parenchymal stain results, and reflux of contrast material into the portal vein can be used to assess portal patency and flow. However, this procedure has fallen into disfavor after reports of resultant segmental hepatic infarction and poor correlation of findings with portal hemodynamics.[1,29]

DIRECT CATHETERIZATION OF SHUNTS

After surgical decompression of the portal venous system, arterial portography may not demonstrate shunt patency well. In such cases, or if direct pressure measurements are desired, direct cannulation of the shunt can be performed. Of course, the type and location of shunt must be known before such a study is attempted.

Any gradient of 5 mm Hg or more across a conventional portocaval or splenorenal shunt is abnormal. If a stenosis is present, it may be dilated with balloon catheters. Ruff and colleagues have successfully treated 20 shunt stenoses as early as 2 weeks postoperatively.[14] In narrow-diameter (8 mm) portocaval shunts, measured gradients between the portal vein and IVC are normally high (up to 13 mm Hg). Catheter infusion of thrombolytic agents has successfully reopened narrow-diameter portocaval shunts thrombosed only days after shunt surgery.[21] Any such catheter intervention must be performed with close monitoring during and after the procedure and with surgical backup for possible shunt rupture or catastrophic bleeding.

FINDINGS

Varices and Other Collateral Veins

In all forms of portal hypertension, disturbances in normal flow patterns may be found. Although arterial portography is not very sensitive, it may still define gastric or esophageal varices. Colonic, rectal, and small bowel varices are potential causes of gastrointestinal blood loss in patients with portal hypertension. Colonic and small bowel varices are almost always associated with prior abdominal surgery and are presumably related to adhesions. Rectal varices may become more of a problem in those whose esophageal varices have been treated by endoscopic sclerotherapy.[30] Enlargement of superior mesenteric or inferior mesenteric veins with associated retrograde flow should alert one to the possibility of such unusual lesions. Opacification of the IVC after injections of contrast material into the superior mesenteric or inferior mesenteric artery also indicates major portosystemic venous communications.[31] Late venous phase films must be carefully examined to detect small bowel or colorectal varices, and oblique projections may occasionally help confirm the diagnosis.

Portal vein thrombosis commonly stimulates development of a collateral network in the porta hepatis that is often erroneously termed "cavernous transformation of the portal vein." Isolated splenic vein thrombosis tends to produce gastric varices in the absence of esophageal varices. The left hepatic vein may be prominent in portal hypertension because it serves as a portosystemic collateral through paraumbilical (*not* umbilical) veins in the ligamentum teres.[32]

In interpreting arterial portography, inflow of unopacified blood and reversal of portal flow can be misinterpreted as partial or complete thrombosis of the portal vein. If an examination is equivocal, simultaneous catheterization and injection of the splenic and superior mesenteric arteries may resolve the issue.

Retrograde (Hepatofugal) Portal Flow

Normally, second- and third-order intrahepatic branches of the portal vein are opacified with arterial portography. As portal flow becomes more stagnant with increasing intrahepatic portal obstruction, opacification diminishes. Portal perfusion has been shown to be an independent prognostic variable in cirrhotic patients, with good antegrade flow associated with long-term survival.[33] In severe portal hypertension, flow becomes hepatofugal, and the portal vein is not opacified by injection of contrast material into the superior mesenteric or splenic artery. In such cases, hepatic arteriography or wedge hepatic venography may demonstrate reversed portal flow. If the major portosystemic outflow is through the left portal vein and paraumbilical collaterals, the main portal vein opacifies in a normal antegrade manner, even though functionally flow is hepatofugal. The same holds true for a patent TIPS. In patients with successful creation of decompressive surgical shunts, portal flow generally reverses, even in those with selective splenorenal shunts.[20] Flow reversal may be less likely to occur in patients with narrow-diameter portocaval shunts.[21] If portal vein patency cannot be resolved by angiography, then duplex ultrasound, contrast material–enhanced computed tomography, and MRI are noninvasive diagnostic alternatives.

Alcoholic Cirrhosis

In advanced alcoholic cirrhosis, the liver may be small, with marked enlargement and corkscrewing of hepatic artery branches. Hepatic arterial flow increases to compensate for loss of normal portal flow, and arterioportal shunting may contribute to portal hypertension. It has been asserted that a corrected WHVP of at least 12 mm Hg is necessary for the development of varices in patients with alcoholic cirrhosis.[13] As noted earlier, any corrected wedge pressure of 5 mm Hg or more represents portal hypertension. Large portosystemic venous collaterals serve to depress the degree of pressure elevation.[31]

Koolpe and Koolpe have found a gradient of 4 mm Hg or more between the IVC and right atrium to be a reliable indicator of alcoholic cirrhosis.[28] They have also observed that in alcoholic cirrhosis, deflation of the balloon of a hepatic vein occlusion catheter results in a slow and irregular drop in pressure over more than 1 second. Patients with alcoholic cirrhosis have hepatofugal portal flow if the ratio of aortic diastolic pressure to hepatic vein wedge pressure is 1.6 or less.[28]

Free hepatic venography shows a normal angle of branch junctions, but irregular fill of branches with peripheral occlusions and a "pruned-tree"

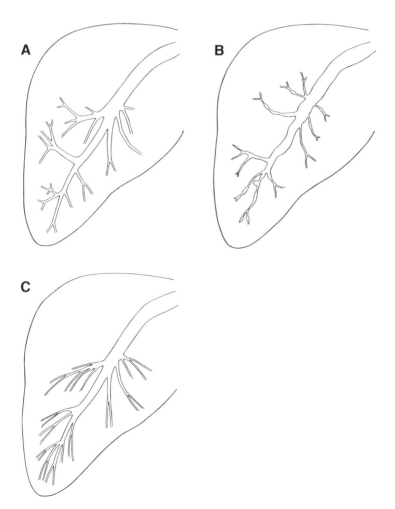

Fig. 5-2   Hepatic venous patterns in healthy (**A**) and diseased (**B** and **C**) livers. **A,** Normal right hepatic vein; **B,** cirrhosis; **C,** Banti's syndrome.

appearance in alcoholic cirrhosis (Fig. 5-2).[34] Venous anastomoses are rarely defined. Wedge hepatic venography produces an irregular parenchymal stain, and portal branches often opacify.[35]

Postnecrotic Cirrhosis
In postnecrotic cirrhosis, arteriographic and venographic findings are similar to those of alcoholic cirrhosis, but tend to be less severe. Balloon deflation in the hepatic vein produces a rapid (less than 1 second) and smooth drop from WHVP to FHVP. There should be no pressure gradient between

abdominal IVC and right atrium.[28] Hepatofugal flow correlates with a ratio of aortic diastolic pressure to WHVP of less than 1.3/1.0.[28]

Noncirrhotic Idiopathic Portal Hypertension
This condition, also known as Banti's syndrome, is rare in the United States but common in Asia.[34] Hepatic venography shows a distinctive, "weeping willow" appearance; hepatic vein branches join together at acute angles (see Fig. 5-2, C). Large communications with other hepatic veins are often evident. Corrected WHVP values and hepatic venograms tend to be normal in the face of multiple occlusions in small and medium-sized portal branches.

PERCUTANEOUS INTERVENTIONS

Embolotherapy
A percutaneous transhepatic route was employed to occlude gastro-esophageal varices in the past. Various agents including gelatin sponge soaked in sodium tetradecyl sulfate (Sotradecol)—a sclerosing agent—coils, bucrylate, and alcohol were used to control acute bleeding.[10,11,36] However, although embolotherapy alone could control bleeding in 76% of patients not responding to other measures, more than two thirds experience bleeding again within a matter of months.[10] High complication rates and low 1-year survival rates of patients treated led to an abandonment of the technique for all but exceptional cases. At Emory University hospitals, transhepatic obliteration of those collaterals diverting flow from the liver has been used to treat patients developing hepatic encephalopathy after portosystemic shunt surgery.[14]

Collins and associates routinely catheterize portocaval shunts in the early postoperative period and occlude any varices not ligated at surgery.[21] Variceal embolization is an integral part of many TIPS procedures, particularly in patients with active hemorrhage. Another application of catheter embolization is in the treatment of arterioportal fistulae associated with hepatocellular carcinoma or trauma causing intractable portal hypertension.[37]

TIPS
An innovative treatment of patients with portal hypertension has been the nonsurgical creation of decompressive shunts. Originally proposed by Rösch, Hanafee, and Snow in 1969,[38] the transjugular intrahepatic portosystemic shunt was applied clinically by Colapinto and colleagues.[39] These early shunts were not practical, for the tracts formed between hepatic vein and portal vein by a transjugular biopsy needle and balloon catheter did not remain consistently open. Only with the development of effective vascular stents could the concept be realized.[40] Stents keep the shunting

tract from collapsing, but unfortunately the growth of tissue within the stents or in the outflow veins commonly produces stenosis and occlusion within 1 or 2 years.[41,42] Thus, TIPS is no panacea for patients with portal hypertension. It has proved quite useful for carrying patients with advanced liver disease through to liver transplantation.[43,44] TIPS placement in those who are not candidates for transplantation is more problematic, and those who need long-term decompression and who are good operative candidates are probably best served by surgical shunting.

TIPS Indications

The primary indication for intervention is continuing or recurrent variceal bleeding refractory to medical or endoscopic control. Preliminary endoscopic examination is mandatory, for bleeding may actually arise from peptic ulcer disease, alcoholic gastritis, esophageal ulcer, Mallory-Weiss tear, or another cause for which portosystemic shunt placement would be inappropriate. Moreover, sclerotherapy or band ligation should be aggressively pursued to stabilize an actively bleeding patient; otherwise, TIPS creation is attended with high morbidity and mortality.[45]

TIPS has also been used to treat massive ascites not responding to diuretics or other conservative measures.[46] Most patients experience great improvement or resolution of their ascites, and post-TIPS diuresis can be dramatic. Patients with hepatic veno-occlusive disease (Budd-Chiari syndrome) have been effectively treated by TIPS. Other benefits of TIPS are less well defined. Portal hypertensive gastropathy may be ameliorated. Renal function may improve in patients with hepatorenal syndrome.[44,47] A drop in intraoperative transfusion requirements and in the duration of liver transplantation surgery has been observed by some investigators but not by others.[44,48]

TIPS Contraindications

Contraindications to TIPS include advanced hepatic encephalopathy (not consequent to recent gastrointestinal hemorrhage), extremely poor hepatic functional reserve, polycystic liver disease, and primary or metastatic malignant tumors. Portal vein thrombosis is a relative contraindication, but percutaneous transhepatic portal vein recanalization combined with TIPS has been successfully applied by Radosevich and associates.[24] However, the need for TIPS in patients with portal vein occlusion but without underlying cirrhosis is unclear. Great caution should be exercised in those with suspected pulmonary hypertension or limited cardiac reserve, for TIPS can place a sudden and severe strain on the heart.[49] We encountered sudden death shortly after TIPS placement in a man who likely had unrecognized pulmonary hypertension. Because of high rates of TIPS stenosis and occlusion over the long term, patients with portal hypertension requiring decom-

Table 5-1   Child-Pugh Classification of Liver Function

Score	1	2	3
Ascites	Absent	Slight to moderate	Severe
Encephalopathy	Absent	Slight to moderate	Severe
Serum albumin	>3.5 g/dl	3–3.5 g/dl	<3 g/dl
Serum bilirubin	<2 mg/dl	2–3 mg/dl	>3 mg/dl
PT prolongation	<4 sec	4–6 sec	>6 sec

Score of 5–6 corresponds to Child-Pugh Class A
Score of 7–11 corresponds to Child-Pugh Class B
Score of 12–15 corresponds to Child-Pugh Class C

PT, Prothrombin time.

pressive shunting who have otherwise mild liver disease (Child-Pugh clinical class A [Table 5-1]) may be better served by a surgical shunt procedure.

TIPS Patient Preparation and Technique
As for any invasive measure, coagulation defects and thrombocytopenia are corrected to the extent possible prior to TIPS. Intravenous administration of broad-spectrum antibiotics at least 1 hour before the procedure is advised. As already noted, the patient should be stabilized and the source of any gastrointestinal bleeding confirmed. Heavy conscious sedation (with intravenous administration of midazolam and fentanyl) is necessary because passage of the needle through hepatic parenchyma and balloon dilation of the tract are quite painful. Adequate monitoring of the patient's vital signs (pulse, respiration, oxygen saturation, blood pressure) ensures safety. In selected cases general anesthesia may be needed.

In planning for TIPS it is useful to have prior images of the portal venous system, whether from duplex sonography, MR angiography, or conventional arterial portography. In this manner portal vein patency and flow direction can be assessed. Also, the presence and size of gastroesophageal varices and other portosystemic collateral channels, as well as liver size, may be defined. TIPS placement may be exceedingly difficult in very small and hard cirrhotic livers; hepatic veins may be diminutive, and anatomic relationships severely distorted. When anatomic definition is obtained with arterial portography, the angiogram may be obtained immediately prior to TIPS. However, performance of arterial portography during a separate session 1 or 2 days before shunt placement minimizes the total duration of the intervention, as well as the patient's acute burden of iodinated contrast medium. Ultrasound imaging can be a helpful adjunct during the procedure. It is commonly used in our institution to mark the location and size of the right internal jugular vein before sterile preparation and draping of the patient's neck. Later, ultrasound may help determine if the selective catheter has entered the right or middle hepatic vein.

The right internal jugular vein is entered and a guidewire advanced to right atrium or IVC. A large working sheath is then introduced. Initial pressure measurements are taken in the right atrium, IVC, and hepatic vein. Venography depicts the size and course of the hepatic vein chosen, most often the right hepatic vein. For the TIPS procedure itself, we at the University of Wisconsin–Madison presently use the five-piece coaxial catheter-needle system described by Rösch and associates.[50] The outer components include a 41-cm-long introducer sheath containing a 52-cm-long 10 Fr Teflon catheter, which itself encloses a 51-cm, 14-gauge curved blunt metal cannula with a distal 15° curve. Through these components are passed a 5 Fr Teflon catheter containing a diamond-tipped stylet, which is flexible in its distal 12 cm. With all components in place in the hepatic vein (the inner components not projecting beyond the outer ones), the 10 Fr catheter is wedged anteroinferiorly against the right hepatic vein wall in about the proximal 1 to 3 cm of the right hepatic vein (Fig. 5-3). Wedging is needed to ensure that the needle does not merely slide along vein wall. The 5 Fr Teflon catheter-stylet combination is quickly advanced 3 to 5 cm through hepatic parenchyma. The stylet is removed, and suction is applied to the catheter as it is slowly withdrawn. When free return of blood is noted, contrast medium is injected to determine if the catheter tip is in a suitable portal branch. The portal bifurcation itself should be avoided, for it is often extrahepatic.[51] Fatal bleeding has been reported after direct portal puncture.[52] Ideally the main right (or left) portal vein is entered, but a more peripheral branch may be adequate for TIPS placement.

If an appropriate portal branch has been entered, a soft-tipped guidewire, such as a Bentson wire, is used to secure access, and the 5 Fr catheter is advanced. The wire is then exchanged for a longer (180 cm or longer) heavy, stiff wire, over which subsequent manipulations are performed. At this point, portal pressure is measured through the 5 Fr Teflon catheter (advanced well into the portal venous system) or through a straight multi-sidehole catheter introduced for portography. Afterwards, the stiff wire is replaced, and its tip is maintained in the superior mesenteric vein or splenic vein during tract dilatation and stenting.

The 10 Fr catheter may sometimes be advanced over the stiff wire into the portal system. In cirrhotic livers this move may be aided by advancing the outer catheter and 14-gauge cannula as a unit. After predilating the parenchymal tract in such a fashion, a 10-mm-diameter Olbert angioplasty balloon catheter is used to prepare the tract for stent placement. The low profile of the Olbert balloon eases its passage through the liver. When possible, the large sheath is then advanced into portal vein and a 10-mm-diameter Wallstent of appropriate length (most commonly 68 mm) is inserted.

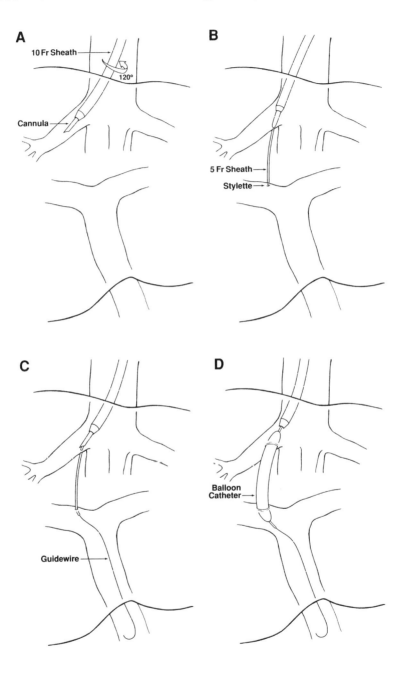

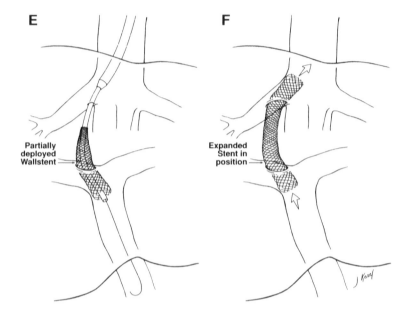

Fig. 5-3 TIPS performed with a Rösch-Uchida set. **A,** Angled directing cannula with sheath placed into right hepatic vein, then rotated anteromedially. **B,** Advancement of sheathed stylet through the directing cannula and hepatic parenchyma into right portal vein. **C,** Insertion of guidewire after removal of stylet. **D,** Balloon dilatation of parenchymal tract. **E,** Deployment of the self-expanding Wallstent as the confining catheter membrane is withdrawn. **F,** TIPS with Wallstent in place.

The large sheath is withdrawn into right atrium, and the stent is deployed, centered on the tract. The balloon catheter is reinserted to maximally expand the stent.

The results of the stent placement are checked by repeat portography and portal pressure measurements. Two guidewires may be placed through the sheath into the portal vein to allow pullback determination of the portosystemic pressure gradient without losing access to the portal vein. A portal vein–hepatic vein (or IVC) pressure gradient of 15 mm Hg or more is satisfactory, for risk of recurrent variceal bleeding at such a gradient is quite low.[53] A gradient of 12 mm Hg or less may be best for prevention of hemorrhage, but too low a gradient might compromise hepatic perfusion.

If tract coverage is marginal or incomplete or if the stent is poorly expanded, additional stent placement or balloon inflation is performed as deemed necessary. Stents should not project into the IVC or more than 1 cm into the portal vein; otherwise, they may interfere with possible later liver transplantation.[54] In a patient with ongoing hemorrhage or in whom very large gastroesophageal varices are present, embolotherapy is used to occlude them by way of the TIPS. Embolization helps maintain flow through the TIPS, for enormous varices can produce a steal phenomenon leading to early shunt occlusion. In most patients, however, embolotherapy is not needed.[55]

When the TIPS placement procedure has been completed, a 9 Fr short Cordis sheath is used to maintain jugular venous access. The long sheath of the TIPS placement set should not be left in place because of the danger of cardiac perforation. Duplex sonography is obtained the next day as a baseline study. If flow through the shunt is shown to be satisfactory, the sheath is removed.

Alternatives and Technical Adjuncts

The procedure described in the previous section is merely one method of placing a typical TIPS. If access via the right internal jugular vein is not available, the left internal jugular or right external jugular can be entered. Other needle systems and other stents may be used, although an inflexible stent, such as the Palmaz, can present difficulties in bridging a curved tract. Patients with marginal hepatic functional reserve and those who are being treated for massive ascites rather than bleeding may have narrower-diameter (8 mm) shunts placed.

Originally, TIPS procedures were performed after percutaneous transhepatic placement of a basket snare into portal vein.[56] This served as a target for advancement of the needle in hepatic vein and secured the guidewire passed into the portal vein. Unfortunately, deaths due to bleeding from the transhepatic puncture were encountered, and such a preliminary procedure has been generally abandoned.[56] However, in certain cases additional localizing procedures can be applied. Harman and colleagues have used ultrasound guidance and 22-gauge needles to place microcoils adjacent to the right portal vein, and create a target for needle advancement.[57] Placement of a fine platinum-tipped guidewire through a 21-gauge needle accomplishes the same.

In one patient for whom TIPS attempts had previously failed because the right hepatic vein and right portal vein were in the same axial plane, we inserted such a wire as a target.[58] With fluoroscopic guidance, the wire was superimposed over a snaring basket positioned in the hepatic vein from a transjugular approach. A hollow 18-gauge needle was advanced percutaneously along the fluoroscopic beam, first into right portal vein (confirmed by injection of iodinated contrast medium) and then into the basket. A long 0.035-inch guidewire was placed through the needle and pulled through the jugular vein by the basket, thus establishing access through a horizontal parenchymal tract. After a sheath was placed from above and pushed through the tract, a second wire could be inserted through it and advanced into the portal venous system. The TIPS was then completed by the customary maneuvers.

Fortunately, in the great majority of patients, portal and hepatic veins do not lie in the same axial plane. Even so, the 15° curve of the cannula may not be appropriate for an individual's anatomy, but the cannula can be bent to a greater angle. When this is done, bending should be performed with the inner components of the access system in place, in order to prevent kinking.[50] One must remember that the middle hepatic vein (unlike the right hepatic vein) is anterior to the major portal branches. Lateral fluoroscopy or ultrasonography can be used to help determine the proper direction of needle advancement.

When a single, adequately expanded stent fails to provide a sufficiently low portosystemic pressure gradient, creation of a second TIPS in parallel may be needed. Haskal and associates found that 10-mm Wallstents did not provide satisfactory portal decompression (less than16 mm Hg residual gradient) in 8 of 93 patients treated.[59] A second TIPS dropped the mean residual gradient from 19 mm Hg to 12 mm Hg in these patients. Presently, 12-mm-diameter Wallstents are available, but it may be difficult to determine a priori which patients may need larger-diameter shunts. An advantage of Palmaz stents is that the diameter can be subsequently increased with balloons of the desired size.[60]

Results and Complications

Successful TIPS placement can be expected in 89% to 100% of patients submitting to the procedure.[44,47,48,61] In one large series, 82% of patients had experienced no rebleeding from varices at 1-year follow-up, and 1-year survival for those having successful TIPS was 100%, 86%, and 73% for patients of Child-Pugh classes A, B, and C, respectively.[61] More than 80% of patients with debilitating ascites have resolution or substantial improvement, usually within 1 week.[44,47,61]

Mortality certainly depends on the clinical status and hemodynamic stability of the patients treated. At the University of Washington, in-hospital mortality was 56% for those bleeding at the time of TIPS.[45] LaBerge and colleagues observed a 30-day mortality of 24% in Child-Pugh class C patients in their series—still less than the mortality of portocaval shunt surgery in similar patients.[47] Then again, Rössle's group had only 3 early deaths among 100 patients, all in individuals who were acutely bleeding at the time of referral. Only one death was directly attributable to the procedure.[61] Fatalities may result from continued gastrointestinal bleeding, bleeding caused by hepatic artery or capsule puncture by the TIPS needle, sepsis, hepatic insufficiency, or multiorgan failure. Puncture of the hepatic artery can lead to infarction or exsanguination.[62]

Most patients maintain grossly stable liver function after TIPS, but close monitoring often reveals some degree of deterioration.[44] Occasionally, hepatic insufficiency becomes rapidly progressive. New hepatic encephalopathy arises in roughly one quarter of those who are followed for weeks to months.[44,47,61] Fortunately, it is usually easily treated and transient. Post-TIPS hemolysis has been documented by systemic laboratory monitoring at our institution. Rarely, it can become a clinical problem, leading to transfusion-dependent anemia.[63,64] We encountered this situation in a patient with parallel TIPS. Percutaneous embolic occlusion of the shunt may be used to reverse intractable encephalopathy or hemolysis. Another reported complication of TIPS is stent migration into the pulmonary circulation.[60,61]

Perhaps the greatest challenge in treating patients with TIPS is shunt obstruction, usually presenting as bleeding or recurrent ascites. Recurrent or unremitting upper gastrointestinal hemorrhage is a problem that must be assessed endoscopically. Bleeding may be from sclerotherapy ulcers or other nonvariceal causes.[44,45] Ultrasonography is well suited for assessment of TIPS function. Changes in intrahepatic flow characteristics and intrastent velocities can detect significant stenoses before shunt thrombosis occurs.[7]

Late post-TIPS stenoses may develop within the stent, portal vein, or, most often, the draining hepatic vein. Stenosis or occlusion has been found in 25% to 37% of patients followed 6 months.[41,42] Mild-to-moderate stenosis does not necessarily progress. Nevertheless, the primary 2-year patency of TIPS was only 32% in one report.[42] Evaluation of a failing or occluded TIPS can be performed from a brachial or femoral venous approach, but right jugular venous access affords the most control for recatheterization. Balloon dilatation alone may be successful in restoring an acceptably low portosystemic pressure gradient, but coaxial placement of a new stent is often required.

At times advancement of a guidewire through a thrombosed shunt from the systemic venous side may be extremely difficult. Use of a large, curved guiding needle or cannula facilitates catheterization.[65] In exceptional circumstances, particularly in the face of severe hepatic vein stenosis or occlusion, percutaneous transhepatic stent puncture can be employed to insert a wire, which is then retrieved through a transjugular sheath with a snare.[66] The sheath can be advanced over the through-and-through wire into the thrombosed stent and a second wire placed through it into the portal vein. TIPS revision can then ensue with balloon expansion and stent placement as needed. At the conclusion of such an intervention the percutaneous transhepatic tract is occluded with coils or gelatin sponge.

REFERENCES

1. Nordlinger BM, Nordlinger DF, Fullenwider JT, et al: Angiography in portal hypertension: Clinical significance in surgery. *Am J Surg* 1980; 139:132–141.

2. Cardella JF, Amplatz K: Preoperative angiographic evaluation of prospective liver recipients. *Radiol Clin North Am* 1987; 25:299–308.

3. Cardella JF, Amplatz K: Postoperative angiographic and interventional radiologic evaluation of liver recipients. *Radiol Clin North Am* 1987; 25:309–321.

4. Ploeg RJ, D'Alessandro AM, Stegall MD, et al: Effect of surgical and spontaneous portasystemic shunts on liver transplantation. *Transplant Proc* 1993; 25:1946–1948.

5. Helton WS, Montana MA, Dwyer DC, Johansen K: Duplex sonography accurately assesses portocaval shunt patency. *J Vasc Surg* 1988; 8:657–660.

6. Williams DM, Eckhauser FE, Aisen A, et al: Assessment of portosystemic shunt patency and function with magnetic resonance imaging. *Surgery* 1987; 102:602–607.

7. Surratt RS, Middleton WD, Darcy MD, et al: Morphologic and hemodynamic findings at sonography before and after creation of a transjugular intrahepatic portosystemic shunt. *Am J Roentgenol* 1993; 160:627–630.

8. Müller MF, Siewert B, Kim D, et al: Rolle der Magnetresonanzangiographie vor transjugulärer Einlage eines portosystemischen Stent-Shunts (TIPS). *Rofo* 1994; 160:312–318.

9. Reuter SR, Redman HC, Cho KJ: Cirrhosis and portal hypertension. In *Gastrointestinal Angiography*. 1986, Philadelphia: WB Saunders. pp 382–445.

10. Benner KG, Keefe EB, Keller FS, Rösch J: Clinical outcome after percutaneous transhepatic obliteration of esophageal varices. *Gastroenterology* 1983; 85:146–153.

11. Joffe SN: Non-operative management of variceal bleeding. *Br J Surg* 1984; 71:85–91.

12. Lebrec D: Long-term management of variceal bleeding: The place of pharmacotherapy. *World J Surg* 1994; 18:229–232.

13. Rikkers LF: Variceal hemorrhage. *Gastroenterol Clin North Am* 1988; 17:289–302.

14. Ruff RJ, Chuang VP, Alspaugh JP, et al: Percutaneous vascular intervention after surgical shunting for portal hypertension. *Radiology* 1987; 164:469–474.

15. Botta GC, Contini S: Endoscopic sclerotherapy as emergency and long-term management of esophageal varices: A changing approach? *Int Angiol* 1988; 7:167–171.

16. Bleeding oesophageal varices: IST, EVL, or TIPS. *Lancet* 1992; 340:515–516.

17. McKee RF, Garden OJ, Carter DC: Injection sclerotherapy for bleeding varices: Risk factors and complications. *Br J Surg* 1991; 78:1098–1101.

18. Planas R, Boix J, Broggi M, et al: Portacaval shunt versus endoscopic sclerotherapy in the elective treatment of variceal hemorrhage. *Gastroenterology* 1991; 100:1078–1086.

19. Rikkers LF, Jin GL, Burnett DA, et al: Shunt surgery versus endoscopic sclerotherapy for variceal hemorrhage: Late results of a randomized trial. *Am J Surg* 1993; 165:27–33.

20. Widrich WC, Robbins AH, Johnson WC, Nabseth DC: Long-term follow-up of distal splenorenal shunts. *Radiology* 1980; 134:341–345.

21. Collins JC, Rypins EB, Sarfeh IJ: Narrow-diameter portacaval shunts for management of variceal bleeding. *World J Surg* 1994; 18:211–215.

22. Zeppa R, Lee PA, Hutson DG, et al: Portal hypertension: A fifteen year perspective. *Am J Surg* 1988; 155:6–9.
23. Foley WD, Stewart ET, Milbrath JR, et al: Digital subtraction angiography of the portal venous system. *Am J Roentgenol* 1983; 140:497–499.
24. Radosevich PM, Ring EJ, Laberge JM, et al: Transjugular intrahepatic portosystemic shunts in patients with portal vein occlusion. *Radiology* 1993; 186:523–527.
25. Brazzini A, Hunter DW, Darcy MD, et al: Safe splenoportography. *Radiology* 1987; 162:607–609.
26. Spigos DG, Tauber JW, Tan WS, et al: Umbilical venous cannulation: A new approach for embolization of esophageal varices. *Radiology* 1983; 146:53–56.
27. Cavaluzzi JA, Sheff R, Harrington DP, et al: Hepatic venography and wedge hepatic vein pressure measurements in diffuse liver disease. *Am J Roentgenol* 1977; 129:441–446.
28. Koolpe HA, Koolpe L: Portal hypertension: Angiographic and hemodynamic evaluation. *Radiol Clin North Am* 1986; 24:369–381.
29. Castañeda-Zuñiga WR, Jauregui H, Rysavy J, et al: Complications of wedge hepatic venography. *Radiology* 1978; 126:53–56.
30. Foutch PG, Sivak MV, Jr: Colonic variceal hemorrhage after endoscopic injection sclerosis of esophageal varices: A report of three cases. *Am J Gastroenterol* 1984; 79:756–760.
31. Burcharth F, Sorenson TIA, Andersen B: Percutaneous transhepatic portography: Relationships between portosystemic collaterals and portal pressure in cirrhosis. *Am J Roentgenol* 1979; 133:1119–1122.
32. Lafortune M, Constantin A, Breton G, et al: The recanalized umbilical vein in portal hypertension: A myth. *Am J Roentgenol* 1985; 144:549–553.
33. Finucci G, Bellon S, Merkel C, et al: Evaluation of splanchnic angiography as a prognostic index of survival in patients with cirrhosis. *Scand J Gastroenterol* 1991; 26:951–960.
34. Futagawa S, Fukazawa M, Musha H, et al: Hepatic venography in non-cirrhotic idiopathic portal hypertension. *Radiology* 1981; 141:303–309.
35. Heeney DJ, Bookstein JJ, Bell RH, et al: Correlation of hepatic and portal wedged venography with histology in alcoholic cirrhosis and periportal fibrosis. *Radiology* 1982; 142:591–597.
36. Yune HY, O'Connor KW, Klatte EC, et al: Ethanol thrombotherapy of esophageal varices: Further experience. *Am J Roentgenol* 1985; 144:1049–1053.
37. Tarazov PG: Intrahepatic arterioportal fistulae: Role of transcatheter embolization. *Cardiovasc Intervent Radiol* 1993; 16:368–373.
38. Rösch J, Hanafee WN, Snow H: Transjugular portal venography and radiologic portacaval shunt: An experimental study. *Radiology* 1969; 92:1112–1114.
39. Colapinto RF, Stronell RD, Gildiner M, et al: Formation of intrahepatic portosystemic shunts using balloon dilatation catheter: Preliminary clinical experience. *Am J Roentgenol* 1983; 140:709–714.
40. Palmaz JC, Sibbitt RR, Reuter SR, et al: Expandable intrahepatic portacaval shunt stents: Early experience in the dog. *Am J Roentgenol* 1985; 145:821–825.
41. Nazarian GK, Ferral H, Castañeda-Zúñiga WR, et al: Development of stenoses in transjugular intrahepatic portosystemic shunts. *Radiology* 1994; 192:231–234.

42. Haskal ZJ, Pentecost MJ, Soulen MC, et al: Transjugular intrahepatic portosystemic shunt stenosis and revision: Early and midterm results. *Am J Roentgenol* 1994; 163:439–444.

43. Ring EJ, Lake JR, Roberts JP, et al: Using transjugular intrahepatic portosystemic shunts to control variceal bleeding before liver transplantation. *Ann Intern Med* 1992; 116:304–309.

44. Martin M, Zajko AB, Orons PD, et al: Transjugular intrahepatic portosystemic shunt in the management of variceal bleeding: Indications and clinical results. *Surgery* 1993; 114:719–727.

45. Helton WS, Belshaw A, Althaus S, et al: Critical appraisal of the angiographic portacaval shunt (TIPS). *Am J Surg* 1993; 165:566–571.

46. Ferral H, Bjarnason H, Wegryn SA, et al: Refractory ascites: Early experience in treatment with transjugular intrahepatic portosystemic shunt. *Radiology* 1993; 189:795–801.

47. LaBerge JM, Ring EJ, Gordon RL, et al: Creation of transjugular intrahepatic portosystemic shunts with the Wallstent endoprosthesis: Results in 100 patients. *Radiology* 1993; 187:413–420.

48. Wojtowycz MM, Schuster MR, Sproat IA, et al: *Influence of TIPS on operative time and intraoperative blood product use in liver transplant surgery.* Presented at the Nineteenth Annual Scientific Meeting of the Society of Cardiovascular and Interventional Radiology, March 1994, San Diego, California.

49. Azoulay D, Castaing D, Dennison A, et al: Transjugular intrahepatic portosystemic shunt worsens the hyperdynamic circulatory state of the cirrhotic patient: Preliminary report of a prospective study. *Hepatology* 1994; 19:129–132.

50. Rösch J, Uchida BT, Barton RE, Keller FS: Coaxial catheter-needle system for transjugular portal vein entrance. *J Vasc Interv Radiol* 1993; 4:145–147.

51. Uflacker R, Reichert P, D'Albuquerque LC, de Oliveira e Silva A: Liver anatomy applied to the placement of transjugular intrahepatic portosystemic shunts. *Radiology* 1994; 191:705–712.

52. Perarnau JM, Rucin B, Schwing D, et al: Transjugular intrahepatic portosystemic shunt (TIPS): Improved technique with the Palmaz stent. *Minimal Invasive Ther* 1992; 1:333–336.

53. Ready JB, Robertson AD, Goff JS, Rector WG, Jr: Assessment of the risk of bleeding from esophageal varices by continuous monitoring of portal pressure. *Gastroenterology* 1991; 100:1403–1410.

54. Rousseau H, Vinel J-P, Bilbao JI, et al: Transjugular intrahepatic portosystemic shunts using the Wallstent prosthesis: A follow-up study. *Cardiovasc Intervent Radiol* 1994; 17:7–11.

55. Zemel G, Becker GJ, Bancroft JW, et al: Technical advances in transjugular intrahepatic portosystemic shunts. *RadioGraphics* 1992; 12:615–622.

56. Rössle M, Richter GM, Nöldge G, et al: Transjugular intrahepatic portosystemic stent shunt: A 2-year follow-up. *Digest Surg* 1992; 9:6–12.

57. Harman JT, Reed JD, Kopecky KK, et al: Localization of the portal vein for transjugular catheterization: Percutaneous placement of a metallic marker with real-time US guidance. *J Vasc Interv Radiol* 1992; 3:545–547.

58. Sproat IA, Wojtowycz MM, Gould MJ: A technical modification of TIPS: The anterior transhepatic approach for the cranially located porta hepatis. *J Vasc Interv Radiol* 1995; in press.

59. Haskal ZJ, Ring EJ, Laberge JM, et al: Role of parallel transjugular intrahepatic portosystemic shunts in patients with persistent portal hypertension. *Radiology* 1992; 185:813–817.

60. Zemel G, Katzen B, Becker GJ, et al: Percutaneous transjugular portosystemic shunt: Preliminary communication. *JAMA* 1991; 266:390–393.

61. Rössle M, Haag K, Ochs A, et al: The transjugular intrahepatic portosystemic stent shunt procedure for variceal bleeding. *N Engl J Med* 1994; 330:165–171.

62. Haskal ZJ, Pentecost MJ, Rubin RA: Hepatic arterial injury after transjugular intrahepatic portosystemic shunt placement: Report of two cases. *Radiology* 1993; 188:85–88.

63. Sanyal AJ, Freedman AM, Purdum PP: TIPS-associated hemolysis and encephalopathy. *Ann Intern Med* 1992; 117:443–444.

64. Riggio O, Ricci G, Zullo A, et al: Intravascular hemolysis and transjugular intrahepatic portosystemic stent shunt. *J Hepatol* 1994; 20:152–153.

65. Gordon RL, LaBerge JM, Ring EJ, Doherty MM: Recanalization of occluded intrahepatic portosystemic shunts: Use of the Colapinto needle. *J Vasc Interv Radiol* 1993; 4:441–443.

66. Wojtowycz MM, Tambeaux RH, Schuster MR: Recanalization of occluded intrahepatic portosystemic shunts: Role of transhepatic stent puncture. *J Vasc Interv Radiol* 1994; 5:377–378.

6

Mesenteric Angiography

KEY CONCEPTS

1. Angiography is indicated for gastrointestinal bleeding that does not resolve with conservative therapy and cannot be localized or treated endoscopically.
2. Identification of the bleeding source allows directed surgical or nonsurgical intervention and minimizes operative mortality.
3. If the activity of bleeding is in question, radionuclide scans are much more sensitive than arteriography for detection of extravasation. A positive scan increases the diagnostic yield of angiography and limits the amount of contrast medium needed.
4. Selective arterial infusion of vasopressin is most effective for gastric bleeding and colonic diverticular hemorrhage.
5. Biplane aortography is needed to evaluate suspected aortoenteric fistula or intestinal angina.
6. Acute mesenteric ischemia has high mortality and can result from arterial embolus, thrombus, low-flow state, or venous occlusion.

INDICATIONS

Since the aggressive use of endoscopy became widespread in the early 1980s, the role of angiography in the diagnosis of gastrointestinal (GI) bleeding has diminished considerably. Still, arteriography remains a valuable study in those patients with recurrent or continued GI hemorrhage whose source has eluded previous endoscopic, radionuclide, and barium studies, especially those whose bleeding has continued after "blind" laparotomy.[1] Lesions of angiodysplasia or other arteriovenous malformations (AVMs) are particularly difficult to identify at surgery, and selective arterial injection of methylene blue can guide resection.[2]

In acute GI bleeding, angiography is most likely to be diagnostic if blood loss exceeds 4 units within 24 hours, if continued intravenous fluids and transfusions are needed to keep the patient stable, and if the nasogastric tube aspirate remains bloody despite lavage with cold saline.[3] When bleeding is intermittent and patient stability permits, radionuclide studies are useful to confirm that extravasation is taking place as well as to guide angiography to the most likely source. Because of their great sensitivity, abnormal red blood cell–labeled scans are associated with angiographic demonstration of active bleeding in over 40% of cases, and a negative scan decreases the likelihood of finding extravasation to about 3%.[4] A not inconsequential number of patients with scans negative for disease *do* have angiographic abnormalities, but catheter studies need not be performed on an emergency basis, and less invasive examinations can be pursued if bleeding has stopped.

Angiography in the face of unrelenting gastric or colonic hemorrhage allows arterial vasopressin infusion or embolization to be performed in selected patients. Operative mortality for emergency surgery is high. Even if focal ischemia results from catheter intervention, the patient's condition may be stabilized prior to any necessary surgery (see Chapter 12 entitled Embolotherapy).

Other indications for mesenteric or celiac angiography include suspected intestinal angina, acute mesenteric ischemia, splenic or other splanchnic artery aneurysm, detection of islet cell tumors not identified by other studies, and trauma. Secreting pancreatic tumors can be localized by transhepatic mesenteric venous sampling. In exceptional cases, angiography may still be requested to determine the resectability of pancreatic carcinoma.

ANATOMIC AND TECHNICAL CONSIDERATIONS

The arterial supply to the stomach comes mainly from the left gastric artery, which usually arises from the celiac trunk and follows the lesser curvature of the stomach to anastomose with the right gastric artery, a much smaller vessel arising from the proper or left hepatic artery. The greater curvature of the stomach is supplied by the gastroepiploic branches of the gastroduodenal and splenic arteries. There are free anastomoses among these various vessels, making it unlikely that occlusion of any single branch will result in ischemia. Short gastric arteries originate along the length of the splenic artery.

The pancreas obtains blood from branches of the gastroduodenal, splenic, and superior mesenteric arteries (SMAs). The pancreaticoduodenal arcades supply the head, and blood flow is provided to the body by way of the pancreatica magna from the splenic artery, and the dorsal pancreatic artery, which may be a branch of the proximal splenic artery or the SMA. These latter vessels join the transverse pancreatic artery, which follows the axis of the organ. The arterial supply to the pancreas is highly variable, and selective angiography is needed for precise definition of anatomy in a given individual.

The SMA provides flow to the entire small intestine beyond the ligament of Treitz. The cecum, right colon, and much of the transverse colon are also supplied by the SMA. The remainder of the colon obtains its blood from the inferior mesenteric artery (IMA). The IMA typically arises from the left anterolateral surface of the aorta at the level of L3.

The ready availability of large collateral pathways between celiac, SMA, and IMA distributions makes chronic arterial insufficiency highly unlikely in the absence of major occlusive disease affecting at least two of the three vessels. Major communications between celiac artery and SMA are present in the pancreaticoduodenal arcades, and transpancreatic flow over other vessels in the body of the organ can also be seen. In a few patients a large central communication between celiac artery and SMA persists from early development as the arc of Bühler. Anastomoses between SMA and IMA circulations occur at the junction of middle colic and left colic arteries. The arcade thus formed proximal to the vasa recta at the edge of the colonic mesentery is called the marginal artery of Drummond. A more central pathway between the SMA and the IMA is the arch of Riolan. These collaterals are commonly filled in elderly patients because the IMA is frequently occluded by atherosclerosis. In some cases of IMA occlusion, the colon may be primarily supplied by the internal iliac arteries over middle rectal–to–superior rectal artery anastomoses.

In performing mesenteric studies, the flow of the vessel should be matched (on the order of 10 ml/second for celiac, 8 ml/second for SMA, and 3 ml/second for IMA) for 6 to 10 seconds. Filming should be rapid during the arterial phase, usually one to two exposures per second, and slowed to a rate of one exposure every 2 to 5 seconds for capillary and venous phases. Imaging should be carried out to at least 30 seconds, to allow appreciation of slow extravasation in cases of GI bleeding and venous filling in patients with portal hypertension or suspected venous occlusion. Digital subtraction techniques are generally of little value in mesenteric studies because of the copious bowel gas often present and the high potential for misinterpreting motion artifact as contrast extravasation. The suspected bleeding vessel should be injected first, and the more selective the catheter placement (e.g., injection of the left gastric artery rather than the celiac axis), the higher the probability that active bleeding will be recognized.

In cases of lower GI hemorrhage, the pelvis should be imaged first (with both IMA and SMA injections), before contrast material accumulates in the bladder. Placement of a Foley catheter prior to angiography is highly recommended. It may be necessary to select each internal iliac artery for a complete study. Because mesenteric angiography often requires multiple injections of large amounts of iodinated contrast medium, the status of the patient's renal function should be known and hydration maintained as well as possible.

Aortography is not routinely needed, except for cases of suspected aortoenteric fistula, intestinal angina, and mesenteric ischemia. Biplane studies are mandatory for these indications. Lateral aortography is also valuable if a major splanchnic vessel cannot be catheterized or identified, a situation that may represent anatomic variation or vascular occlusion.

GASTROINTESTINAL HEMORRHAGE

The great majority of GI bleeding stops spontaneously, and most episodes do not recur. It is persistent or recurrent massive hemorrhage that accounts for the 8% to 10% mortality of acute GI bleeding.[3] A clinical distinction must be made between upper GI and lower GI hemorrhage. Up to 90% of all GI bleeding is from a lesion proximal to the ligament of Treitz, and most patients have bloody nasogastric tube aspirates.[5] However, absence of a positive aspirate does not exclude duodenal ulcer as a cause of melena or hematochezia. Fortunately, endoscopy performed within 6 hours of hospital admission can positively identify bleeding points in all but a few patients with upper GI hemorrhage.[6] Endoscopy is important both for excluding lesions not ordinarily needing angiographic diagnosis or amenable to catheter interventions (such as gastroesophageal varices, nasopharyngeal abnormalities, or anorectal lesions) and for treating upper GI bleeding unresponsive to conservative measures.[3,7]

Hemorrhage that stops, only to recur at intervals, is a particular problem if endoscopy and barium studies are repeatedly negative. Evaluation of such bleeding can be time-consuming, frustrating, and expensive. Angiography and intraoperative endoscopy are the diagnostic measures most likely to be fruitful in this situation.[1,8] In some cases computed tomographic scans and ultrasonography may enable one to detect parenchymal abnormalities responsible for GI hemorrhage (such as hepatic aneurysms, arterioportal fistulae, pseudoaneurysms from pancreatitis, and tumors) and thus select patients for directed arterial study.[9]

Upper Gastrointestinal Bleeding

The most common cause of upper GI blood loss is peptic ulcer disease, followed in frequency by gastroesophageal varices.[5,7] (For a discussion of the latter, see Chapter 5 entitled Portal Venography, Portal Hypertension, and TIPS). Stress gastritis was once a major clinical problem, but with improvements in medical therapy and prophylaxis it has virtually disappeared as an indication for emergency gastric surgery.[5] Other less common causes of hemorrhage include various benign and malignant neoplasms, aortoenteric fistula (which should *always* be suspected if the patient has an aortic graft in place), pancreatitis, hemobilia, AVMs, and splanchnic arterial aneurysms. Mesenteric venous thrombosis has produced upper GI hemorrhage in isolated cases.[10]

In an otherwise healthy patient, a standard indication for operative intervention is loss of at least 6 units of blood within 24 hours. Mortality for emergency surgery in cases of upper GI tract bleeding is as high as 23%.[5] Precise identification of the bleeding site and prompt treatment are of paramount importance. Reports of angiographic accuracy have ranged from 60% to 86%, and angiography is indicated when endoscopy fails or is unavailable, as long as the patient is not grossly unstable.[3]

Endoscopic electrocoagulation, thermal and laser coagulation, and mucosal injection of ethanol or epinephrine are techniques capable of controlling many gastric bleeds, but endoscopy cannot reliably treat hemorrhage from vessels larger than 2 mm in diameter.[6] Large bleeding vessels are often amenable to occlusion with embolic particles. Catheter embolization is more effective for gastric bleeding than for duodenal lesions, because of patterns of collateral arterial supply (see Chapter 12 entitled Embolotherapy). Smaller vessel bleeding or diffuse gastritis may be treated with selective vasopressin infusion (see the section entitled Arterial Infusion of Vasopressin later in this chapter). However, even in the absence of arteriographic abnormality or extravasation, Lang and Wittich recommend embolization of the left gastric artery over vasopressin infusion as a more effective treatment for those at risk of multiorgan failure as a consequence of renewed bleeding.[11]

Lower Gastrointestinal Bleeding

Only 1 patient in 10 with GI bleeding is found to have a source in jejunum, ileum, or colon.[5] An upper GI source must always be excluded before melena or bloody stools are attributed to a more distal abnormality. Patients with lower GI bleeding tend to be more elderly than those with gastric or duodenal lesions.

Acute Hemorrhage

In acute lower GI hemorrhage, the role of endoscopy is not well established. If bleeding is massive and continuing, angiography is a primary diagnostic measure. In such a situation, angiographic accuracy is only 40% to 48%, but this is still considerably better than undirected surgical resection, which finds the underlying cause in only 30%.[2,3] Localization of a bleeding source is of great importance, because limiting the extent of emergency surgery can drop operative mortality from 40% associated with subtotal colectomy to 13% with segmental resection.[2]

Colonic Diverticula

Colonic diverticula are responsible for roughly half of all cases of lower GI hemorrhage. Although most diverticula are found in the left colon, the great majority of bleeding diverticula are in the right colon. Diverticular bleeds are typically abrupt in onset, massive, and painless, and they are unlikely to recur.[12]

Angiodysplasia

Angiodysplasia is another common cause of acute bleeding. Although it is more commonly found in those over 60 years of age, angiodysplasia has been described in much younger patients as well. These lesions, often multiple, are properly termed *telangiectasias,* for they represent dilation of preexisting vascular structures. They are vascular tangles of dilated mucosal or submucosal venules most commonly found in cecum or ascending colon. It has been postulated that angiodysplasia is caused by intermittent obstruction of venous outflow, but ischemia or toxic effects of bowel contents have also been implicated in its pathogenesis.[13]

For a positive diagnosis of bleeding from angiodysplasia to be made, actual extravasation must be seen. Up to 27% of all elderly patients may have angiodysplasia, but half of these also have colonic diverticula.[2] If extravasation is not detected, carcinoma or another lesion must always be excluded.

Meckel's Diverticulum

This embryologic remnant, present in distal ileum, has a prevalence of 2% in the adult population.[12] Because ectopic gastric mucosa is found in a large number of Meckel's diverticula, about one fourth of patients eventually present with lower GI hemorrhage. Bleeding is more common in children but can develop at any age. Technetium pertechnetate radionuclide scans have been used to detect bleeding diverticula with good success.[3] The vitelline artery, a separate branch of the SMA, is a vessel specific to Meckel's diverticulum, but in 80% of diverticula this vessel has involuted and been replaced by a distal ileal branch.[14]

Other Lesions
Endoscopic polypectomy is an iatrogenic cause of acute bleeding. Carcinoma, polyps, or other tumors can bleed spontaneously, but such blood loss is more likely to be chronic and intermittent rather than massive. Inflammatory bowel disease and small bowel or colonic ulcers must also be considered in the differential diagnosis.

Chronic Lower Gastrointestinal Bleeding
Barium and endoscopic examinations uncover all but a few neoplastic or inflammatory causes of intermittent, recurrent, or low-grade hemorrhage. Even so, about 5% of patients do not have a diagnosis made by conventional means.[15] Small bowel lesions are responsible for many of these cases, with angiodysplasia or AVMs eventually uncovered in 20% to 35%.[15,16] Angiography is worth performing, and Lau and associates have reported high accuracy for lower GI hemorrhage of obscure origin.[1] Even in patients with initally negative studies, they found that repeat arteriographic examination could reliably establish the bleeding source. Rösch and colleagues have injected boluses of heparin and streptokinase to unmask bleeding sites in particularly refractory cases, but such intervention is risky and should be avoided.[17]

   When a vascular malformation is present, the cather should be left in place as the patient is taken to the surgery. Arterial injection of methylene blue is a valuable aid in the surgical localization of such lesions. Resected vascular malformations must be marked by a surgical suture because they can be easily overlooked by the pathologist.[8] Ideally, surgical specimens are examined histologically after arterial injection of a silicone or other polymer.

Angiographic Findings in Gastrointestinal Bleeding
The sine qua non of bleeding is extravasation of contrast material, which is seen as a puddling or staining that persists beyond the capillary and venous phases. Delayed films sometimes clearly show intestinal folds, if bleeding is brisk enough. Occasionally, the extravasated contrast may accumulate between two folds and appear radiographically as a "pseudovein." For extravasation to be detectable, bleeding must exceed 0.5 ml/min.[18]

   Few lesions responsible for hemorrhage have characteristic angiographic findings. Aneurysms, pseudoaneurysms, and frank AVMs such as those of the Rendu-Osler-Weber syndrome are easily recognized. Angiodysplasia, however, can be quite subtle in appearance. Criteria for diagnosis include vascular tufts appearing in the arterial phase of injection, early opacification of a draining vein, and delayed emptying of a dilated and tortuous intramural vein.[13] Aortoenteric fistula is not often diagnosed angiographically, but observation of a nipplelike projection or a pseudoaneurysm in the presence of a vascular graft is presumptive evidence of a fistula.[3]

Ulcerations, inflammatory lesions, diverticula, and neoplasms usually present nonspecific angiographic findings. Intestinal leiomyomas and leiomyosarcomas are hypervascular and typically have an intense capillary stain.[19] Similar findings may be seen in patients with acquired immunodeficiency syndrome (AIDS) with intestinal lesions of Kaposi's sarcoma.[20] Venous-phase films must always be inspected for signs of portal or mesenteric vein thrombosis. Unsuspected esophageal or mesenteric varices can be detected on late films. Because bleeding can be very intermittent and spasm can prevent opacification of the extravasating vessel, repeat injection or repeat angiography may be warranted.[1]

Role of Radionuclide Studies

Radionuclide studies are not indicated in patients with massive continuous bleeding. However, if there is a question as to whether bleeding has stopped or if hemorrhage is intermittent, scans are quite useful. A red blood cell scan or sulfur colloid scan that is negative for disease is highly unlikely to be followed by an arteriogram showing extravasation.[4,21] Also, a positive scan can guide angiography directly to the area and vessel most likely to be bleeding, minimizing the amount of contrast medium necessary. In a patient who may have hypotension or renal compromise, contrast dose is an important consideration.

Technetium-labeled sulfur colloid scans can enable one to detect rates of bleeding as low as 0.05 ml/min.[21] Because the tracer is rapidly extracted by liver and spleen, blood pool circulation time is only 12 to 15 minutes (still good in comparison with the few seconds iodinated contrast medium has to demonstrate a bleeding site). Background activity is quickly cleared, but the high number of counts originating in liver and spleen makes the study useless in cases of upper GI hemorrhage, and extravasation at the colonic flexures may be hard to detect.

Technetium-labeled red blood cell studies take more time to prepare, and they detect only greater amounts of bleeding, but they are still more sensitive than angiography.[4] Upper GI hemorrhage can be detected, and blood pool circulation lasts for many hours. At least 85% of positive studies require more than 1 hour of imaging.[4] One potential drawback is that, if early imaging does not detect the bleeding site, activity found at a later time may represent blood that has entered bowel and has been propelled away from the bleeding source by peristalsis.

Technetium pertechnetate scanning is used when a Meckel's diverticulum is suspected to be bleeding. Tracer accumulates in gastric mucosa. Because a bleeding Meckel's diverticulum contains ectopic gastric tissue, a technetium scan is positive in up to 75% of cases.[3]

Arterial Infusion of Vasopressin

Direct arterial infusion of vasopressin has been used to treat various causes of GI bleeding. Once employed for variceal hemorrhage, selective infusion has given way to intravenous vasopressin, which is equally effective for acutely bleeding gastroesophageal varices.[22] Vasopressin has been particularly effective for bleeding of gastric origin; it achieves control with selective left gastric artery infusion in 82% of cases.[23] As noted earlier, some advocate early use of embolization for gastric bleeding to minimize the risk of recurrence.[11] Infusion of the celiac axis or gastroduodenal arteries is much less likely to produce benefit.

Vasopressin is also useful for colonic diverticular bleeds, with control obtained in the great majority of patients. However, up to half of those controlled acutely are likely to bleed again.[2] Because emergency colonic surgery carries a high mortality, even temporary stabilization of the patient can reduce operative risk. Patients with angiodysplasia or bleeding of small bowel origin are less likely to respond to vasopressin infusion.[24]

When used intraarterially, vasopressin should be started at 0.2 unit/min and the angiographic results checked at 20 minutes. If vasoconstriction is not excessive and bleeding persists, the dose can be increased to 0.4 unit/min. After bleeding stops, the infused dose should be tapered gradually over several hours to avoid a rebound hyperemia.[3] Saline may be infused for some time before the catheter is removed to allow immediate retreatment should bleeding resume.

Vasopressin must be avoided in patients with ischemic heart disease. Therapy is associated with a 9% rate of serious complications, including cardiac, mesenteric, and acral ischemia; hyponatremia; and cerebral edema.[25] If the left gastric artery is being infused, particular attention must be paid to cardiac dysrhythmias because phrenic branches of the left gastric artery can supply pericardium.[3] Vasopressin must also be avoided after embolotherapy, for bowel infarction is a possible result.

Therapeutic Embolization in Gastrointestinal Hemorrhage

Arterial embolization has been used with success in the gastric and colonic circulations in cases of bleeding not responding to other measures.[25,26] Embolization has been safely applied to a number of lesions of the small bowel as well.[24] The minimum number of particles needed to stop hemorrhage should be injected as selectively as possible, and embolization in conjunction with vasopressin infusion is not recommended.[25] Gelatin sponge, a temporary occluder, has been the most commonly used material, but Guy and associates have had success and minimal complications with polyvinyl alcohol particles placed into the arteria recta supplying the bleeding site.[27] Presence of coagulopathy is associated with a poor prognosis, but embolotherapy can still be effective.[28] The major risks of bowel embolization are ischemia and stricture formation, but these risks must be balanced against the high mortality rate of emergency surgery.[29] Risk of ischemia is higher in patients with severe atherosclerosis or prior bowel surgery. Embolotherapy is especially useful in the treatment of bleeding pancreatic or hepatic pseudoaneurysms (see Chapter 12 entitled Embolotherapy).[9,30,31]

MESENTERIC ISCHEMIA

Inadequate perfusion of the bowel can lead to a variety of symptoms. If there is chronic arterial insufficiency, the syndrome of intestinal angina is produced. Arteriography is an essential part of diagnostic evaluation, as it is in cases of acute arterial ischemia, whether from embolus, in situ thrombus, or a low-flow state. Mesenteric vein thrombosis is more difficult to diagnose clinically than acute arterial ischemia, and the angiographic findings are usually indirect.

Intestinal Angina

Patients with intestinal angina complain of postprandial pain, nausea, vomiting, and diarrhea. Weight loss is marked, and many patients are cachectic in appearance. Symptoms may be so severe that the patient has a fear of eating. Unfortunately, complaints are not so clear-cut in many cases.

Chronic arterial insufficiency of bowel typically requires occlusion of at least two of the three celiac and mesenteric vessels, and the third must often be stenotic for symptoms to arise. Such extensive occlusive disease must be present because of the rich network of collateral vessels that is normally available. Atherosclerosis is commonly the underlying disease, but Takayasu's arteritis, systemic lupus erythematosus, Wegener's granulomatosis, and a variety of other inflammatory conditions have also produced intestinal angina.[32]

Duplex sonography and magnetic resonance angiography may become screening measures, but more work must be done to establish their value.[33,34] When conventional arteriography is ordered for suspected intestinal angina, biplane abdominal aortography is indispensable. Injection is made at or above the level of the celiac axis at T12. The lateral view best demonstrates the origins of the celiac and superior mesenteric arteries. A steep left posterior oblique projection may show the orifice of the IMA, if it is not well seen on the biplane study. Note should be made of patterns of filling and of development or absence of collaterals. A severe narrowing of the proximal celiac associated with angulation of the vessel (the so-called median arcuate ligament compression syndrome) is a common finding in healthy individuals, and its significance in symptomatic patients is questionable.

With proper patient selection, surgical revascularization has a 70% success rate but a 3% to 8% mortality.[35] Odurny and colleagues have used balloon angioplasty to produce relief of symptoms for up to 2 years, but lesions recurred in many of their patients.[35] Median arcuate ligament compression and ostial lesions are not amenable to dilatation.

Acute Arterial Ischemia
Symptoms of acute ischemia include severe pain, nausea, vomiting, and diarrhea (with or without gross blood). Although acute mesenteric ischemia is an uncommon cause of hospital admission, mortality is quite high: 70% to 90%.[32] Angiography should be done early if the diagnosis is suspected and symptoms have persisted at least 2 hours. In one series, expeditious mesenteric arteriography lowered mortality to 53%.[36] Most have arterial occlusion from thrombus or embolus (onset of pain is usually very abrupt in the latter case), and surgical intervention is indicated. However, 20% to 32% of patients are found to have nonocclusive mesenteric ischemia.[9,36]

Nonocclusive ischemia is associated with low cardiac output, with use of digitalis, ergot alkaloids, propranolol, or vasoconstricting drugs, and with hypovolemia.[32] Patients are typically quite elderly. Angiographic findings consist of slow flow and prominent arterial spasm. Catheter infusion of papaverine directly into the SMA (30 to 60 mg/hour) has provided some benefit, but patients must be closely observed for signs of peritonitis. Surgery should be reserved for those developing bowel necrosis.

Mesenteric Vein Thrombosis
Mesenteric ischemia of venous origin is much less common than acute arterial ischemia. It also tends to have a more gradual onset and better prognosis, with mortality under 40%.[9] As mentioned previously, upper GI bleeding may be seen, a symptom not found in ischemia of arterial cause. Patients with a condition predisposing to thrombosis, such as use of oral contraceptives, antithrombin III or protein C deficiency, neoplasm, or cirrhosis, generally do not do as well as those with no underlying disease.

Angiography may be nondiagnostic. Slow arterial flow, spasm, poor filling, and failure of venous opacification are typical findings.[32] Computed tomography (CT) scanning or duplex ultrasonography can be used to confirm the diagnosis.[37] It is anticipated that spiral CT-angiography will be especially valuable when this condition is suspected.

Veins extending from the marginal mesenteric arcades are usually involved, so thrombectomy is of little value. Standard treatment consists of bowel resection and anticoagulation. There should be wide margins in the resection because early recurrent ischemia is a common postoperative problem.[9]

PANCREATIC ANGIOGRAPHY

Computed tomography has proved quite accurate for staging pancreatic carcinomas, and angiography need not be performed in the great majority of cases; in fact, pancreatic angiography may be misleading.[38,39] Encasement of major arterial or portal venous branches makes a tumor unresectable. Care should be taken that focal spasm is not misinterpreted as encasement.

Angiography is still used for evaluation of patients with suspected islet cell tumors. These neoplasms tend to be slow-growing and small. Aside from insulinomas, most endocrine pancreatic tumors are malignant.[40] Although many lesions can be identified by means of CT and ultrasonography, their accuracy is limited by the small tumor size. Arteriography is most valuable when other imaging has been negative or equivocal, and arteriography can enable detection of multiple lesions, hepatic metastases, and vascular encasement.

Islet cell tumors tend to be circumscribed and have a dense, homogeneous capillary blush.[40] Technique is critical in their demonstration, and superselective catheterization and distention of the stomach with gas are recommended to improve accuracy. Intestinal mucosal blushes and accessory spleens are potential sources of confusion. Oblique projections can be helpful; CT-angiography can provide additional information when angiographic findings are equivocal. Even so, it has been found that all but a few tumors detected angiographically can be palpated at surgical exploration.[41] Intraoperative ultrasound may be able to localize lesions that cannot be palpated, so the application of angiography for islet cell tumors may diminish in the future. Preoperative localization may be restricted to patients submitting to reexploration.

MESENTERIC VENOUS SAMPLING FOR ISLET CELL TUMORS

An invasive examination that in some hands has been even more accurate than arteriography for islet cell tumor localization is selective mesenteric venous sampling for hormonal assay.[41] The approach is identical to transhepatic cannulation of the portal vein for direct portography, but the catheter tip is advanced into the splenic vein. Blood samples are obtained at 10- to 15-mm intervals as the catheter is withdrawn toward the liver. Accuracy is greatest if small tributary veins from the pancreas are sampled and the hormone levels are carefully mapped.[40] With the advent of intraoperative ultrasound, such invasive sampling is now rarely needed for localization.

MISCELLANEOUS CONDITIONS

Splenic Artery Aneurysms

The most common nonaortoiliac aneurysms in the abdomen are splenic artery aneurysms, but the incidence is less than 1 in 1000 in the general population.[42] They are relatively more common in younger women than other aneurysms. Splenic artery aneurysms may rupture, embolize, or thrombose. Because of the high mortality from rupture, all symptomatic lesions should be resected, and asymptomatic aneurysms exceeding 5 cm diameter in patients under 60 years of age should also be treated. Patients at great risk for surgery may be managed by catheter embolization.[43] Aneurysms in pregnant women or women of childbearing age pose particular hazards for rupture; they should be aggressively treated.

Splenic Trauma

Angiography is reserved for suspected cases of primary vascular injury. The spleen often shows a mottled parenchymal blush, which should not be confused with contusion or laceration. Barely half of lesions found at surgical pathologic examination are detected by splenic angiography.[44] However, catheterization allows bleeding to be controlled by embolotherapy if extravasation is found. Embolization should be very selective in such instances, with as much splenic pulp preserved as possible.

REFERENCES

1. Lau WY, Ngan H, Chu KW, Yuen WK: Repeat selective visceral angiography in patients with gastrointestinal bleeding of obscure origin. *Br J Surg* 1989; 78:226–229.
2. Leitman IM, Paull DE, Shires GT: Evaluation and management of massive lower gastrointestinal hemorrhage. *Ann Surg* 1989; 209:175–180.
3. Kadir S, Ernest CB: Current concepts in angiographic management of gastrointestinal bleeding. *Curr Probl Surg* 1983; 20:281–343.
4. Winzelberg GG, McKusik KA, Froelick JW, et al: Detection of gastrointestinal bleeding with 99m Tc-labeled red blood cells. *Semin Nucl Med* 1982; 12:139–146.
5. Greenburg AG, Saik RP, Bell RH, Collins GM: Changing patterns of gastrointestinal bleeding. *Arch Surg* 1985; 120:341–344.
6. Gostout CJ: Acute gastrointestinal bleeding: A common problem revisited. *Mayo Clin Proc* 1988; 63:596–604.
7. Petrini JL, Jr: Endoscopic therapy for gastrointestinal bleeding. *Postgrad Med* 1988; 84:239–244.
8. Schwartz RW, Hagihara PF, Griffin WO, Jr: Intraoperative endoscopy for recurrent gastrointestinal bleeding. *South Med J* 1988; 81:1106–1108.
9. Savastano S, Feltrin GP, Miotto D, et al: Vascular parenchymal sources of upper gastrointestinal bleeding. *Acta Radiol* 1989; 30:39–43.
10. Clavien P-A, Dürig M, Harder F: Venous mesenteric infarction: A particular entity. *Br J Surg* 1988; 75:252–255.
11. Lang EV, Wittich G: Therapeutic and prophylactic transcatheter therapy in patients with massive arterial upper gastrointestinal haemorrhage. *Minimal Invasive Ther* 1993; 2:173–180.

12. Lawrence MA, Hooks VH, Bowden TA, Jr: Lower gastrointestinal bleeding: A sytematic approach to classification and management. *Postgrad Med* 1989; 85:89–100.
13. Hemingway AP: Angiodysplasia: Current concepts. *Postgrad Med J* 1988; 64:259–263.
14. Bree RL, Reuter SR: Angiographic demonstration of a bleeding Meckel's diverticulum. *Radiology* 1973; 108:287–288.
15. Thompson JN, Hemingway AP, McPherson GAD, et al: Obscure gastrointestinal haemorrhage of small-bowel origin. *Br Med J* 1984; 288:1663–1665.
16. Monk JE, Smith BA, O'Leary JP: Arteriovenous malformations of the small intestine. *South Med J* 1989; 82:18–22.
17. Rösch J, Feller FS, Wawrukiewicz AS, et al: Pharmacoangiography in the diagnosis of recurrent massive lower gastrointestinal bleeding. *Radiology* 1982; 145:615–619.
18. Peterson WL: Obscure gastrointestinal bleeding. *Med Clin North Am* 1988; 72:1169–1176.
19. Valls C, Sancho C, Bechini J, et al: Intestinal leiomyomas: Angiographic imaging. *Gastrointest Radiol* 1992; 17:220–222.
20. Sharma VS, Valji K, Bookstein JJ: Gastrointestinal hemorrhage in AIDS: Arteriographic diagnosis and transcatheter treatment. *Radiology* 1992; 185:447–451.
21. Alavi A: Detection of gastrointestinal bleeding with 99mTc-sulfur colloid. *Semin Nucl Med* 1982; 12:126–138.
22. Joffe SN: Non-operative management of variceal bleeding. *Br J Surg* 1984; 71:85–91.
23. Eckstein MR, Kelemouridis V, Athanasoulis CA, et al: Gastric bleeding: Therapy with intraarterial vasopressin and transcatheter embolization. *Radiology* 1984; 152:643–646.
24. Palmaz JC, Walter JF, Cho KJ: Therapeutic embolization of the small-bowel arteries. *Radiology* 1984; 152:377–382.
25. Uflacker R: Transcatheter embolization for treatment of acute lower gastrointestinal bleeding. *Acta Radiol* 1987; 28:425–430.
26. Rösch J, Keller FS, Kozak B, et al: Gelfoam powder embolization of the left gastric artery in treatment of massive small-vessel gastric bleeding. *Radiology* 1984; 151:365–370.
27. Guy GE, Shetty PC, Sharma RP, et al: Acute lower gastrointestinal hemorrhage: Treatment by superselective embolization with polyvinyl alcohol particles. *Am J Roentgenol* 1992; 159:521–526.
28. Encarnacion CE, Kadir S, Beam CA, Payne CS: Gastrointestinal bleeding: Treatment with gastrointestinal arterial embolization. *Radiology* 1992; 183:505–508.
29. Mitty HA, Efremidis S, Keller RJ: Colonic stricture after transcatheter embolization for diverticular bleeding. *Am J Roentgenol* 1979; 133:519–521.
30. Tegtmeyer CJ, Bezirdjian DR, Ferguson WW, Hess CE: Transcatheter embolic control of iatrogenic hematobilia. *Cardiovasc Intervent Radiol* 1981; 4:88–92.
31. Huizinga WKJ, Kalideen JM, Bryer JV, et al: Control of major haemorrhage associated with pancreatic pseudocysts by transcatheter arterial embolization. *Br J Surg* 1984; 71:133–136.

32. Hunter GC, Guernsey JM: Mesenteric ischemia. *Med Clin North Am* 1988; 72:1091–1115.
33. Moneta GL, Lee RW, Yeager RA, et al. : Mesenteric duplex scanning: A blinded prospective study. *J Vasc Surg* 1993; 17:79–86.
34. Li KCP, Whitney WS, McDonnell CH, et al: Chronic mesenteric ischemia: Evaluation with phase-contrast cine MR imaging. *Radiology* 1994; 190:175–179.
35. Odurny A, Sniderman KW, Colapinto RF: Intestinal angina: Percutaneous transluminal angioplasty of the celiac and superior mesenteric arteries. *Radiology* 1988; 167:59–62.
36. Boos S: Angiographie der Arteria mesenterica 1976 bis1991: Wandel der Indikationen bei der mesenterialen Durchblutungsstörung? *Radiologe* 1992; 32:154–157.
37. Mildenberger P, Jenny E, Schild H: Nachweis einer thrombose der vena mesenterica superior nach splenektomie mittels real-time- und doppler-sonographie. *Radiologe* 1988; 28:395–398.
38. Jafri SZH, Aisen AM, Glazer GM, Weiss CA: Comparison of CT and angiography in assessing resectability of pancreatic carcinoma. *Am J Roentgenol* 1984; 142:525–529.
39. Murugiah M, Windsor JA, Redhead DN, et al. : The role of selective visceral angiography in the management of pancreatic and periampullary cancer. *World J Surg* 1993; 17:796–800.
40. Rossi P, Allison DJ, Bezzi M, et al. : Endocrine tumors of the pancreas. *Radiol Clin North Am* 1989; 27:129–161.
41. Proye C, Boissel P: Preoperative imaging versus intraoperative localization of tumors in adult surgical patients with hyperinsulinemia: A multicenter study of 338 patients. *World J Surg* 1988; 12:685–689.
42. Greene DR, Gorey TF, Tanner WA, et al: The diagnosis and management of splenic artery aneurysms. *J R Soc Med* 1988; 81:387–388.
43. Baker KS, Tisnado J, Cho S-R, Beachley MC: Splanchnic artery aneurysms and pseudoaneurysms: Transcatheter embolization. *Radiology* 1987; 163:135–139.
44. Casarella WJ, Martin EC: Angiography in the management of abdominal trauma. *Semin Roentgenol* 1984; 19:321–327.

7

Thoracic Aortography and Bronchial Angiography

KEY CONCEPTS

1. Aortic laceration should be suspected in anyone with major deceleration injury and mediastinal widening. Normal findings on high-quality mediastinal computed tomographic scan virtually exclude significant aortic injury.
2. The most common sites of aortic injury are the aortic isthmus, ascending aorta, and diaphragmatic hiatus.
3. Dissection is the most common acute primary aortic disease, with an incidence two to three times that of ruptured abdominal aortic aneurysm.
4. In 13% of aortic dissections, no false lumen or intimal flap can be identified on aortography. Flattening of the true lumen and wall thickening are indirect signs.
5. Atherosclerotic aneurysms less than 5 cm in diameter are unlikely to rupture, but patients with Marfan's syndrome, mycotic aneurysms, or luetic aneurysms should have elective repair of even small, asymptomatic lesions.

INDICATIONS

Thoracic aortography remains the definitive diagnostic study for the detection of acute and chronic aortic injury, as well as for the preoperative delineation of aortic aneurysms and dissections. It defines the relationship of aortic abnormalities to the heart and branch vessels as no cross-sectional imaging technique can. Thoracic angiography is also used to clarify the nature of paraaortic masses that might represent aortic diverticula, pulmonary sequestrations, or, in rare cases, invading neoplasms.

Bronchial/intercostal arteriography is mainly reserved for determining the source of recurrent and massive hemoptysis, with embolization as a treatment option. Occasionally it is employed in the preoperative evaluation of chronic pulmonary embolism.

AORTIC TRAUMA

Clinical Aspects

The thoracic aorta is susceptible to injury by rapid deceleration or crushing, and aortic tears are a common cause of death in high-speed motor vehicle accidents.[1,2] The majority of those with aortic rupture do not survive to reach medical care. However, those patients who are admitted with acute injury are at a 40% to 50% risk of exsanguination within the first 24 hours, if the diagnosis is not made and surgical treatment begun.[1,3] Risk of death is as high as 90% by 1 month after injury.[4] Although some may survive hospitalization and be discharged without aortic injury suspected, they are prone to developing chronic pseudoaneurysms that may enlarge and rupture as long as 49 years later.[5,6]

Aortic disruption may be limited to the intima, or it may involve the entire thickness of the vessel wall. Extent of injury ranges from only a discrete portion of the aortic circumference to complete transection. The site of tear most likely to be diagnosed angiographically is at the aortic isthmus, where the ligamentum arteriosus joins the pulmonary artery and aorta. Here the relatively mobile aortic arch joins the descending aorta, which is fixed by investing fascia. In the past the mechanism of injury was generally held to be the great shear stress arising at this junction. More recently an alternate mechanism has been proposed: the sternum is severely depressed by striking an object during sudden deceleration, traps the aorta on the spine, and lacerates it.[7,8] Of all aortic disruptions diagnosed, 80% to 86% are found at the isthmus.[2,4,9] The next most likely site of angiographically diagnosed disruption is the aortic root, with an incidence of about 9%.[9] The number of traumatic injuries to the ascending aorta is actually higher, but such injuries are more likely to be fatal, and fewer patients come to aortography. A small number of tears occur at the level of the diaphragm, and imaging studies should always extend to this area.

Plain Radiographic Findings

A large number of signs have been described as suggesting aortic injury on chest radiographs. Chief among these is mediastinal widening, measured as a ratio of superior mediastinal to chest wall width.[3] A ratio of 0.25 to 0.28 on a supine chest film should raise the suspicion of aortic injury. Greater ratios are more specific (but less sensitive) for aortic rupture. Care must be taken in interpreting films with any degree of patient rotation. Many apparent cases of mediastinal widening resolve on an anteroposterior view of the chest with the patient upright and leaning several degrees forward, but such a study is not always possible to obtain. It should be noted that only a minority of mediastinal hematomas are actually related to aortic laceration.

Other plain radiographic signs reported include shift of a nasogastric tube to the right, depression of the left bronchus, tracheal deviation, and presence of an apical cap. Pneumothorax, hemothorax, pulmonary contusion, and rib or clavicular fractures are indicative of major trauma but do not have specific value in predicting aortic injury.[3] None of the signs listed has high accuracy alone, but in 49 confirmed cases of disruption, Stark and colleagues observed that not a single chest radiograph was within normal limits.[2] Nevertheless, there have been well-documented cases of aortic laceration associated with entirely normal chest radiographs.[10] The consequences of a missed diagnosis are so grave that, if any chest abnormality is seen or if clinical suspicion is high enough, aortography is justified. Over the years, experience has dictated that one should expect to perform eight or nine negative studies for every positive arteriogram in order to avoid missing the diagnosis in anyone.[2,3] The number of negative aortograms is likely to decrease, now that computed tomography (CT) scanning and transesophageal ultrasonography are available.

The place of CT in evaluation of suspected aortic injury has been hotly debated in the past few years. Raptopoulos and associates examined 131 patients with trauma and compared chest radiographic, CT, and angiographic findings.[11] They found that chest CT had a 100% negative predictive value (meaning no patient had aortic laceration in the face of a normal CT scan), better than the 99% negative predictive value of a normal chest radiograph. At the same time, 19% of patients with mediastinal or other abnormality on CT had positive aortograms; of all those with abnormal chest radiographs, only 6% had positive aortograms. Chest CT was felt to be an appropriate measure in all clinically stable patients who would otherwise have a diagnostic aortogram (excepting those with clearly abnormal chest radiographs). The number of aortograms for trauma might be cut in half without affecting sensitivity. The experience of other investigators has been supportive of this conclusion.[12,13] Spiral CT should be very well suited for this indication, while minimizing the amount of contrast medium needed for an intravenous bolus injection.

Transesophageal echocardiography (TEE) has recently been employed to examine trauma victims in the emergency department, and it appears to be very sensitive for lacerations at the isthmus or in the descending thoracic aorta. In the series reported by Kearney and colleagues, 7 of 69 patients were found to have aortic tears, all subsequently confirmed at surgery or autopsy.[14] TEE took half the time of conventional aortography to perform. No matter what imaging strategy is considered in thoracic trauma, an unstable patient should be taken immediately to the operating room!

Arteriographic Technique

Thoracic aortography should be performed with a high-flow pigtail catheter, 6 Fr or larger, placed within 1 to 2 cm of the aortic valve. Injection should be of sufficient rate and volume to ensure that the valve cusps are well defined on filming (30 ml/second for 2 seconds is adequate for most adults). Filming must be rapid (two to three exposures per second) and should be carried out well into the washout phase to detect persistent puddling or extravasation. Biplane filming is advantageous because *at least two views of the aorta are mandatory* before a laceration can be excluded. If there is any question of intimal irregularity or transection, other views must be obtained. Although rapid-frame digital subtraction angiography has been successfully applied in cases of aortic injury,[1] the large field of view, maximum spatial resolution, and capability for biplane study make conventional film arteriography the standard for diagnosis. It remains to be seen if rotational digital angiography will be of any additional value.

If a femoral approach is used for catheter placement, any resistance to advancement of catheter or wire should raise concern, and in the absence of other disease such resistance is diagnostic of aortic disruption.[15] Deaths have been reported after power injection of contrast directly into traumatic pseudoaneurysms.

Findings of aortic trauma range from minimal wall irregularity representing intimal tear to complete transection with contained or uncontained extravasation from the lumen. Bronchial artery origins and atherosclerotic or other mural irregularities sometimes pose diagnostic problems. Usually these can be resolved angiographically, but at times thoracic exploration is unavoidable. A ductus bulge or diverticulum has a fairly characteristic appearance and should not be a cause for confusion (see the following sections). When a true tear is discovered, all films must be carefully examined. Multiple arterial lacerations are not rare, especially if the aortic injury is at a site other than the isthmus.[4]

Chronic Aortic Pseudoaneurysms

Patients with this condition may present with pain, hoarseness, or dyspnea months to years after injury.[5] Many chronic aortic pseudoaneurysms are discovered incidentally on chest radiographs. A focal bulge from the ventral aspect of the proximal descending thoracic aorta is characteristic, but some pseudoaneurysms can affect the ascending aorta.[9] Wall calcification is common, but mural thrombus is not.[5] Review of radiographs from the time of trauma usually shows mediastinal widening in retrospect. Because of the distinct tendency of these lesions to rupture and the low operative mortality for elective repair, it is generally recommended that all chronic pseudoaneurysms of the thoracic aorta be treated surgically.

AORTIC DIVERTICULA

There are various forms of aortic diverticula. One consists of a bulbous widening to the origin of an aberrant right subclavian artery, which represents incomplete regression of the primitive right aortic arch.[16] A much rarer diverticulum is the mirror image of this variant in a right aortic arch. The most common aortic diverticulum is thought by most to be a remnant of the ductus arteriosus, seen as a bulge at the anteromedial aspect of the

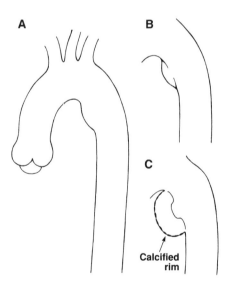

Fig. 7-1 Angiographic bulges at the aortic isthmus. **A,** Ductus "bump," a normal variant. The wall is smoothly continuous with the normal aorta. **B,** One manifestation of acute aortic laceration, an "ulcer" with overhanging or irregular edges. **C,** Ductus aneurysm demonstrating wall calcification and mural thrombus.

aortic isthmus. It is a variant of normal in infants, regressing with time so that a focal bulge at the isthmus persists into adulthood in only 9% of the general population.[17] Ductus diverticula are distinguished from aortic lacerations and pseudoaneurysms by their smooth margins and lack of a delay in washout of iodinated contrast material (Fig. 7-1).

The differential diagnosis of masses in the aortopulmonary window must include ductus arteriosus aneurysm.[18] Ductus aneurysms are likely to contain mural thrombus, a feature distinguishing them from the chronic pseudoaneurysms of trauma.[19] Like chronic pseudoaneurysms, they often show peripheral calcification. Diagnosis is important, for untreated ductus aneurysms incur a high mortality.

AORTIC DISSECTION

Predisposing Factors and Clinical Presentation

Aortic dissection is the most common acute disease affecting the aorta, and its incidence is two to three times that of ruptured abdominal aortic aneursym.[20] In fact, up to 5% of patients admitted with a clinical diagnosis of acute myocardial infarction may actually be suffering aortic dissection. The great majority of patients have a history of hypertension. Those rare cases presenting under age 40 tend to have Marfan's syndrome or coarctation of the aorta or to involve pregnant women. Aortic dissection is also a recognized complication of cocaine abuse.[21]

Cystic medial necrosis, a degenerative condition of the aortic wall, was long thought responsible for dissection. However, Wilson and Hutchins reviewed the autopsies of more than 204 individuals with aortic dissection and found that only 10% had evidence of cystic medial necrosis.[22] Others have done case-control studies, finding that those with aortic dissection are no more likely than patients dying from other causes to have cystic medial necrosis. Pathogenesis of dissection is no doubt complex and multifactorial. Biomechanical stress in those with hypertension or iatrogenic trauma can cause intimal disruption. Abnormal connective tissue in conditions such as Marfan's syndrome has been implicated. More than 10% of cases may not have *any* tear found at autopsy, and dissection may possibly be initiated by bleeding into vasa vasorum in these instances.

Typical symptoms include severe chest pain of abrupt, rather than gradual, onset. However, pain may be localized to the back, abdomen, or neck. Patients may complain of dyspnea, hoarseness, nausea and vomiting, or anuria. Those with extension of dissection into the aortic root may have systolic murmurs of aortic insufficiency. Peripheral pulses can be unequal, damped, or absent. Death results from pericardiac tamponade, secondary myocardial or cerebral infarction, rupture, or mesenteric or renal ischemia.

Dissection versus Aneurysm versus Pseudoaneurysm

The widely used term *dissecting aneurysm* is a misnomer because most acute dissections occur in an aorta of normal size (i.e., one that is *not* aneurysmal). Dissection is just that—a dissection or separation of arterial wall layers. Separation of aortic wall layers is most likely to occur in the outer third of the media.[20] Pusatile blood works to extend a dissection.

An aneurysm is focal dilatation of a vessel. All three layers of aortic wall (intima, media, and adventitia) are intact in an uncomplicated aortic aneurysm (Fig. 7-2). A pseudoaneurysm is a disruption of the arterial wall. This may be limited to intima (without the layer separation found in dissection) with bulging of the other layers, or it may involve all layers. In the latter case, the pseudoaneurysm can also be termed a *contained hematoma*.

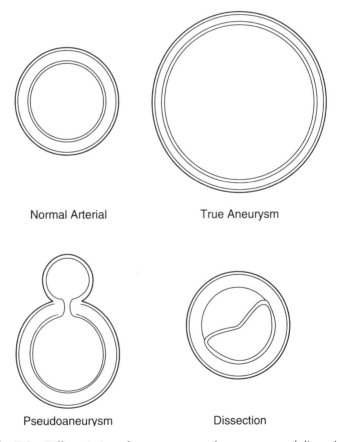

Normal Arterial   True Aneurysm

Pseudoaneurysm   Dissection

Fig. 7-2 Differentiation of aneurysm, pseudoaneurysm, and dissection.

Classification and Treatment of Dissections

The traditional classification of aortic dissection was proposed by deBakey: type I, both ascending and descending thoracic aorta involved; type II, confined to ascending aorta and arch; type III, only descending or abdominal aorta affected. A more practical modification was proposed by Daley in 1970: type A, dissections involving ascending aorta, type B, all other aortic dissections[20] (Fig. 7-3). Daley's classification is more relevant to treatment because proximal dissections are rapidly fatal if not treated surgically, usually by graft placement. Those with uncomplicated type B dissections respond much better to medical management with propranolol and other antihypertensive medications, and 90% now survive to be discharged from the hospital.[23] With the drop in surgical mortality from increased experience and improved technique, some advocate surgery even for type B patients because long-term conservative treatment can result in aneurysm, rupture, or redissection.

The great majority of dissections arise from a tear in the ascending aorta or arch. However, in defining the type of dissection present, *location of an intimal tear is irrelevant.* For example, a dissection can propagate in a retrograde fashion from a tear in the descending aorta to involve the aortic root

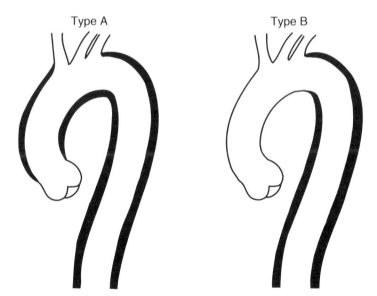

Fig. 7-3 Simplest clinically relevant classification of aortic dissections. *Type A* involves ascending aorta or arch, whether or not the dissection extends into the descending aorta. *Type B* involves descending aorta *only.*

or great vessel origins. It is the extension of a dissection into the great vessels, coronary arteries, or pericardium that determines prognosis. Resection or repair of a tear does not play a critical role in surgical treatment.[20]

Noninvasive Imaging

The most common plain film finding in aortic dissection is mediastinal widening. There may be an increased diameter to the aortic knob, "double density," or deviation of the trachea.[24] Pleural effusion or cardiac enlargement may represent rupture into the pleural space or pericardium. Separation of intimal calcification from the margin of the aortic knob by more than 4 mm is a sign suggestive of, but not entirely specific for, dissection. An unequivocally normal chest film makes the diagnosis less likely but does not exclude it. About 6% of cases show no abnormality on plain radiographs.[25]

Echocardiography can assist one in making the diagnosis of dissection when it involves the aortic root, and in many patients a length of the descending aorta can also be evaluated.[26,27] Still, spurious echoes have been misinterpreted as intimal flaps.[26,28] Transesophageal echocardiography has greatly extended the length of aorta that may be reliably imaged and can improve diagnostic accuracy.

Computed tomographic scan is a very reliable noninvasive study, allowing more complete depiction of the aorta than sonography. The protocol of Thorsen and colleagues specifies rapid injection of intravenous contrast medium and repeated scanning (angio-CT) at three levels: aortic root, mid-ascending aorta, and aortic arch.[29] They found CT to be more accurate than angiography in the diagnosis of dissection. Spiral CT permits the thoracic aorta to be imaged rapidly and in continuity during a single intravenous contrast material bolus. Magnetic resonance imaging (MRI) is also well suited to evaluating patients with suspected aortic dissection, particularly with the multiplicity of imaging planes possible. As does CT, MR allows the diagnosis of aortic dissection, even in the absence of an intimal tear or opacification of the false lumen.[30,31] Even so, although it may soon be matched by MR angiography, catheter aortography remains the best procedure for demonstrating occlusion of branch vessels and aortic regurgitation, both important for planning surgery.

Angiographic Findings and Accuracy

Aortography can be performed by a femoral route in patients with preserved femoral pulses. The pigtail catheter must be positioned above the aortic valve to demonstrate any possible regurgitation or coronary artery occlusions consequent to dissection. Rapid injection of contrast material with rapid biplane filming remains the standard for diagnosis. Filming should be carried out at least 12 to 15 seconds after injection to allow for delayed filling or slow washout of either true or false lumen. If a test injection shows slow flow, the power injection rate should be modified accordingly. Multiple projections are mandatory, for an intimal flap or multiple lumina may not be recognized in one projection. Digital subtraction arteriography is more appropriate for postoperative or long-term follow-up of patients with known dissection.[32] If thoracic aortography fails to confirm the presence of a dissection, biplane abdominal study should still be performed because primary abdominal dissections do occur.

The sine qua non of aortic dissection is the demonstration of an intimal flap, separating true and false lumen. The lumina may opacify sequentially or simultaneously. In the review of Earnest and associates, the false lumen opacified in 87% of aortograms.[24] Even when the false lumen fails to fill, if the true lumen is compressed or if widening of the extraluminal border exceeds 10 mm, the diagnosis can be made with reasonable certainty. However, an aneurysm with mural thrombus or with leakage into the mediastinum can have a similar appearance. Abnormal position of the angiographic catheter (which should follow the outside curve of the aorta) may suggest aortic dissection. Dissections tend to follow the outer curve of the aorta, and they commonly extend into the left renal artery when the abdominal aorta is involved. Care must be taken that prolonged washout of dependent iodinated contrast media in the descending aorta of a patient with isolated aortic insufficiency is not misinterpreted.[33] At times a dissection may have the appearance of a mural "ulcer."[33,34]

False lumen injection will not opacify the sinuses of Valsalva in a type A dissection. Power injection into a false lumen does not appear to present any extraordinary risk, but, as noted earlier, the injection rate should be modified to match observed flow. Precise differentiation of false lumen as opposed to true lumen generally has little bearing on diagnosis or treatment. The false lumen often provides blood to kidneys or other viscera. In this regard, it should be noted that therapy is directed at prevention of extension rather than obliteration of the false lumen. Repeated observations have shown that a distal false channel commonly persists after proximal surgical intervention.[6,35] In selected cases of renal or visceral ischemia, fenestration techniques using atherectomy catheters or angioplasty balloons to disrupt intima can be attempted to improve perfusion.

Accuracy of arteriography for acute dissection has been cited as 95% to 99%.[36] In their review of 55 aortograms determined to be negative, Eagle and colleagues found that many patients were ultimately determined to have primary myocardial infarction, aneurysm, aortic valve disease, or pericarditis.[37] However, four patients were found to have dissections, and the lower limit of angiographic false-negative studies was calculated to be 2% to 4%. The diagnosis of chronic dissection can be problematic if the false lumen has thrombosed, and many cases may be angiographically indistinguishable from aneurysms. Whether the condition is acute or chronic, if angiographic findings are equivocal, angio-CT or MRI can often resolve the issue.[38]

Transluminal techniques may soon be applied in the treatment of some dissections. Stents or intraluminal grafts may be used to stabilize aortic wall and prevent propagation of the process.

ANEURYSMS OF THE THORACIC AORTA

Atherosclerotic Aneurysms

Intrathoracic aneurysms most often affect the descending aorta, and most true aneurysms are atherosclerotic in origin. As with lesions in other arteries, thoracic aneurysms may produce symptoms by compression of adjacent structures, distal embolization of mural thrombus, occlusion, or rupture. Among the various clinical presentations are pain, stridor, dysphagia, superior vena cava syndrome, hoarseness, or aortic insufficiency.[6] In rare cases, hemoptysis may be due to aneurysm-induced aortobronchopulmonary fistula.[39] Risk of rupture is related to size in atherosclerotic lesions, almost negligible in those aneurysms smaller than 5 cm, but more than 40% if the aneurysm exceeds 10 cm in diameter.[6] The size and stability of thoracic aneurysms can be economically and noninvasively assessed by serial chest radiographs.

Thoracic or thoracoabdominal aneurysms are much more difficult to treat than abdominal aortic aneurysms, and surgical mortality remains high. One of the greatest risks in elective surgery for descending thoracic lesions (whether they are aneurysms, dissections, or traumatic lesions) is spinal cord ischemia and paraplegia. The artery of Adamkiewicz usually arises between the T8 and L1 levels. Reattachment of large intercostal or lumbar vessels during graft placement can decrease the incidence of paraplegia to about 16% in extensive resections.[40] Still, identification and reimplantation of vessels feeding the spinal cord have not decreased the incidence of spinal ischemia in comparison to those in whom such vessels are not found on angiography.[41,42] Other intraoperative measures may prove to be much more important. Acher and associates found that a combination of cerebrospinal fluid drainage and naloxone resulted in a rate of postoperative neurologic deficit that was less than 2%, significantly lower than the 22% encountered in the control group.[43]

Penetrating Atherosclerotic Ulcers

Penetrating aortic ulcer is an entity gaining increased recognition.[44] These focal lesions are associated with thickening of the aortic wall and commonly present with chest or back pain or distal embolization. They usually involve the descending thoracic aorta, although they have also been described in the arch and in the abdominal aorta. Many patients have aneurysmal disease, either at the site of the ulcer or in other vessels. With time, penetrating atherosclerotic ulcers progress to saccular or fusiform aneurysms with some risk of rupture or, rarely, dissection.[44] Initial treatment is control of hypertension in those with pain. Ulcers producing emboli or leading to aortic enlargement may be resected.

Mycotic, Luetic, and Other Aneurysms

Mycotic aneurysms are typically eccentric saccular lesions that often involve the aortic root and have a high tendency to rupture. They usually represent a complication of bacterial endocarditis or other distant infection. Organisms most commonly implicated are staphylococcal, streptococcal, or enterococcal species.[45] Syphilitic aneurysms, much more common in the preantibiotic era, tend to affect the ascending aorta and arch. Because aneurysms due to syphilis and other microorganisms may enlarge suddenly and rupture, prompt elective repair is indicated, even if the lesions are small and asymptomatic.

Marfan's syndrome predisposes not only to aortic dissection but also to true aneurysms of the ascending aorta. Surgery is recommended as soon as dilatation becomes evident. Sinus of Valsalva aneurysms are associated with a subendocardial cushion defect and high ventriculoseptal defect.[6] They most often arise in the right sinus and must be distinguished from mycotic lesions.

TAKAYASU'S AORTITIS

Patients with Takayasu's arteritis are relatively young, more often women, and likely to have symptoms and serologic abnormalities suggesting inflammatory disease.[46] The condition is a panarteritis of unknown cause that affects the vasa vasorum of elastic arteries. Although it is one of the most common vascular diseases in Asia, its incidence in North America and Europe is low.

About one third of patients have irregular lesions difficult to distinguish angiographically from atherosclerosis. More typically, long, smooth, concentric, segmental stenoses of the thoracic aorta are present. Proximal portions of the brachiocephalic vessels are also usually involved, as are the abdominal aorta, superior mesenteric artery, and renal arteries.[47] The pulmonary circulation is often affected by the disease, and many patients demonstrate abnormalities on perfusion scans.

Aside from stenoses, mild ectasia and small cystic protrusions from the arterial wall can be seen. Renovascular hypertension is a common complication of Takayasu's arteritis, and it poses the greatest risk from the disease. Remarkably, cerebral and mesenteric ischemia are rare.[47]

PULMONARY SEQUESTRATION

Pulmonary sequestration is a developmental anomaly in which a portion of the lung is partially or completely isolated from the pulmonary circulation (with or without a separate pleural investment). The most common location for a sequestration is on the left side in the vicinity of the posterior basal segment.[48] Pulmonary sequestration can present as an asymptomatic paraaortic mass, rarely containing calcification.[49] Symptomatic lesions are commonly infected, and resection is indicated for these cases.

Arterial supply generally comes from the aorta, sometimes from below the diaphragm. Multiple arteries may be seen in 20%, and the vessels usually traverse the pulmonary ligment.[50] Aortography is recommended, both to confirm the diagnosis and to delineate the supplying and draining vessels.

BRONCHIAL AND INTERCOSTAL ANGIOGRAPHY

Bronchial and intercostal arteriography are most useful in the diagnosis and embolic treatment of refractory massive hemoptysis (see Chapter 12

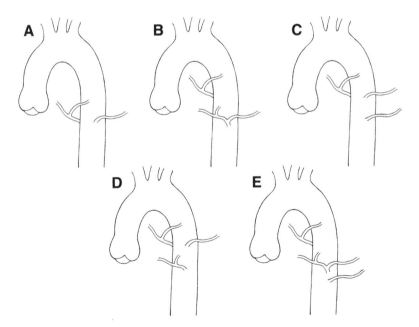

Fig. 7-4 The major variations in bronchial artery distribution. **A** and **B** are found in about half of the population; **C, D,** and **E** are present in another 30%. (Modified from Uflacker R, Kaemmerer A, Picon PD, et al: Bronchial artery embolization in the management of hemoptysis. *Radiology* 1988; 157:637–644; with permission.)

entitled Embolotherapy). Tuberculosis, sarcoidosis, cystic fibrosis, aspergilloma, and bronchiectasis are among the disorders responsible for such hemoptysis. Systemic arterial branches can also enlarge to provide collateral supply to areas of lung affected by chronic pulmonary embolism, and angiography is useful prior to surgical treatment of such disease.[51]

Bronchial arteries have a highly variable distribution (Fig. 7-4). Most commonly there is a single right intercostobronchial trunk and one or two left bronchial arteries, but this pattern is present in fewer than half of patients.[52] The bronchial arteries usually originate from the descending thoracic aorta near the level of T5 or T6, and they are not normally seen peripheral to the hilum.[53] Cobra, Simmons, or Mikaelsson catheter configurations are most useful for selective catheterization of intercostal or bronchial arteries.

Low-osmolar contrast media and careful injections of small volumes are advised in the study of these vessels. Although the risk of spinal cord injury is low, the anterior spinal artery can originate from bronchial or intercostal arteries. Paraplegia remains a possible complication.

REFERENCES

1. Mirvis SE, Pais SO, Gens DR: Thoracic aortic rupture: Advantages of intraarterial digital subtraction angiography. *Am J Roentgenol* 1986; 146:987–991.
2. Stark P, Cook M, Vincent A, Smith DC: Traumatic rupture of the thoracic aorta: A review of 49 cases. *Radiologe* 1987; 27:402–406.
3. Mirvis SE, Bidwell JK, Buddemeyer EU, et al: Imaging diagnosis of traumatic aortic rupture: A review and experience at a major trauma center. *Invest Radiol* 1987; 22:187–196.
4. Fleckenstein JL, Schultz SM, Miller RH: Serial aortography assesses stability of "atypical" aortic arch ruptures. *Cardiovasc Intervent Radiol* 1987; 10:194–197.
5. Heystraten FM, Rosenbusch G, Kingma LM, Lacquet LK: Chronic posttraumatic aneurysm of the thoracic aorta: Surgically correctable occult threat. *Am J Roentgenol* 1986; 146:303–308.
6. Althaus U, Marincek B: Thorakale aortenaneurysmen. *Schweiz Med Wochenschr* 1984; 114:1547–1559.
7. Crass JR, Cohen AM, Motta AO, et al: A proposed new mechanism of traumatic aortic rupture: The osseous pinch. *Radiology* 1990; 176:645–649.
8. Cohen AM, Crass JR, Thomas HA, et al: CT evidence for the osseous pinch mechanism of traumatic aortic injury. *Am J Roentgenol* 1992; 159:271–274.
9. Lundell CJ, Quinn MF, Finck EJ: Traumatic laceration of the ascending aorta: Angiographic assessment. *Am J Roentgenol* 1985; 145:715–719.
10. Cohen AM, Crass JR: Traumatic lacerations of the aorta and great vessels with a normal mediastinum at radiography. *J Vasc Interv Radiol* 1992; 3:541–544.
11. Raptopoulos V, Sheiman RG, Phillips DA, et al: Traumatic aortic tear: Screening with chest CT. *Radiology* 1992; 182:667–673.

12. Morgan PW, Goodman LR, Aprahamian C, et al: Evaluation of traumatic aortic injury: Does dynamic contrast-enhanced CT play a role? *Radiology* 1992; 182:661–666.
13. Agee CK, Metzler MH, Churchill RJ, Mitchell FL: Computed tomographic evaluation to exclude traumatic aortic disruption. *J Trauma* 1992; 33:876–881.
14. Kearney PA, Smith W, Johnson SB, et al: Use of transesophageal echocardiography in the evaluation of traumatic aortic injury. *J Trauma* 1993; 34:696–703.
15. LaBerge JM, Jeffrey RB: Aortic lacerations: Fatal complications of thoracic aortography. *Radiology* 1987; 165:367–369.
16. Salomonowitz E, Edwards JE, Hunter DW, et al: The three types of aortic diverticula. *Am J Roentgenol* 1984; 142:673–679.
17. Goodman PC, Jeffrey RB, Minagi H, et al: Angiographic evaluation of the ductus diverticulum. *Cardiovasc Intervent Radiol* 1982; 5:1–4.
18. Traughber PD, Wojtowycz M, Karwande SV, et al: Roentgenologic CPC: Enlarging mediastinal mass. *Invest Radiol* 1987; 22:240–243.
19. Mitchell RS, Seifert FC, Miller DC, et al: Aneurysm of the diverticulum of the ductus arteriosus in the adult. *J Thorac Cardiovasc Surg* 1983; 86:400–408.
20. Anagnostopoulos CE: *Acute Aortic Dissections.* 1975, Baltimore: University Park Press. pp 1–249.
21. Grannis FW, Jr, Bryant C, Caffaratti JD, Turner AF: Acute aortic dissection associated with cocaine abuse. *Clin Cardiol* 1988; 11:572–574.
22. Wilson SK, Hutchins GM: Aortic dissecting aneurysms: Causative factors in 204 subjects. *Arch Pathol Lab Med* 1982; 106:175–180.
23. Nienaber CA, von Kodolitsch Y: Metaanalyse zur Prognose der thorakalen Aortendissektion: Letalität im Wandel der letzten vier Jahrzehnte. *Herz* 1992; 17:398–416.
24. Earnest F, Muhm JR, Sheedy PF, Jr: Roentgenographic findings in thoracic aortic dissection. *Mayo Clin Proc* 1979; 54:43–50.
25. Kaufman SL, White RI, Jr: Aortic dissection with "normal" chest roentgenogram. *Cardiovasc Intervent Radiol* 1980; 3:103–106.
26. Victor MF, Mintz GS, Kotler MN, et al: Two dimensional echocardiographic diagnosis of aortic dissection. *Am J Cardiol* 1981; 48:1155–1159.
27. Come PC: Improved cross-sectional echocardiographic technique for visualization of the retrocardiac descending aorta in its long axis. *Am J Cardiol* 1983; 51:1029–1032.
28. Kolettis M, Toutouzas P, Avgoustakis D: False echocardiographic diagnosis of aortic root dissection in case of abdominal aortic dissection. *Br Heart J* 1981; 45:602–604.
29. Thorsen MK, SanDretto MA, Lawson TL, et al: Dissecting aortic aneurysms: Accuracy of computed tomographic diagnosis. *Radiology* 1983; 148:773–777.
30. Yamada T, Shimpei T, Harada J: Aortic dissection without intimal rupture: Diagnosis with MR imaging and CT. *Radiology* 1988; 168:347–352.
31. Wolff KA, Herold CJ, Tempany CM, et al: Aortic dissection: Atypical patterns seen at MR imaging. *Radiology* 1991; 181:489–495.

32. Guthaner DF, Miller DC: Digital subtraction angiography of aortic dissection. *Am J Roentgenol* 1983; 141:157–161.

33. Shuford WH, Sybers RG, Weens HS: Problems in the aortographic diagnosis of dissecting aneurysm of the aorta. *N Engl J Med* 1969; 280:225–231.

34. Hekali P, Velt P, Gutierrez O, et al: Radiology of aortic dissection: Pitfalls in diagnosis. *Eur J Radiol* 1986; 6:314–318.

35. Pinet F, Froment JC, Guillot M, et al: Prognostic factors and indications for surgical treatment of acute aortic dissections: A report based on 191 observations. *Cardiovasc Intervent Radiol* 1984; 7:257–266.

36. DeSanctis RW, Doroghazi RM, Austen WG, Buckley MJ: Aortic dissection. *N Engl J Med* 1987; 317:1060–1067.

37. Eagle KA, Quertermous T, Kritzer GA, et al: Spectrum of conditions initially suggesting acute aortic dissection but with negative aortograms. *Am J Cardiol* 1986; 57:322–326.

38. Akins EW, Carmichael MJ, Hill JA, Mancuso AA: Preoperative evaluation of the thoracic aorta using MRI and angiography. *Ann Thorac Surg* 1987; 44:499–507.

39. Coblentz CL, Sallee DS, Chiles C: Aortobronchopulmonary fistula complicating aortic aneurysm: Diagnosis in four cases. *Am J Roentgenol* 1988; 150:535–538.

40. Pokela R, Karkola P, Tarkka M, et al: Surgery of thoracoabdominal aortic aneurysms. *Scand J Thorac Cardiovasc Surg* 1984; 18:179–189.

41. Fereshetian A, Kadir S, Kaufman SL, et al: Digital subtraction spinal cord angiography in patients undergoing thoracic aneurysm surgery. *Cardiovasc Intervent Radiol* 1989; 12:7–9.

42. Savader SJ, Williams GM, Trerotola SO, et al: Preoperative spinal artery localization and its relationship to postoperative neurologic complications. *Radiology* 1993; 189:165–171.

43. Acher CW, Wynn MM, Hoch JR, et al: Combined use of cerebral spinal fluid drainage and naloxone reduces the risk of paraplegia in thoracoabdominal aneurysm repair. *J Vasc Surg* 1994; 19:236–248.

44. Harris JA, Bis KG, Glover JL, et al: Penetrating atherosclerotic ulcers of the aorta. *J Vasc Surg* 1994; 19:90–99.

45. Castañeda-Zuñiga WR, Nath PH, Zollikofer C, et al: Mycotic aneurysm of the aorta. *Cardiovasc Intervent Radiol* 1980; 3:144–149.

46. Yamato M, Lecky JW, Hiramatsu K, Kohda E: Takayasu arteritis: Radiographic and angiographic findings in 59 patients. *Radiology* 1986; 161:329–334.

47. Liu YQ: Radiology of aortoarteritis. *Radiol Clin North Am* 1985; 23:671–688.

48. Khalil KG, Kilman JW: Pulmonary sequestration. *J Thorac Cardiovasc Surg* 1975; 70:928–937.

49. Wojtowycz M, Gould HR, Atwell DT, Pois A: Calcified bronchopulmonary sequestration. *CT: J Computed Tomography* 1984; 8:171–173.

50. Bolman RM, Wolfe WG: Bronchiectasis and bronchopulmonary sequestration. *Surg Clin North Am* 1980; 60:867–882.

51. Mills SR, Jackson DC, Sullivan DC, et al: Angiographic evaluation of chronic pulmonary embolism. *Radiology* 1980; 136:301–308.

52. Cadotte R, Leger C, Harel C, Belanger R: Bronchial angiography: A report of 21 patients. *J Can Assoc Radiol* 1986; 37:22–24.
53. North LB, Boushy SF, Houk VN: Bronchial and intercostal arteriography in non-neoplastic pulmonary disease. *Am J Roentgenol* 1969; 107:328–342.

8

Upper Extremity Angiography

KEY CONCEPTS

1. Manifestations of upper extremity arterial disease include claudication, ulcers, and Raynaud's phenomenon.
2. Raynaud's phenomenon without fixed vascular occlusion does
   not pose the threat of tissue loss.
3. Unilateral Raynaud's phenomenon signals an underlying arterial
   lesion.
4. Embolization from proximal plaques or aneurysms can lead to
   amputation.
5. Arterial spasm in the hand is countered by extremity warming
   and direct injection of vasodilators; the pain of contrast injection
   is minimized by low-osmolar agents and digital subtraction
   angiography.
6. Thoracic outlet syndrome is responsible for most cases of intermittent venous obstruction and spontaneous thrombosis.

INDICATIONS

Angiography of the upper extremities is used to evaluate arterial insufficiency, aneurysms, arteriovenous malformations, venous occlusion, and traumatic, thermal, or electrical injuries. Arteriography is much less often needed in the upper than in the lower extremities, for only about 5% of all cases of limb ischemia involve the arms.[1–3] A tendency for spasm to affect the vessels of the hand makes Raynaud's phenomenon a prominent feature in many cases of ischemia, and spasm calls for special techniques of examination. Claudication and gangrene can also be features of arterial occlusive disease in the arms.

Primary distal arterial disease must be differentiated from that produced by more proximal lesions. Noninvasive studies may fail to uncover an aneurysm or nonocclusive plaque giving rise to small emboli, and a majority of patients with digital ischemia actually have a proximal lesion responsible for their symptoms.[4] Thoracic outlet compression of arteries or veins and involvement of hand vessels by connective tissue disorders and systemic vasculitis are among the factors that distinguish upper extremity disease from common lower extremity disorders.[3, 5–7] Unlike the foot, the hand is prone to ischemic complications from repetitive trauma.[8,9] Because of the often confusing clinical presentation of upper extremity vascular problems, angiography is valuable for both diagnosis and treatment planning.

ARTERIAL EXAMINATION TECHNIQUE

As a rule, the arterial supply to the extremity should be delineated completely, from the origin of the innominate or subclavian artery through the digital vessels. This is best done from a femoral approach, but in cases of severe proximal disease or systemic atherosclerosis, axillary or brachial artery puncture may be needed. In relatively young patients without tortuous vessels, an H1H configuration catheter is well adapted for the catheterization of brachiocephalic vessels from the femoral artery. A sidewinder or Simmons catheter is a better choice for most older individuals. Stenoses involving the origins of vessels arising from the aortic arch may be missed on a single projection, and attention must be paid to the presence of collateral arterial channels or reversed flow in the vertebral artery.

Once the intrathoracic arteries are examined, the catheter is advanced over a guidewire into the axillary artery for more distal injections. If possible, the tip is placed into the distal brachial artery for examination of the hand. Up to 15% of people have a high origin to the radial artery, which sometimes bifurcates from the axillary artery, a potential source of error if proximal imaging is neglected.[4,10]

The injection of iodinated contrast medium into upper extremity arteries can be extremely painful. Fortunately, the availability of low-osmolar agents and digital subtraction angiography has improved the tolerability of arteriography considerably. Lidocaine should not be mixed with contrast agent because of the possibility of reflux into the vertebral artery.

Methods of Countering Spasm

Because of the difficulties posed by spasm, various schemes for vasodilatation have been tested to provide optimal filling of palmar and digital vessels. Although it has been suggested that contrast media cause a vasodilatation that can be used to improve flow for an early second injection, this has not been confirmed in practice.[11,12] Oral administration of alcohol and brachial plexus block with lidocaine yield unpredictable results.[10,12] General anesthesia produces rapid and complete fill of digital vessels, but it is not commonly employed or desired for angiography in the United States. Tolazoline (15 to 25 mg), phentolamine (2 to 4 mg), and reserpine (0.5 mg in 10 ml of saline injected slowly) have been injected intraarterially to increase flow.[4,10,13] With tolazoline or phentolamine, filming should be performed within 30 seconds to several minutes of injection. Reserpine produces its greatest effect 40 minutes after administration.[10]

Effects of Temperature

Temperature is a prime factor affecting vascular tone, and normal digital blood flow correlates with a fingertip temperature above 31°C.[10,11] The extremity may be warmed directly, or a large heating pad can be used to increase body core temperature. A brachial artery catheter–to-wrist flow time of 4 seconds or less indicates effective ablation of any vasospasm. Arneklo-Nobin and colleagues recommend body warming and phentolamine in combination as the best routine preparation for hand arteriography.[10]

ANATOMIC CONSIDERATIONS

Proximal arterial occlusions alone rarely lead to tissue necrosis because of rich collateral networks available around the shoulder and elbow. The forearm and hand are supplied by the radial, ulnar, and interosseous arteries. The radial artery continues as the deep (proximal) palmar arch (Fig. 8-1). The ulnar artery becomes the superficial palmar arch, which provides the primary vascular supply to the fingers. If there is a major anastomosis between the ulnar and radial circulations, a palmar arch is called *complete.* The deep palmar arch is complete in 95% of the population, whereas the superficial arch is complete in only about 80%.[4] The variations in palmar anatomy are responsible for the individual differences in the ability to tolerate arterial occlusions in the forearm and wrist. A clinical assessment of

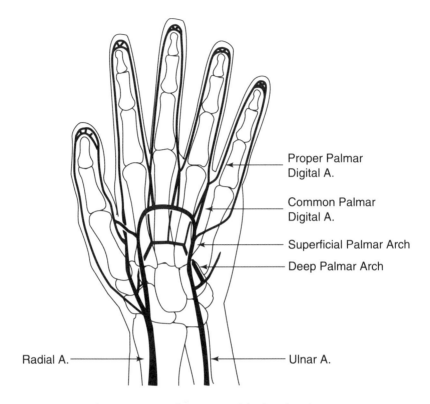

Fig. 8-1 Arterial anatomy of the hand and wrist.

the adequacy of collateral circulation can be made by the Allen test: compression of radial and ulnar arteries at the wrist with observation of the reversal of finger blanching by the sequential release of compression.

ARTERIAL DISORDERS

Raynaud's Phenomenon
The symptoms first described by Raynaud in the late nineteenth century are precipitated by cold or other sympathetic stimuli: the affected digits become blanched, cold, and numb and later turn cyanotic and ruborous with an attendant burning, throbbing pain. Although the lower extremities may be affected, symptoms are more common and more pronounced in the fingers and hands. The syndrome may be primary (Raynaud's disease) if no underlying vascular lesion or systemic disease can be found to account for the symptoms. If an underlying condition is established, the clinical manifestations are called *secondary Raynaud's phenomenon*.

Primary Raynaud's Phenomenon

Besides absence of other illness to account for arterial insufficiency, the following conditions must be met to make the diagnosis of primary Raynaud's phenomenon: bilateral episodes, absence of gangrene, and presence of symptoms for at least 2 years.[4] Leppert and colleagues have found the prevalence of Raynaud's phenomenon to be 16% among Swedish women, which is in line with similar surveys.[14] The prevalence among men appears to be less than half this figure. There is a small but significant association with smoking, and patients with extremity symptoms are also more likely to suffer recurrent headaches, muscle pains, and joint pain.[14]

Although vasospasm is strongly implicated, the reasons for heightened vascular sensitivity to stimuli in primary Raynaud's phenomenon remain controversial.[3,15,16] Surgical sympathectomy and numerous medical treatments have been tried with only limited success, but there is evidence that nifedipine may decrease the incidence and severity of attacks.[16]

Because primary Raynaud's phenomenon is unlikely to result in tissue loss, arteriography is rarely indicated and should be reserved for those with evidence of arterial occlusion. Noninvasive studies such as segmental blood pressure measurements, Doppler, and plethysmography are excellent screens for fixed obstructions down to the level of the fingertips.[10] Those with uncomplicated primary Raynaud's phenomenon have normal resting digital arterial pressures. Magnetic resonance imaging (MRI) may become an excellent means of ascertaining the presence or absence of fixed obstructions in the digital arteries in the near future.[17]

Secondary Raynaud's Phenomenon

Raynaud's phenomenon is often the first manifestation of a variety of disorders, and connective tissue diseases may become evident only years later.[2,18] Fixed digital artery occlusions are responsible for ulcers and gangrene, but tissue breakdown seldom occurs before other systemic signs of scleroderma, rheumatoid arthritis, systemic lupus erythematosus, or mixed connective tissue disease appear.[4] Raynaud's phenomenon has also been observed in such diverse conditions as chronic renal failure, hypothyroidism, and occult malignant disease.[16] Angiography is not particularly useful for making the diagnosis of collagen vascular disease or for distinguishing among its various forms. Hematologic, pulmonary, and gastrointestinal studies are more productive in this regard.

Arteriography has greater value in evaluating *unilateral* Raynaud's symptoms. These may be consequent to thoracic outlet compression, aneurysm, radiation therapy, chronic or repetitive trauma, iatrogenic brachial artery injury, or emboli from a cardiac source. In such cases surgical vascular reconstruction and/or cervical sympathectomy can prevent tissue loss.[5,19,20]

Atherosclerosis

Atherosclerosis predominantly involves proximal vessels, and many innominate or subclavian artery lesions remain asymptomatic unless they produce emboli. If flow is reversed in the vertebral artery (subclavian steal), symptoms, if present, are more likely to relate to central nervous system ischemia than to the arm. When ischemia does complicate upper extremity atherosclerosis, amputation is the ultimate result in up to 22%.[7] If the only forearm vessel intact is the interosseous artery, the prognosis is poor.[21] As noted, proximal plaques producing emboli can be difficult to detect. Multiple views and pullback pressure measurements improve diagnostic yield.[13]

Some subclavian or axillary artery aneurysms are caused by extrinsic compression at the thoracic outlet and development of poststenotic dilatation (see the section on Thoracic Outlet Syndrome later in this chapter). However, most true aneurysms at this location are caused by atherosclerosis, and many patients also have abdominal aortic, femoral, or other peripheral aneurysms.[22] These lesions characteristically contain mural thrombus, and although they can rupture, the greatest threat they pose is from distal embolization.

Thromboangiitis Obliterans (Buerger's Disease)

This disease often produces painful ischemic ulcers of the fingertips, as well as in the feet. At times the lesions of thromboangiitis obliterans are difficult to distinguish angiographically from atherosclerosis. However, they are generally more distal, with concomitant forearm and hand arterial occlusions.[7] In their most typical appearance, occlusions are long and are bridged by paralleling corkscrew collaterals. Arterial spasm is not a prominent finding. Patients are relatively young and almost invariably male, and there is a strong association with tobacco use. The risk of major upper extremity amputation is very low, less than 2%[23] (see Chapter 2 entitled Angiography of the Abdominal Aorta, Pelvis, and Lower Extremities).

Embolization from a Cardiac Source

Most emboli lodging in the upper extremity come from the heart, and atrial fibrillation is a predisposing factor. They are more likely to occlude the axillary and brachial arteries than vessels of the forearm and hand.[24] Onset of symptoms is typically abrupt, and a filling defect or sharp cutoff is found at angiography. However, a sharp arterial cutoff is not specific to embolization, and other causes of occlusion cannot be excluded by angiographic criteria alone.

Vasculitides

A great number of systemic diseases affect upper extremity vessels, and only a few are specifically addressed here.

Connective Tissue Disorders

Raynaud's phenomenon accompanies many cases of scleroderma, systemic lupus erythematosus, rheumatoid arthritis, and related diseases and—as noted earlier—frequently constitutes the initial clinical presentation. Occlusive disease is typically distal and bilaterally symmetric in its distribution.[1,25] Collateral vessels are usually inadequately developed, and filling beyond the obstructed segments is poor.[7] Giant cell arteritis (temporal arteritis) differs from the other connective tissue disorders in that it affects larger vessels, such as the subclavian and axillary arteries, and rarely causes digital vessel occlusions.[26] Both angiographically and histologically, giant cell arteritis may be difficult to distinguish from Takayasu's arteritis.

Surgical sympathectomy has been advocated as a treatment for distal occlusive disease, but results of standard cervical or thoracic procedures have been poor in patients with scleroderma and related illnesses.[2,27,28] Alternative interventions proposed include digital sympathectomy and intraarterial injection of reserpine, but symptomatic relief obtained is more often than not incomplete and temporary.[15,27,29] In connective tissue disorders, the activity of disease in the hands usually parallels disease progression or regression seen elsewhere. Recurrent tissue loss and ulceration are more likely in those with connective tissue diseases than in patients with small vessel occlusions from other causes.[1]

Takayasu's Arteritis

This vasculitis primarily affects the aorta, its major branches, and the pulmonary arteries. It is a giant-cell necrotizing arteritis, and it commonly compromises the subclavian arteries.[30] Stenotic lesions are characteristically smooth, with normal appearance to those arterial segments unaffected by the disease. Most patients have symptoms of fever and malaise, suggesting an active inflammatory process.

Hypersensitivity and Toxic Vasculitis

Hypersensitivity angiitis is characterized by rapid onset of small vessel occlusions. The process is usually self-limited, and ulcers respond to local care.[1] In many cases an inciting agent is never identified.

Use of ergotamine (an α-adrenergic blocking agent) for migraine headaches can sometimes elicit pronounced peripheral arterial constriction and occlusion.[31] Symptoms are usually acute in onset, and both upper and lower extremities can be affected. Arteriography shows long segments of severe narrowing.

Chronic occupational exposure to vinyl chloride has been associated with arterial wall thickening, perivascular inflammation, and Raynaud's phenomenon.[32] Stenoses and occlusions are limited to digital arteries, sparing the palmar arches. Angiography can confirm the diagnosis before the bony changes of acro-osteolysis become evident.

Arterial Injury

As in the lower extremities, blunt or penetrating trauma can produce occlusion, hemorrhage, pseudoaneurysm, or arteriovenous fistula. Examination technique and findings in acute trauma are similar (see Chapter 2).

Repetitive Trauma

The hand and wrist are particularly sensitive to recurrent vibration or occupational trauma from tools. Motions involving twisting or striking with the palm, even apparently trivial, have been implicated in vascular occlusion or aneurysm formation. The ulnar artery is particularly susceptible to trauma where it passes over the hamate bone, superficial to the carpal ligament.[9] The clinical presentation of hypothenar hammer syndrome is usually insidious, with ischemia typically affecting the fourth and fifth fingers of the dominant hand.

Because of its relatively protected position and the complete formation of the deep palmar arch in most people, the radial artery is less likely to suffer trauma from pressure on the thenar eminence. Still, cases of occlusion have been described.[8] One must be aware of these effects of repetitive trauma in order to elicit the necessary history, which may not be volunteered or considered relevant by the patient.

Long-term use of axillary-support crutches poses a risk for axillary artery aneurym.[33] Presenting symptoms of acute or chronic ischemia are the result of distal embolization. Early detection and aneurysm repair can prevent limb loss in this situation.

Iatrogenic Trauma

Widespread use of the brachial artery for catheterization, particularly for cardiac angiography, has currently made iatrogenic trauma one of the most common causes of upper extremity arterial insufficiency. In a survey of more than 12,000 patients having cardiac studies performed with 8 Fr catheters in a single institution, McCollum and Mavor found that 0.9% needed surgical repair of the puncture site.[34] A more recent report of patients undergoing angiography with 4 Fr and 5 Fr catheters from a brachial approach noted a thrombectomy rate of 4%, despite the routine use of heparin during angiography.[35] No doubt the tendency of the brachial artery to go into spasm predisposes it to postcatheterization complications.

Other Injuries

Intraarterial injection of illicit drugs can produce multiple digital artery occlusions, mycotic aneurysms, and arteriovenous fistulas. Severe electrical injuries are associated with segmental stenoses or occlusions, and angiography is instrumental in determining the level of any necessary amputation.[7] Angiography serves the same function in cases of frostbite.[36]

THE THORACIC OUTLET SYNDROME

The narrow costoclavicular space, bounded inferiorly by the first rib, superiorly by clavicle, posteriorly by the scalenus medius muscle, and anteriorly by the costoclavicular ligament, forms a functional bottleneck for the vessels to the upper extremity. Anomalous ribs, muscles, and fascial slips can compress the brachial plexus, subclavian artery, or subclavian vein. Local radiation therapy, clavicular fractures, and osteomyelitis can evoke perivascular fibrosis and cause an acquired thoracic outlet syndrome.[5] It has been postulated that some cases are caused by a cervical stretch injury followed by prolonged muscle contraction and hypertrophy. The great majority of thoracic outlet problems arise from brachial plexus compression, and only about 3% of cases have signs of arterial or venous obstruction.[37]

Most patients with arterial compression have an associated fusiform aneurysm, but the presence of mural thrombus may obscure the abnormality on arteriography. Machleder recommends examination with arm abduction and external rotation to elicit compression.[4] However, this challenge and others that have been recommended are nonspecific, and many people without clinical symptoms can obliterate their brachial pulses by such maneuvers.[38]

Venous compression (or the "thoracic inlet syndrome") can produce intermittent symptoms or acute thrombosis. The most common surgical treatment of arterial or venous compression is resection of the first rib or clavicle, but in cases of venous obstruction recurrent symptoms can arise from postoperative scarring.[37]

UPPER EXTREMITY VENOGRAPHY

Venography is used to diagnose venous obstruction in patients suffering arm swelling and pain. Thrombosis must be distinguished from lymphedema, hemorrhage, and other conditions that present in a similar fashion. Venous thrombosis may be a primary condition, or it may be secondary to central venous catheterization (for a discussion of the latter, see Chapter 9 entitled Dialysis Access, Central Venous Catheters, and Other Central Venous Problems). When thrombosis arises spontaneously, a hypercoagulable condition or central obstructing tumor must be excluded diagnostically.

Primary axillary-subclavian vein thrombosis (Paget-Schroetter syndrome) typically affects young men, usually in the dominant arm. A recent history of vigorous or unusual exercise can often be obtained.[39] If the clot is detected early, thrombolysis or thrombectomy is recommended, for long-term morbidity is a common consequence of conservative treatment.[39,40] Thoracic outlet syndrome is implicated in 80% of cases of spontaneous venous occlusion.[4]

The majority of patients with signs of venous obstruction from thoracic outlet compression have intermittent symptoms relieved by rest and do not demonstrate thrombosis.[41] Hyperabduction (to 180°) may produce occlusion on venography, but this sign is not very specific. Color-flow duplex sonography can be employed in the detection of intermittent or positional obstruction.[42] Schubart and associates have used venous pressure measurements to assess the significance of obstruction induced by abduction and external rotation, finding normal resting pressure to be 5 mm Hg and a rise of 10 mm Hg or more to indicate disease.[41]

THERAPEUTIC VASCULAR INTERVENTIONS

In selected cases, thrombolytic therapy is quite helpful in distal arterial occlusions of the upper extremity.[43] As in experience with other vessels, best results are obtained with relatively acute thromboses. Thrombolysis of primary venous thrombosis has also been successful, but any underlying external compression must be treated surgically.[37,44] Balloon angioplasty has been applied to subclavian artery stenoses with good results (see Chapter 10 entitled Percutaneous Angioplasty, Recanalization, and Vascular Stents). Experience with transluminal angioplasty in the more distal arteries of the upper extremity has been sparsely reported.

In the past, angiographers have been called upon to treat Raynaud's phenomenon with intraarterial injection of reserpine. Slow injection of 1 mg into the brachial artery has produced objective and subjective signs of improvement for up to 13 months in some patients.[15,27] However, injectable reserpine is no longer available in the United States.

REFERENCES

1. Mills JL, Friedman EI, Taylor LM, Jr, Porter JM: Upper extremity ischemia caused by small artery disease. *Ann Surg* 1987; 206:521–527.
2. Welling RE, Cranley JJ, Krause RJ, Hafner CD: Obliterative arterial disease of the upper extremity. *Arch Surg* 1981; 116:1593–1595.
3. Kobinia GS, Olbert F, Russe OJ, Denck H: Chronic vascular disease of the upper extremity: Radiologic and clinical features. *Cardiovasc Intervent Radiol* 1980; 3:25–41.
4. Machleder H: Vaso-occlusive disorders of the upper extremity. *Curr Probl Surg* 1988; 25:7–67.
5. Bouthoutsos J, Morris T, Martin P: Unilateral Raynaud's phenomenon in the hand and its significance. *Surgery* 1977; 82:547–551.

6. Adler J, Hooshmand A: The angiographic spectrum of the thoracic outlet syndrome with emphasis on mural thrombosis and emboli and congenital vascular anomalies. *Clin Radiol* 1973; 24:35–42.

7. Erlandson EE, Forrest ME, Shields JJ, et al: Discriminant arteriographic criteria in the management of forearm and hand ischemia. *Surgery* 1981; 90:1025–1036.

8. Wandtke JC, Spitzer RM, Olsson HE, Welch E: Traumatic thenar ischemia. *Am J Roentgenol* 1976; 127:569–571.

9. Pineda CJ, Weisman MH, Bookstein JJ, Saltzstein SL: Hypothenar hammer syndrome: Form of reversible Raynaud's phenomenon. *Am J Med* 1985; 79:561–570.

10. Arneklo-Nobin B, Albrechtsson U, Eklöf B, Tylén U: Indications for angiography and its optimal performance in patients with Raynaud's phenomenon. *Cardiovasc Intervent Radiol* 1985; 8:174–179.

11. Rösch JF, Antonovic R, Porter JM: The importance of temperature in angiography of the hand. *Radiology* 1977; 123:323–326.

12. Viehweger G, Plötz J: Vergleichende angiographische untersuchungen in lokal-, regional- und allgemein-anästhesie an der oberen extremität. *Rofo* 1974; 121:303–310.

13. Maiman MH, Bookstein JJ, Bernstein EF: Digital ischemia: Angiographic differentiation of embolism from primary arterial disease. *Am J Roentgenol* 1981; 137:1183–1187.

14. Leppert J, Åberg H, Ringqvist I, Sörensson S: Raynaud's phenomenon in a female population: Prevalence and association with other conditions. *Angiology* 1987; 38:871–877.

15. Romeo SG, Whalen RE, Tindall JP: Intra-arterial administration of reserpine. *Arch Intern Med* 1970; 125:825–829.

16. Smith CR, Rodeheffer RJ: Treatment of Raynaud's phenomenon with calcium channel blockers. *Am J Med* 1985; 78:39–42.

17. Blackband SJ, Chakrabarti I, Gibbs P, et al: Three-dimensional MR imaging and angiography with a local gradient coil. *Radiology* 1994; 190:895–899.

18. Dale WA, Lewis MR: Management of ischemia of the hand and fingers. *Surgery* 1970; 67:62–79.

19. Mesh CL, McCarthy WJ, Pearce WH, et al: Upper extremity bypass grafting: A 15-year experience. *Arch Surg* 1993; 128:795–802.

20. Nehler MR, Dalman RL, Harris EJ, et al: Upper extremity arterial bypass distal to the wrist. *J Vasc Surg* 1992; 16:633–642.

21. Gross WS, Flanigan DP, Kraft RO, Stanley JC: Chronic upper extremity arterial insufficiency. *Arch Surg* 1978; 113:419–423.

22. Pairolero PC, Walls JT, Payne WS, et al: Subclavian-axillary artery aneurysms. *Surgery* 1981; 90:757–762.

23. Ohta T, Shionoya S: Fate of the ischaemic limb in Buerger's disease. *Br J Surg* 1988; 75:259–262.

24. Janevski B: Arterial embolism of the upper extremities. *Rofo* 1986; 145:431–434.

25. Wallner B, Kratzsch G, Friedrich JM, Roth J: Die intraarterielle DSA der Handarterien in der Diagnostik entzündlicher Bindegewebserkrankungen. *Rofo* 1989; 151:565–568.

26. Mickley V, Friedrich JM, Sunder-Plassmann L: Angiographische Diagnose bei Riesenzellarteriitis der Armarterien. *Rofo* 1992; 157:579–583.

27. Nilsen KH, Jayson MI: Cutaneous microcirculation in systemic sclerosis and response to intra-arterial reserpine. *Br Med J* 1980; 280:1408–1411.

28. Van de Wal HJ, Skotnicki SH, Wijn PF, Lacquet LK: Thoracic sympathectomy as a therapy for upper extremity ischemia: A long-term follow-up study. *Thorac Cardiovasc Surg* 1985; 33:181–187.

29. Flatt AE: Digital artery sympathectomy. *J Hand Surg* 1980; 5:550–556.

30. Sano K, Aiba T, Saito I: Angiography in pulseless disease. *Radiology* 1970; 94:69–74.

31. Bagby RJ, Cooper RD: Angiography in ergotism: Report of two cases and a review of the literature. *Am J Roentgenol* 1972; 116:179–186.

32. Falappa P, Magnavita N, Bergamaschi A, Colavita N: Angiographic study of digital arteries in workers exposed to vinyl chloride. *Br J Ind Med* 1982; 39:169–172.

33. Abbott WM, Darling RC: Axillary artery aneurysms secondary to crutch trauma. *Am J Surg* 1973; 125:515.

34. McCollum CH, Mavor E: Brachial artery injury after cardiac catheterization. *J Vasc Surg* 1986; 4:355–359.

35. Grollman JH, Jr, Marcus R: Transbrachial arteriography: Techniques and complications. *Cardiovasc Intervent Radiol* 1988; 11:32–35.

36. Gralino BJ, Porter JM, Rösch J: Angiography in the diagnosis and therapy of frostbite. *Radiology* 1976; 119:301–305.

37. Roos DB: Thoracic outlet syndromes: Update 1987. *Am J Surg* 1987; 154:568–573.

38. Warrens AN, Heaton J: Thoracic outlet compression syndrome: The lack of reliability of its clinical assessment. *Ann R Coll Surg Engl* 1987; 69:203–204.

39. Becker GJ, Holden RW, Rabe FE, et al: Local thrombolytic therapy for subclavian and axillary vein thrombosis. *Radiology* 1983; 149:419–423.

40. Smith-Behn J, Althar R, Katz W: Primary thrombosis of the axillary/subclavian vein. *South Med J* 1986; 79:1176–1178.

41. Schubart PJ, Haeberlin JR, Porter JM: Intermittent subclavian venous obstruction: Utility of venous pressure gradients. *Surgery* 1986; 99:365–367.

42. Longley DG, Yedlicka JW, Molina EJ, et al: Thoracic outlet syndrome: Evaluation of the subclavian vessels by color duplex sonography. *Am J Roentgenol* 1992; 158:623–630.

43. Coulon M, Goffette P, Dondelinger RF: Local thrombolytic infusion in arterial ischemia of the upper limb: Mid-term results. *Cardiovasc Intervent Radiol* 1994; 17:81–86.

44. Machleder HI: Evaluation of a new treatment strategy for Paget-Schroetter syndrome: Spontaneous thrombosis of the axillary-subclavian vein. *J Vasc Surg* 1993; 17:305–317.

9

Dialysis Access, Central Venous Catheters, and Other Central Venous

KEY CONCEPTS

1. Hemodialysis access fistulae and grafts have a limited lifetime, usually no more than 2 years.
2. Early detection and treatment of stenoses can prolong the use of shunts by 6 months or more.
3. Catheter-related thrombosis is the most common complication of prolonged central venous catheterization.
4. Many cases of catheter-induced central thrombosis go unrecognized, but the incidence of pulmonary embolism may be as high as 12%.
5. Fluoroscopic guidance of percutaneous central venous catheter placement eases introduction and expands options for access.
6. If not removed, embolized fragments of venous catheters, pacer wires, and other foreign bodies can cause fatal complications, but most can be snared percutaneously.

INTRODUCTION

With the increasing use of hemodialysis in the treatment of chronic renal failure and the increasing reliance on central venous catheters in administration of long-term cancer chemotherapy, antibiotics, and parenteral alimentation, radiologists are seeing a growing number of patients with problems arising from such vascular access devices. Although catheters and fistulae have a limited lifetime, a number of interventions can be performed percutaneously to prolong their usefulness or to guide the surgical correction of complications. For those patients who need treatment for an indefinite period of time, each loss of vascular access is a major setback, making future care more difficult. Therefore, the early recognition of dysfunction, often remediable by relatively minor radiologic or surgical procedures, is of great clinical importance. Radiologic guidance of central venous catheter placement is particularly useful when prior difficulties in obtaining vascular access have been encountered.

DIALYSIS FISTULAE AND SHUNTS

The number of patients undergoing hemodialysis for chronic renal failure in the United States increased dramatically in the 1980s, exceeding 90,000 in 1987.[1,2] One sixth of hospital stays among end-stage renal disease patients are associated with vascular access–related morbidity with a mean hospital stay of 7 days.[3] Maintenance of vascular access in these patients presents a major problem requiring a great commitment of resources, the annual cost estimated to exceed $150 million.[3]

Permanent peripheral hemodialysis access can be created by direct anastomosis of vein to the side of an artery or by placement of a graft bridging artery and vein. The introduction of the Brescia-Cimino forearm fistula in the 1960s was a breakthrough in the care of dialysis patients. It remains the procedure of choice because of its better long-term patency and lower complication rate when compared to dialysis grafts.[2] However, thrombosis of antecubital veins after repeated venipuncture or atherosclerotic disease involving the upper extremity limits the application of surgical fistulae. In such cases, synthetic or bovine vein grafts can be placed in straight or looped configurations. Bovine grafts have not proved very suitable, and most dialysis grafts are now made of polytetrafluoroethylene. Although arteriovenous (AV) shunts have been created in the lower extremities, they predispose a patient to sepsis, and upper extremity dialysis access is the generally preferred route.[4] Mean patency of AV grafts is 1.7 years versus 2.8 years for forearm fistulae.[2]

Complications of Dialysis Access

Potential problems with grafts and fistulae include failure of maturation, thrombosis, stenosis, infection, pseudoaneurysm formation, and vascular steal.

In a fistula, 4 to 6 weeks are needed for the vein to respond to increased flow by enlargement and mural thickening. A fistula cannot be used for hemodialysis until it has matured (shunts formed by grafts can be used earlier, and no maturation interval is necessary). The maturation of a dialysis fistula is impaired if flow is diminished by anastomotic or arterial stenosis, or if a single unimpeded outflow vein is absent.

Difficulties acquired after maturation and use often manifest themselves prior to thrombosis by poor flow, increased venous resistance (in outflow problems), or generation of negative pressures during dialysis (in arterial inflow problems). Venous anastomotic or more proximal (central) stenoses are *much* more common than arterial lesions, with an incidence ratio of about 15:1.[1] Neointimal hyperplasia and fibrosis account for most stenotic lesions.

Occlusions may result from stenoses, or they may occur with prolonged compression after removal of dialysis needles, hypovolemia, other low-flow states, infection, or hypercoagulability. Pseudoaneurysms and infection are rare in Brescia-Cimino fistulae (present in 1% to 2%), but they are fairly common complications of synthetic grafts: with 10% and 15% occurrences, respectively.[2]

The diversion of blood flow from the distal extremity through a shunt can cause pain and ischemia. This vascular steal commonly results from too large an anastomosis. The incidence of this problem has diminished with the increasing experience of vascular surgeons and introduction of grafts tapered to 4 mm at their arterial ends.[1]

Preoperative Venography

In most cases clinical examination can determine if an extremity is suitable for AV fistula or graft. However, there have been patients in whom prior use of a subclavian venous catheter has resulted in clinically inapparent stenosis or occlusion, which becomes symptomatic only after the placement of a dialysis shunt.[5,6] If there is any indication of upper extremity venous insufficiency or history of prolonged central venous catheterization, preliminary venography may be indicated. If a fistula or graft has failed, the surgeon may request a venogram to define remaining veins and to exclude a central abnormality.

Venography is performed through a needle placed in a hand or distal forearm vein, with a proximal tourniquet or blood pressure cuff inflated above venous pressure. The study is best performed with large-format spot films (two- or three-on-one multiexposure format), with the patient's forearm placed in various positions to obtain multiple projections of the veins when filled. Filling should be documented centrally into the superior vena cava (SVC) after the tourniquet is removed. The central portion of the examination is facilitated by digital subtraction imaging (DSA). Inflow of unopacified blood from jugular veins or contralateral innominate vein must not be confused with clot. Filling of collateral veins is a very reliable sign of obstruction. Opacification of such veins in the absence of an obvious lesion should alert the examiner to a subtle stenosis needing additional views for delineation.

Imaging and Evaluation of Dialysis Shunts
Duplex Sonography
Improvements in vascular sonography have led to its use in evaluating dialysis access. Duplex ultrasound can be used to identify mechanical kinks, stenoses, and thromboses with high accuracy.[7,8] However, the examination procedure is more involved and time-consuming and requires more technical expertise than conventional studies with contrast material. Ultrasound does not present a "global" view of the fistula or graft, and acceptance of scanning results by the referring clinician may be limited. Because conventional studies are relatively simple, inexpensive, and minimally invasive, ultrasound can be reserved for conditions in which it may be more accurate than angiography, such as suspected pseudoaneurysm or vascular steal.[8] Duplex sonography can also be applied to patients with a history of hypersensitivity to contrast material or in whom angiography reveals an equivocal abnormality.

Contrast Media Examinations
Early approaches to examination with contrast material involved selective arteriography or brachial artery puncture.[9,10] Time and experience have shown, however, that direct puncture of the shunt presents extremely low risk and provides good diagnostic information with a much less cumbersome technique.

Angiography should be performed at the first sign of dysfunction, for cannulation of an occluded fistula will not uncover an underlying abnormality unless thrombolysis is pursued. Performance and interpretation are helped by knowledge of the type of fistula or graft in place, including location of anastomoses. The graft or venous limb of a fistula can be examined through a dialysis needle left in place or by puncture with a 21-gauge butterfly infusion needle. From a diagnostic standpoint, it makes no difference if the needle is directed retrograde or antegrade. Free return of blood indicates proper position, but this is confirmed by a test injection of contrast material under fluoroscopy.

Digital subtraction angiography, 100-mm spot films, or cut-film angiography can all be used, but DSA permits rapid evaluation of a shunt with dilute contrast medium. Initial injections are made without cuff occlusion of venous outflow, and these define flow, venous anastomosis, and proximal veins. If the patient has clinical signs of outflow obstruction (diffuse edema and high venous resistance during dialysis) and no abnormality is discovered, additional projections must be obtained. Should a distal obstruction to outflow be found, the examination should not be concluded before more central flow through subclavian vein, innominate vein, and SVC is defined. Many outflow obstructions involve multiple sites.[11,12]

Examination of the graft or vessel upstream from the needle, as well as the arterial anastomosis, calls for occlusion of outflow by a blood pressure cuff. The cuff is inflated above arterial pressure immediately before filming, and the pressure is released immediately after the injected contrast material fills both the arterial and venous sides of the graft or fistula. Again, use of DSA simplifies evaluation by allowing immediate assessment of the degree of filling attained. Also, because reflux of contrast material into the arteries of the upper extremity can be extremely painful, DSA adds to patient comfort by allowing use of very dilute contrast media. Definition of the arterial anastomosis is particularly important in cases of suspected steal or if poor flow or pressures during dialysis indicate obstructed inflow. Rarely is standard catheter arteriography needed to rule out a proximal arterial lesion. In fact, most arterial anastomoses and feeding vessels can be readily demonstrated by IV-DSA.[11]

All injections of iodinated contrast media may be performed manually or mechanically. The volume and rate chosen depend on the flow observed during test injections. Generally, volumes of 10 to 25 ml administered at 1 to 5 ml/second are adequate for each field imaged. An exposure rate of at least one frame per second should be used, except in central studies of poor venous outflow. A rapid frame rate is essential for appreciating the pattern of arm and forearm collateral venous filling in the presence of focal outflow obstruction.

Interventions

Because thrombectomy and surgical revision can extend dialysis access lifetime by an average of 4 to 8 months, prolongation of graft or AV fistula use by at least 6 months can be considered a successful intervention.[1] By this criterion, combined use of thrombolysis and/or balloon angioplasty has succeeded in treating graft thrombosis or poor flow in 53% to 76% of such attempts.[10,13–15] The importance of early intervention is underscored by the considerably better 6-month patency attained by angioplasty of stenotic, but still patent, shunts: 76% to 82% versus 36% to 62% for occlusions treated in these same reports.

Percutaneous Angioplasty and Vascular Stents

Percutaneous transluminal angioplasty (PTA) can proceed either through the graft, through the venous limb of the fistula, or, in cases of proximal (central) venous stenoses, through a femoral venous approach. Risk of pseudoaneurysm from placement of a balloon through graft appears to be minimal, and puncture site compression with surgical collagen sponge promotes hemostasis.[13]

As mentioned previously, most stenoses in dialysis access shunts are due to intimal hyperplasia, which is felt to be incited by the turbulence and shear stresses resulting from high blood flow.[15] Intimal hyperplasia seems to be particularly severe at venous anastomoses, and successful dilatation often requires prolonged inflation (minutes at a time) with high-pressure balloons. Especially refractory lesions have been opened with coaxial Teflon fascial dilators.[10] Because dilatation can be quite painful in these patients, infiltration of lidocaine about the site of the lesion before PTA is advisable.[10,13]

Some have found that central venous stenoses in the presence of dialysis shunts are quite readily treated by PTA.[6,15] Reports with longer-term follow-up, however, describe a high recurrence rate.[16,17] Lesions in central vessels are dilated with larger balloons, up to 20 mm in diameter. Arm and forearm stenosis within grafts or veins usually requires balloons 6 to 10 mm in diameter. Arterial inflow lesions may be treated with 4-mm balloons. As in any PTA procedure, balloon size is predicated on the size of the vessel to be treated, allowing for a small amount of overdilatation.

Although early response tends to be good, most vessels that stay open for 6 months have recurrent stenosis within 1 year. Still, dialysis fistula or graft PTA can be repeated with good results.[15] Some patients apparently have a predisposition to intimal hyperplasia and have early restenosis whether they are treated percutaneously or by surgical revision.[14]

Expandable metal stents are useful in selected patients with central venous stenoses, especially those with lesions showing elastic rebound after PTA.[16] Primary patency rates may be improved, but many still need periodic and repeated interventions.[16,17] Central venous stenting may be justified in patients with limited alternatives, but placement in the costoclavicular segment of the subclavian vein should be avoided because of the risk of stent collapse.[18] Also, the patient and attending medical personnel must be made aware of the device and its location in order to prevent stent puncture during attempted subclavian venous catheter placement.[17] Stents should not be used in more peripheral upper extremity veins, for they may interfere with subsequent surgery.

Stenoses in fistulae that have failed to mature are not amenable to percutaneous angioplasty, and they may be prone to rupture.[10,15,19] A narrowing that extends over more than 4 cm in length is also unlikely to respond to balloon dilatation.[13,15]

Thrombolysis

Earlier experience with graft declotting by infusion of streptokinase was disappointing, and treatment was often complicated by bleeding through the graft or hemodialysis puncture sites.[4,20] More rapid administration of the fibrinolytic agent, mechanical disruption of the clot, and use of urokinase have allowed better control of lysis and greater success.[4,14] Even if a lesion not treatable by angioplasty is uncovered, surgical revision can often be more limited than it would have been without lytic therapy. Still, use of thrombolysis is not universally accepted. Schuman and associates did not find any substantial advantage in cost, time, or success rates to catheter thrombolysis versus surgical thrombectomy.[21] Moreover, recent studies suggest that urokinase or other thrombolytic enzymes are not needed for successful percutaneous declotting of dialysis grafts (see later in this chapter).[12,22]

The original pharmacothrombolytic technique described by Davis and colleagues involves puncture of occluded grafts near arterial and venous anastomoses, with the placement of crossing hook-tipped catheters.[14] Entry into the lumen is indicated by the return of a small amount of serosanguinous fluid or easy insertion of a soft-tipped guidewire. Each catheter is slowly rotated and withdrawn from the respective anastomosis, while a concentrated dose (25,000 units/ml) of urokinase is injected into the clot. The total dose so administered is 100,000 to 150,000 units. A heparin bolus of 2000 to 3000 units is also given, followed by an intravenous heparin drip. One catheter tip is then positioned near the arterial anastomosis and the other left in midgraft, each infusing 2000 units/min until pulse or bleeding from needle puncture sites is noted. With flow reestablished, an angioplasty balloon is used to compress residual thrombus and to dilate any stenosis found. The short duration of infusion by this technique allows the patient to be observed in the angiography suite throughout the procedure. Any bleeding that arises can be immediately controlled by direct compression.

Further refinements by this same San Diego group include the addition of heparin (500 units/ml) to the first vial of urokinase solution and use of multi-sidehole or multislit catheters designed for a pulse-spray technique (Fig. 9-1).[23] Such catheters permit the entire graft to be treated simultaneously by tuberculin syringes forcefully injecting 0.2 ml aliquots at 30-second intervals. Thrombolysis should be attempted only if a guidewire and catheter can be passed centrally to the right atrium. Before pulse-spray injection of the clot is initiated, pullback venography and balloon dilatation of any venous stenosis may be performed. Results of treatment are checked by injection of iodinated contrast medium after one vial of urokinase has been administered. A lysis-resistant plug is often present near the arterial anastomosis, and it is most effectively removed by pulling it back

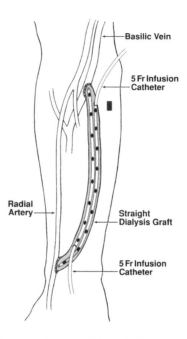

Fig. 9-1 Crossed-catheter technique of thrombolysis in a straight forearm dialysis shunt. The degree of overlap of catheters is not critical, as long as there is some overlap to permit delivery of fibrinolytic agent to all parts of the clotted graft.

with an occlusion balloon catheter after some flow through the graft has been restored. With this refined protocol, Roberts and colleagues have now decreased the time needed for lysis to under 30 minutes and the total dose of urokinase administered to a mean of 330,000 units, while restoring flow in 94% of the grafts attempted.[23]

In a remarkable prospective randomized study of 103 clotted dialysis grafts, Beathard compared a similar pulse-spray urokinase technique with pulse-spray clot disruption using heparinized saline alone.[12] Treatment succeeded in 94% and 93% of the grafts, respectively, and patency rates on follow-up were also equivalent.

Another recent report describes using percutaneously introduced balloon thrombectomy catheters to displace clot into the central venous circulation.[22] Such purely mechanical methods may avoid the expense of the thrombolytic enzyme, but issues of repeated application must be resolved. Although no clinical evidence of pulmonary embolism was found in either of these studies, irreversible compromise to the pulmonary vascular capacity can be postulated and further investigations are needed. In any case, mechanical declotting with central displacement of thrombus should be avoided in patients with any degree of respiratory insufficiency or pulmonary hypertension.

CENTRAL VENOUS CATHETERS

Large-bore central venous catheters have been applied increasingly for long-term administration of cancer chemotherapy, antibiotics, hyperalimentation, dialysis, and blood withdrawal. These catheters may be partially or totally implanted and have a longer useful lifetime than conventional, smaller-bore central catheters. Catheters with subcutaneous infusion chambers have been reported to remain functional for a mean of 6 months or more, in comparison to subcutaneously tunneled Hickman catheters, which have a mean lifetime of 40 to 110 days.[24,25] Patency is maintained by regular flushing with heparinized saline when the lines are not in use. Serious complications with these devices are quite rare, with sepsis, endocarditis, catheter fracture, and embolization representing the major life-threatening problems.

Fibrin Sheaths and Mechanical Problems with Catheters
There is more than a trivial incidence of mechanical malfunctioning of catheters or of central venous thrombosis requiring radiologic evaluation and possible intervention. In several recent series, 22% to 54% of patients with various infusion catheters experienced problems at some point.[24–26] Most commonly, a fibrin sheath forms about the catheter, making blood withdrawal difficult or impossible. If the sheath is complete, it may cause infusate to track back along the catheter into the soft tissues of the chest wall. This must be differentiated from catheter breakage or disconnection causing extravasation. Fibrin deposits occur on virtually all long-term catheters, but, when difficulties arise, the majority of catheters can be reopened by direct instillation of low-dose thrombolytic agents.[26] Those lines not responding to 5000-unit aliquots of urokinase can usually be restored to function by a 6-hour infusion of urokinase, given 40,000 units/hour (5000 units/ml).[27]

Fibrin sheaths may be seen as thin membranes about the catheter, with or without associated pericatheter clot. On a normal catheter injection, contrast material should flow freely from the port being injected, with rapid flow of unopacified blood diluting the contrast stream. Retrograde flow is abnormal, and it may be the only appreciable sign of a fibrin sheath.

Among the other mechanical problems that have been described are catheter malposition, catheter tip abutting the wall of the SVC and preventing aspiration, tight sutures causing occlusion, back-migration of the catheter into the subcutaneous tract, and local infection. Catheter malpo-

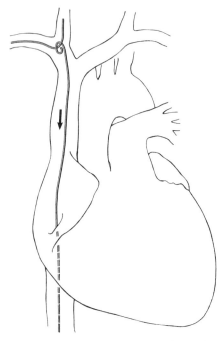

Fig. 9-2   Use of an angiographic pigtail catheter placed from a femoral venous approach to reposition a malpositioned central venous catheter. The catheter tip is pulled from the internal jugular vein down into the superior vena cava.

sition can sometimes be corrected by percutaneous transvenous manipulation (Fig. 9-2) similar to that used to remove embolized catheter fragments (see the section on Percutaneous Removal of Intravascular Foreign Bodies later in this chapter).

Totally implanted systems, which have access through a subcutaneous silicone membrane, must be punctured *only* by specially designed needles;[25] otherwise, the membranes may be damaged, leading to premature failure of the catheter. When the proper needles are used, many cases of extravasation are due to poor needle placement rather than to a problem intrinsic to the infusion port.

Catheter-Related Central Venous Thrombosis
Thrombosis of central veins as a result of long-term infusion catheters has been said to be a rare complication, presenting clinically in fewer than 1% of patients, according to some.[5,28] However, others quote an occult rate of thrombosis between 17% and 40%.[28–31] It is clear that such occlusions usually do not present acute or long-term problems, and venous insufficiency or claudication is less likely to result from secondary subclavian

vein thrombosis than it is with primary venous occlusion.[28] Still, occlusion must be recognized and treated in those patients who are entirely dependent on venous hyperalimentation for nonmalignant conditions or who need long-term hemodialysis. Progressive loss of central venous access in such patients is a serious problem.

One underappreciated consequence of catheter-related central venous thrombosis is pulmonary embolism, which may be fatal. Multiple reports indicate an incidence of about 12% of this complication in patients with catheter-related clots.[29,30]

When symptoms of venous occlusion do arise, standard therapy has been removal of the catheter and anticoagulation by heparin.[30] Before any such measures are taken, venous thrombosis should be confirmed radiographically, because hematoma, trauma, tumor, and lymphedema can present with similar symptoms. Not only should the catheter be injected with iodinated contrast material, but an upper extremity venogram must also be acquired to define the extent of thrombosis. Venous Doppler systems are not sensitive as a screening measure because of flow through collateral veins, and most Doppler studies do not permit detection of occlusion.[28,30] It remains to be seen if duplex sonography will play a useful role.

Although catheter removal and anticoagulation are generally advised for thrombosis, full anticoagulation alone has resolved symptoms in patients without signs of infection.[29] It is unclear how many patients with clinical improvement actually have recanalization of their veins. No doubt a portion of them, perhaps the majority, have chronic thrombosis and development of adequate flow through collaterals. A more aggressive approach involves the use of thrombolysis.

Fraschini and associates have described 81% success with local urokinase infusion of clots present for less than 1 week by patient history.[31] In most cases they did not find catheter removal necessary. Success was highly correlated with *direct* infusion of clot; infusion of a peripheral vein in the arm was almost uniformly unproductive. They recommend a urokinase dose of 1000 to 2000 units/kg per hour and have found fibrinogen levels to be the best test for predicting puncture site bleeding complications (which correlate with serum fibrinogen levels of less than 100 mg/dl). Those with residual thrombus after recanalization are prone to reocclusion, and these patients may best be treated with long-term anticoagulation. Otherwise, a short course of intravenous heparin after successful lysis may be all that is necessary for a good result. Patients with active phlebitis should not undergo infusion until their inflammatory symptoms subside.[31] In another report, 33 of 38 central venous catheters were salvaged by a comparable technique, after a mean duration of urokinase infusion of 2.4 days.[32]

Radiologic Catheter Placement

Most long-term infusion catheters can be placed under local anesthesia, and many procedures have been performed bedside. Selby and colleagues have used initial bilateral upper extremity venography to guide Seldinger puncture of the subclavian vein for insertion of 11 Fr double-lumen dialysis catheters.[33] After blood return from the needle and confirmation of appropriate entry by contrast material injection, the tract is widened with Teflon dilators that are advanced over a standard angiographic guidewire. A DSA roadmapping technique would be a useful adjunct to the method they describe.

Hickman catheters, originally implanted by way of cephalic vein cutdown, have been placed percutaneously under fluoroscopic guidance in 51 patients by Robertson and associates.[34] They give their patients 1 g of cefoxitin intravenously 1 hour prior to catheter placement. In the procedure they describe, the skin inferior to the junction of the mid and distal thirds of the clavicle is sterilely prepared, and a 21-gauge needle attached to an aspirating syringe is advanced from this spot, taking care to avoid the periosteum of rib or clavicle. Once the subclavian vein is entered, an 0.018-inch mandril guidewire is passed, and a transition dilator is used to introduce a larger wire. The tract chosen to tunnel the catheter is liberally anesthetized with lidocaine, and the tunneling device supplied with the catheter is inserted through a second incision toward the site through which the needle has entered the vein. The Hickman catheter is attached to the tunneling tool and pulled back through the tract and out of the second incision. The Dacron cuff of the catheter (important for prevention of bacterial colonization and infection) should lie about 3 cm within the tunnel. Before the intravenous portion of the catheter is inserted through a peelaway sheath, that end of the catheter is trimmed to an appropriate length, ideally allowing the tip to lie at the junction of the SVC and right atrium. By Food and Drug Administration guidelines, a central venous catheter tip should not enter the right atrium because of the risk of inducing cardiac rhythm disturbances or the very rare, but potentially fatal risk of perforating myocardium and producing cardiac tamponade.[35] After proper positioning is confirmed by chest radiography, the remaining exposed catheter is buried and the incisions sutured. Robertson and associates have had 100% success in catheter placement and a low complication rate with this technique.[34] Others have used ultrasound to guide entry into the subclavian vein, which avoids the complications of pneumothorax and hemothorax encountered with "blind" surgical procedures.[36]

An alternate approach for long-term venous access is through the upper extremity with insertion of a peripherally inserted central catheter (PICC). In the technique of Andrews and colleagues, the basilic or other upper arm vein is punctured under fluoroscopic guidance during opacification by contrast medium injected from a more peripheral site.[37] In isolated patients with severe hypersensitivity to iodinated contrast media or in whom peripheral access for the guiding venogram cannot be established, a femorally introduced catheter or wire snare can be advanced into the basilic vein to serve as a target for the puncturing needle. A peel-away sheath is introduced, allowing insertion of the soft Silastic catheter. After confirmation of appropriate tip position, the catheter is flushed and fixed with skin sutures. The external port should not project below the elbow, and the nondominant arm is used whenever possible. At the University of Wisconsin–Madison nearly 400 PICCs are being inserted annually, and some catheters have been functioning up to 10 months.

Although PICC catheters with subcutaneous ports are available, non-tunneled catheters can be maintained with an infection rate as low as 0.13 per 100 catheter days, comparable to that of implanted Hickman catheters.[38] Catheters must be placed with meticulous antisepsis; 2% chlorhexidine for site preparation, as well as for cleansing before dressing changes, is recommended.[39] One theoretical advantage of PICCs is avoidance of the central venous stenosis commonly associated with the trauma of direct subclavian catheterization.

In patients with progressive loss of vascular access, there are various unconventional alternatives. Although long-term insertion of central venous catheters from a femoral approach is often complicated by infection and thrombosis, Treiman and Silberman have reported acceptable results with tunneled catheters placed through proximal saphenous venotomies.[40] Translumbar insertion into the inferior vena cava (IVC) is also an option.[41] If the femoral vein is open, a pigtail catheter advanced from below can serve as a target; otherwise, the lumbar spine is used as a landmark. At the University of Wisconsin, we have placed a hyperalimentation catheter trans-hepatically, through a hepatic vein into the right atrium. This radical approach was necessary after surgical implantation into the azygos vein was complicated by infection and the IVC was not available, having been surgically occluded at an earlier time. In such desperate situations, thrombolysis, recanalization, and vascular stent placement may also be considered.

VENAE CAVAE RECANALIZATION

Superior vena cava syndrome (swelling of the neck and upper extremities from venous congestion) may result from tumor, granulomatous disease, or central venous catheter–induced thrombosis. Tumor-induced obstruction of the SVC has caused pulmonary embolism when anticoagulation has not been instituted, and high mortality has been reported for SVC occlusion.[42,43] Still, symptoms often resolve with heparin and/or warfarin (Coumadin) therapy and treatment of any underlying disorder. In isolated

REFERENCES

1. Bell DD, Rosental JJ: Arteriovenous graft life in chronic hemodialysis. *Arch Surg* 1988; 123:1169–1172.
2. Zibari GB, Rohr MS, Landreneau MD, et al: Complications from permanent hemodialysis vascular access. *Surgery* 1988; 104:681–686.
3. Feldman HI, Held PJ, Hutchinson JT, et al: Hemodialysis vascular access morbidity in the United States. *Kidney Int* 1993; 43:1091–1096.
4. Zeit RM, Cope C: Failed hemodialysis shunts: One year of experience with aggressive treatment. *Radiology* 1985; 154:353–356.
5. Davis D, Petersen J, Feldman R, et al: Subclavian vein stenosis: A complication of subclavian dialysis. *JAMA* 1984; 252:3404–3406.
6. Ingram TL, Reid SH, Tisnado J, et al: Percutaneous transluminal angioplasty of brachiocephalic vein stenoses in patients with dialysis shunts. *Radiology* 1988; 166:45–47.
7. Pieterman H, Tordoir JHM: Non-invasive evaluation of prosthetic dialysis shunt in asymptomatic patients. *Rofo* 1986; 145:541–546.
8. Middleton WD, Picus DD, Marx MV, Melson GL: Color doppler sonography of hemodialysis vascular access: Comparison with angiography. *Am J Roentgenol* 1989; 152:633–639.
9. Glanz S, Bahist B, Gordon DH, et al: Angiography of upper extremity access fistulas for dialysis. *Radiology* 1982; 143:45–52.
10. Hunter DW, Castañeda-Zuñiga WR, Coleman CC, et al: Failing arteriovenous dialysis fistulas: Evaluation and treatment. *Radiology* 1984; 152:631–635.
11. England REM, Jackson A: Imaging of dialysis access: A review of 67 failing fistulas investigated by intravenous digital subtraction angiography. *Br J Radiol* 1993; 66:32–36.
12. Beathard GA: Mechanical versus pharmacomechanical thrombolysis for the treatment of thrombosed dialysis access grafts. *Kidney Int* 1994; 45:1401–1406.
13. Glanz S, Gordon D, Butt KMH, et al: Dialysis access fistulas: Treatment of stenoses by transluminal angioplasty. *Radiology* 1984; 152:637–642.
14. Davis GB, Dowd CF, Bookstein JJ, et al: Thrombosed dialysis grafts: Efficacy of intrathrombotic deposition of concentrated urokinase, clot maceration, and angioplasty. *Am J Roentgenol* 1987; 149:177–181.
15. Saeed M, Newman GE, McCann RL, et al: Stenoses in dialysis fistulas: Treatment with percutaneous angioplasty. *Radiology* 1987; 164:693–697.
16. Kovalik EC, Newman GE, Suhocki P, et al: Correction of central venous stenoses: Use of angioplasty and vascular Wallstents. *Kidney Int* 1994; 45:1177–1181.
17. Shoenfeld R, Hermans H, Novick A, et al: Stenting of proximal venous obstructions to maintain hemodialysis access. *J Vasc Surg* 1994; 19:532–539.
18. Bjarnason H, Hunter DW, Crain MR, et al: Collapse of a Palmaz stent in the subclavian vein: Case report. *Am J Roentgenol* 1993; 160:1123–1124.
19. Bourne EE: Late venous rupture after angioplasty of an arteriovenous dialysis fistula. *Am J Roentgenol* 1988; 150:797–798.
20. Young AT, Hunter DW, Castañeda-Zuñiga WR, et al: Thrombosed synthetic hemodialysis access fistulas: Failure of fibrinolytic therapy. *Radiology* 1985; 154:639–642.

21. Schuman E, Quinn S, Standage B, Gross G: Thrombolysis versus thrombectomy for occluded hemodialysis grafts. *Am J Surg* 1994; 167:473–476.
22. Trerotola SO, Lund GB, Scheel PJ, et al: Thrombosed dialysis access grafts: Percutaneous mechanical declotting without urokinase. *Radiology* 1994; 191:721–726.
23. Roberts AC, Valji K, Bookstein JJ, Hye RJ: Pulse-spray pharmacomechanical thrombolysis for treatment of thrombosed dialysis access grafts. *Am J Surg* 1993; 166:221–226.
24. Repelaer van Driel OJ, Kuin CM, van de Velde CJH: Surgically implanted subcutaneous venous access devices in cancer patients. *Neth J Surg* 1988; 40:97–99.
25. Lorenz M, Hottenrott C, Seufert RM, Encke A: Total implantierbarer dauerhafter zentralvenöser zugang: Langzeiterfahrung mit subcutanen infusionskammern. *Langenbecks Arch Chir* 1988; 373:302–309.
26. Cassidy PF, Jr, Zajko AB, Bron KM, et al: Noninfectious complications of long-term central venous catheters: Radiologic evaluation and management. *Am J Roentgenol* 1987; 149:671–675.
27. Haire WD, Lieberman RP: Thrombosed central venous catheters: Restoring function with six-hour urokinase infusion after failure of bolus urokinase. *J Parenter Enter Nutr* 1992; 16:129–132.
28. Smith VC, Hallett JW, Jr: Subclavian vein thrombosis during prolonged catheterization for parenteral nutrition. *South Med J* 1983; 76:603–606.
29. Anderson AJ, Krasnow SH, Boyer MW, et al: Thrombosis: The major Hickman catheter complication in patients with solid tumor. *Chest* 1989; 95:71–75.
30. Horattas MC, Wright DJ, Fenton AH, et al: Changing concepts of deep venous thrombosis of the upper extremity: Report of a series and review of the literature. *Surgery* 1988; 104:561–567.
31. Fraschini G, Jadeja J, Lawson M, et al: Local infusion of urokinase for the lysis of thrombosis associated with permanent central venous catheters in cancer patients. *J Clin Oncol* 1987; 5:672–678.
32. Seigel EL, Jew AC, Delcore R, et al: Thrombolytic therapy for catheter-related thrombosis. *Am J Surg* 1993; 166:716–719.
33. Selby JB, Tegtmeyer CJ, Amodeo C, et al: Insertion of subclavian hemodialysis catheters in difficult cases: Value of fluoroscopy and angiographic techniques. *Am J Roentgenol* 1989; 152:641–643.
34. Robertson LJ, Mauro MA, Jaques PF: Radiologic placement of Hickman catheters. *Radiology* 1989; 170:1007–1009.
35. McGee WT, Ackerman BL, Rouben LR, et al: Accurate placement of central venous catheters: A prospective, randomized, multicenter trial. *Crit Care Med* 1993; 21:1118–1123.
36. Laméris JS, Post PJM, Zonderland HM, et al: Percutaneous placement of Hickman catheters: Comparison of sonographically guided and blind techniques. *Am J Roentgenol* 1990; 155:1097–1099.
37. Andrews JC, Marx MV, Williams DM, et al: Technical note: The upper arm approach for placement of peripherally inserted central catheters for protracted venous access. *Am J Roentgenol* 1992; 158:427–429.

38. Raad I, Davis S, Becker M, et al: Low infection rate and long durability of non-tunneled Silastic catheters: A safe and cost-effective alternative for long-term venous access. *Arch Intern Med* 1993; 153:1791–1796.

39. Maki DG, Ringer M, Alvarado CJ: Prospective randomised trial of povidone-iodine, alcohol, and chlorhexidine for prevention of infection associated with central venous and arterial catheters. *Lancet* 1991; 338:339–343.

40. Treiman GS, Silberman H: Chronic venous access in patients with cancer: Selective use of the saphenous vein. *Cancer* 1993; 72:760–765.

41. Lund GB, Lieberman RP, Haire WD, et al: Translumbar inferior vena cava catheters for long-term venous access. *Radiology* 1990; 174:31–35.

42. Adelstein DJ, Hines JD, Carter SG, Sacco D: Thromboembolic events in patients with malignant superior vena cava syndrome and the role of anticoagulation. *Cancer* 1988; 62:2258–2262.

43. Smith NL, Ravo B, Soroff HS, Khan SA: Successful fibrinolytic therapy for superior vena cava thrombosis secondary to long-term total parenteral nutrition. *J Parenter Enter Nutr* 1985; 9:55–57.

44. Ali MK, Ewer MS, Balakrishnan PV, et al: Balloon angioplasty for superior vena cava obstruction. *Ann Intern Med* 1987; 107:856–857.

45. Dyet JF, Nicholson AA, Cook AM: The use of the Wallstent endovascular prosthesis in the treatment of malignant obstruction of the superior vena cava. *Clin Radiol* 1993; 48:381–385.

46. Yamada R, Sato M, Kawabata M, et al: Segmental obstruction of the hepatic inferior vena cava treated by transluminal angioplasty. *Radiology* 1983; 149:91–96.

47. Yang XL, Chen CR, Cheng TO: Nonoperative treatment of membranous obstruction of the inferior vena cava by percutaneous balloon transluminal angioplasty. *Am Heart J* 1992; 124:405–412.

48. Sholar PW, Bell WR: Thrombolytic therapy of inferior vena cava thrombosis in paroxysmal noctural hemoglobinuria. *Ann Intern Med* 1985; 103:539–541.

49. Grabenwoeger F, Dock W, Pinterits F, Appel W: Fixed intravascular foreign bodies: A new method for removal. *Radiology* 1988; 167:555–556.

50. Yedlicka JW, Carlson JE, Hunter DW, et al: Nitinol gooseneck snare for removal of foreign bodies: Experimental study and clinical evaluation. *Radiology* 1991; 178:691–693.

51. Mocellin R: Transluminale extraktion intrakardial embolisierter katheterfragmente bei kindern. *Z Kinderchir* 1987; 42:343–345.

10

Percutaneous Angioplasty, Recanalization, and Vascular Stents

KEY CONCEPTS

1. Percutaneous transluminal angioplasty (PTA) is a safe and effective treatment for short arterial stenoses and occlusions. Atherectomy devices have not shown any clear advantage over balloons for uncomplicated lesions.
2. PTA enlarges the vessel lumen by disrupting plaque, intima, and media in a controlled manner.
3. For prevention of early thrombosis, platelet aggregation inhibitors must be started prior to PTA. Nitroglycerin, nifedipine, and heparin are other essential adjunct medications.
4. A guidewire should be maintained across a lesion until the dilation procedure is deemed to be completed.
5. Failure or complication of PTA very rarely adversely affects a patient's clinical status or surgical options.
6. Vascular stents can be used to treat lesions refractory to PTA or post-PTA dissections. Other indications are less clearly defined and under continuing investigation.

In 1964 Dotter and Judkins introduced a new method of treating vascular occlusive disease, a technique that has become known as percutaneous transluminal angioplasty (PTA).[1] Initially, a system of stiff coaxial catheters was used to open stenoses and occlusions. Unfortunately, the resulting arteriotomy matched the diameter of the vessel lumen produced. The large catheters also caused extensive endothelial trauma, leading to high rates of early thrombosis, restenosis, and generally poor long-term results.

Various investigators experimented with balloon catheters, but Grüntzig and Hopff succeeded in developing a balloon that would reliably inflate to a predetermined diameter and not beyond.[2] The Grüntzig balloon permitted the widespread application of PTA not only to the peripheral arteries but also to renal, coronary, and other central vessels. Since the dissemination of the technique in the late 1970s, much progress has been made in balloon and catheter materials, guidewires, and adjuvant medical therapy. As a result, PTA has become widely accepted as a safe alternative or complement to surgical intervention for many patients with vascular disease. Early skepticism and the reluctance of many vascular surgeons to refer patients are slowly being overcome by data, such as those from the Veterans Administration Cooperative study, confirming that if PTA is initially successful, clinical results are as good and as durable as those of bypass surgery.[3] Moreover, failed or complicated PTA is unlikely to worsen the patient's condition or hinder attempts at reconstructive surgery.[3,4]

Nevertheless, the limitations of balloon angioplasty have prompted the investigation of novel recanalization devices and percutaneously placed vascular stents. Comparison of surgery, balloon angioplasty, and the newer endovascular devices has been hampered by inconsistencies in definition of disease, reporting of results, and long-term follow-up. To this end, reporting standards as proposed by Rutherford and Becker are being applied with greater frequency, allowing easier interpretation of published clinical trials (Tables 10-1 to 10-3).[5]

Initial enthusiasm for laser-assisted angioplasty was tempered by experience showing unacceptable late results in the face of high cost with no clear advantage over balloon recanalizations.[6,7] Laser angioplasty has essentially been abandoned in clinical practice and is an unfortunate demonstration of the dissemination of an expensive, unproven technology in the absence of solid supporting data. Atherectomy catheters of varying designs continue to be applied and evaluated.[8–12] Expandable vascular stents are the most promising of the new endovascular devices, but indications for placement remain to be well defined.[13–16] Most recently, covered stents have been developed for percutaneous vascular graft insertion.[17] Nevertheless, all methods of recanalization or bypass face similar problems in maintaining patency. A major breakthrough in the biochemical or

Table 10-1   Clinical Categories of Acute Limb Ischemia

Category	Description	Capillary Return	Muscle Weakness	Sensory Loss	Doppler Signals	
					Arterial	Venous
Viable	Not immediately threatened	Intact	None	None	Audible AP more than 30 mm Hg	Audible
Threatened	Salvageable if promptly treated	Intact, slow	Mild, partial	Mild, incomplete	Inaudible	Audible
Irreversible	Major tissue loss, amputation required regardless of treatment	Absent (marbling)	Profound, paralysis (rigor)	Profound, anesthetic	Inaudible	Inaudible

AP = Ankle pressure.
From Rutherford RB, Becker GJ: Standards for evaluation and reporting the results of surgical and percutaneous therapy for peripheral arterial disease. J Vasc Interv Radiol 1991; 2:169–174; with permission.

Table 10-2 Clinical Categories of Chronic Limb Ischemia

Grade	Category	Clinical Description	Objective Criteria
	0	Asymptomatic, no hemodynamically significant occlusive disease	Normal results of treadmill* stress test
I	1	Mild claudication	Treadmill exercise completed, postexercise AP is greater than 50 mm Hg but more than 25 mm Hg less than normal
	2	Moderate claudication	Symptoms between those of categories 1 and 3
	3	Severe claudication	Treadmill exercise cannot be completed, postexercise AP is less than 50 mm Hg
II	4	Ischemic rest pain	Resting AP is 40 mm Hg or less, flat or barely pulsatile ankle or metatarsal plethysmographic tracing, toe pressure less than 30 mm Hg
III	5	Minor tissue loss, nonhealing ulcer, focal gangrene with diffuse pedal ischemia	Resting AP of 60 mm Hg or less, ankle or metatarsal plethysmographic tracing flat or barely pulsatile, toe pressure less than 40 mm Hg
	6	Major tissue loss, extending above transmetatarsal level, functional foot no longer salvageable	Same as for category 5

AP = Ankle pressure
*Five minutes at 2 mph on a 12° incline
From Rutherford RB, Becker GJ: Standards for evaluation and reporting the results of surgical and percutaneous therapy for peripheral arterial disease. J Vasc Interv Radiol 1991; 2:169–174; with permission.

Table 10-3 Standard Definitions of Vascular Patency

Term	Definition
Primary patency	Maintained without any intervention near the previously treated arterial segment/anastomosis
Assisted primary patency	Intervention (surgery, balloon angioplasty, or other) in the previously treated segment before thrombosis
Secondary patency	Patency reestablished (by thrombectomy, thrombolysis) after occlusion

immunologic prevention of myointimal hyperplasia will probably be needed to provide any substantial improvement over the present results of conventional balloon angioplasty.

INDICATIONS FOR BALLOON ANGIOPLASTY

Leaving aside the use of PTA in the coronary circulation and the heart, the prime indication for balloon angioplasty is lower extremity occlusive disease. Most patients with uncomplicated claudication improve on an exercise program with conservative management. Persistent limiting claudication, pain at rest, or gangrene indicates the need for revascularization. After history, clinical evaluation, and noninvasive studies confirm the presence of vascular occlusive disease, angiography is mandatory to determine its level and extent. At the University of Wisconsin–Madison we have found that magnetic resonance angiography can serve as a valuable screening study for selecting patients with lesions amenable to PTA.

Although PTA is best suited for treating relatively isolated disease, it can be applied successfully to more extensive lesions in limb salvage situations, particularly in those patients with high operative risk.[18] If the length of stenosis does not exceed 7 cm, if an occlusion is no longer than 10 to 12 cm, and if the lesion can be safely approached percutaneously, PTA should be considered a primary treatment option. Best results are obtained for short iliac or aortic bifurcation obstructions, with femoropopliteal disease somewhat less likely to respond. However, technical advances have made the effective treatment of even tibial vessels possible.[19–21] A more controversial suggested indication for balloon angioplasty is the blue toe syndrome.[22,23]

For the abdomen, PTA is recognized as the treatment of choice for renal fibromuscular dysplasia and renal transplant arterial stenosis, even by the most skeptical surgeons.[24] It is also appropriate for many patients with atherosclerotic stenoses implicated in renovascular hypertension or azotemia, including those patients with solitary kidneys.[25–28]

Balloon angioplasty has also been employed in upper extremity ischemia, subclavian steal syndrome, mesenteric ischemia, dialysis access stenoses, and central venous obstructions.[29–32] Clinical efficacy has ranged from very good to poor, depending on the indication. However, the low morbidity of balloon angioplasty has led to its application in situations where long-term success is not likely to be good, because in some individuals a major surgical procedure may be postponed or avoided altogether.

PATIENT PREPARATION

As mentioned previously, the relationship of a patient's complaints to vascular compromise must be established by history, physical examination, and such noninvasive studies as segmental Doppler blood pressure measurements, pulse volume recordings, or duplex ultrasound. The presence and relative strength of peripheral pulses must be assessed and recorded. Note should be made of hypertension, coagulation status, cardiac and cerebrovascular disease, diabetes, renal insufficiency, and patient medications. A bed must be available on a ward where nursing and other support personnel are experienced in monitoring and treating patients after PTA. In many cases, such as after renal artery dilatation, scheduled admission to an intensive care or telemetry monitored unit must be arranged. Although outpatient angioplasty has been described, its use has not been widely accepted in the United States.[33,34]

After the patient is examined, the procedure is explained. Attendant risks (including limb loss and death) are presented, and a realistic appraisal of potential benefits is given. Alternative treatment, whether surgical or conservative, is described. The necessity of strict bed rest after PTA, with 12- to 18-hour immobilization of the extremity through which the catheter is placed, is made clear. If a recent diagnostic arteriogram is not available, the patient is informed that a treatment decision may be made at the conclusion of angiography in consultation with the referring physician and the patient.

Standard preangiography orders are written, including intravenous hydration and restriction of oral intake to clear fluids after midnight prior to the procedure. Unless there is a contraindication, platelet aggregation inhibitors (125 to 325 mg of aspirin orally, with or without dipyridamole 75 mg three times daily) should be given prior to PTA and continued for 3 to 6 months afterward. There is compelling evidence that lack of antiplatelet premedication increases the rates of platelet deposition at angioplasty sites and early thrombosis.[20,35,36] For renal, popliteal, and trifurcation PTA, nifedipine 10 mg may be given orally the evening before and again the morning of the procedure in order to prevent spasm. Ideally, angioplasty procedures are performed early in the day to ensure optimal monitoring and patient care, as well as to allow diabetics to resume their diets as soon as possible.

A good working relationship with one's vascular surgical colleagues is absolutely necessary for the radiologist performing percutaneous angioplasty. Many patients with "angioplastiable" lesions may be treated at the conclusion of diagnostic angiography, and the referring surgeon can be called to review the films before the diagnostic catheter is removed. If the surgeon concurs that PTA is appropriate, the patient's hospitalization can be shortened and the additional expense of a separate catheter procedure may be avoided. For this reason, we routinely include "possible percutaneous angioplasty" in the consent obtained from patients undergoing runoff angiography. Otherwise, the administration of sedatives during the diagnostic examination interferes with the ability of the patient to provide informed consent. Delaying PTA after diagnostic arteriography presents the risk that a limited stenosis may become a long occlusion, making catheter intervention more difficult or unfeasible.[37]

At our institution, we insist that all patients having angiography for peripheral vascular disease be evaluated by a vascular surgeon to ensure that a given patient is a candidate for revascularization. Surgical backup is particularly important for aortic, iliac, subclavian, and renal artery PTA. Although major complications are uncommon, the potential consequences of arterial rupture or occlusion in central vessels demand the availability of prompt operative intervention. For patients with transplanted or other solitary kidneys, a surgical team and operating room on standby may be warranted.[4]

RISKS

The hazards of PTA include all the risks of selective angiography, including hypersensitivity reaction to iodinated contrast media, renal failure, and vascular injury related to catheterization. In addition to these basic risks, PTA, by the directed focal trauma it induces as well as by the larger hole needed at the percutaneous entry site and concurrent anticoagulation, presents a greater chance of bleeding at the entry site, acute arterial dissection, thrombosis, and distal embolization. Rarely, the artery dilated may rupture.[38,39] Long-term use of corticosteroids may predispose a patient to PTA-induced vessel rupture. Death from the procedure, albeit rare, is most commonly due to rupture or hypotension with myocardial infarction.

The risk of complication is dependent on the patient's general condition, the difficulty of approaching and crossing the lesion in question, and the experience of the operator. According to four large series in which data from 352 to 4380 patients undergoing a variety of PTA procedures were analyzed, hospital mortality associated with angioplasty ranges from 0.07% to 0.4%.[38,40–42] Limb loss attributable to PTA has occurred in 0.4% of procedures.[41] Complications needing prompt surgical attention or more extensive surgery than would have been performed otherwise are cited in 1% to 4% of balloon angioplasties.[38,40–42] Major problems are most often uncontrollable bleeding at the puncture site, acute arterial occlusion, and distal embolization. Local thrombolysis can often be used to treat the last two of these conditions. Local application of new collagen puncture-tract plugs may decrease the number of major hematomas in the future.[43] Septic complications are highly unusual but potentially life-threatening, and they have been associated with repeated use of the same groin puncture site for vascular access.[44,45]

The complication rate of femoropopliteal PTA may vary from less than 1% in younger claudicants to 32% in patients over 65 with threatened limb loss.[46] Total morbidity of PTA generally varies from 5% to 19%, depending on the vessels treated.[38] Most complications are minor and do not require any directed therapy or prolongation of hospitalization. Risks specific to certain treated sites are addressed in greater detail later.

To place the hazards of PTA in perspective, one should be aware of the morbidity and mortality of surgery for similar indications. Several recent surgical series have reported mortality of 0.8% to 3.1% for lower extremity bypass grafts, early occlusion or surgical reexploration in 3% to 11%, and wound infection complicating 13% to 19% of in situ saphenous vein grafts.[3,47–49]

BASIC TECHNIQUE AND AVAILABLE MATERIALS

Vascular Access

One of the most important technical factors in determining the success and safety of a planned percutaneous angioplasty is vascular access. This usually means a patent common femoral artery providing an antegrade or retrograde approach to the lesion. The procedure can be performed through axillary artery catheterization, and this may be the only practical approach for some stenoses, particularly in mesenteric or renal arteries. However, the greater difficulty in controlling postprocedural puncture site bleeding and the possible neurologic consequences of major hematoma in the arm argue against the axillary approach. The popliteal artery has been used by some for percutaneous recanalization of superficial femoral arteries, but this approach is quite unconventional.[50] It should kept in mind that smaller arteries are more prone to spasm and occlusion.

Vascular Sheaths

Sheaths are invaluable for PTA because they limit the amount of puncture site trauma from manipulation, make the procedure less uncomfortable for the patient, and permit the reinsertion of a smaller angiographic catheter after balloon removal for postangioplasty arteriography. When antegrade puncture is performed, progress of the procedure may be monitored through intermittent injection of contrast media via the sideport of the sheath. Also, many high-pressure balloons form stiff "wings" when they are forcefully deflated, projections that could lacerate the puncture site during removal. Use of a sheath removes this theoretical hazard. Before inserting a sheath, check that the balloon to be used will pass easily through the sheath and its valve. The size of sheath needed is usually 1 Fr to 1.5 Fr greater than the shaft of the balloon catheter.

Passing the Obstruction

Guidewires

After obtaining vacular access, passage of a guidewire beyond the obstruction is the most critical step in PTA. Rarely, a stenosis may be crossed by the catheter alone, with intermittent injections of small amounts of contrast medium during advancement;[51] however, standard practice is to probe the stenosis or occlusion gently with a soft-tipped guidewire. For very narrow stenoses, a straight or tight (1.5-mm curve) J-tip wire is preferable. A Bentson wire, which is extremely floppy, is often helpful. If the tip of this wire engages a plaque, a loop can be formed by further advancement of the wire. The loop often seeks the lumen of the vessel and secures passage of the obstruction. Other wires that are quite useful include the various torque-control floppy-tipped guidewires. Hydrophilic polymer-coated guidewires, by their extremely slippery nature when wet, have proved invaluable in difficult lesions.

Digital Roadmap

When probing the lesion, a digital vascular roadmap, a feature available on many digital subtraction angiographic units, can be used to direct the manipulations. A roadmap is obtained by contrast medium injection and storage of the resulting image for real-time subtraction during later fluoroscopy. This feature is helpful both for wire placement and for balloon introduction and inflation.[52] If no roadmap is available, forceps or towel clips placed adjacent to the lesion can be used as reference points during PTA.

Predilatation

A slight curve or hook to the catheter tip, such as is present in Berenstein or H1H catheters, helps engage eccentric stenoses. Once a wire traverses the obstruction, the catheter can be advanced through it. This maneuver serves to "predilate" the lesion and allows the operator to safely exchange the wire for a heavier, stiffer one, as necessary. In some particularly resistant or calcified lesions, passage of a tapered Teflon van Andel catheter can open the lumen to a 7 Fr size, easing placement of the dilatation balloon.

Dissection or Perforation

If at any point during the manipulations subintimal dissection or perforation is suspected, a sidearm Y-adapter can be attached to the catheter hub, and its O-ring tightened about the guidewire. Contrast medium can be injected through the sidearm, although the pressure needed for injection around the guidewire may be great. If the tip of the catheter is at the suspected perforation or beyond, the wire may be removed and the catheter hub checked for backflow of blood. A small amount of contrast material is injected during fluoroscopy to clarify the situation. If a sheath has been used in an antegrade puncture, the sidearm can be injected to check intra-luminal placement of catheter or wire.

When an intimal flap has been raised, the lesion can rarely be tra-versed. Occasionally the true lumen may still be successfully cannulated, but Bolia and colleagues have actually used deliberate subintimal wire and catheter passage to recanalize long or difficult femoropopliteal occlu-sions.[53] They have employed 7 Fr catheters and 1.5-mm J-wires for such procedures, finding that reentry of true lumen often occurs beyond the obstruction without additional manipulations. When spontaneous reentry is not achieved, a curved catheter and stiff end of a guidewire are helpful; care must be taken not to extend the dissection beyond the level of the original occlusion. With this technique, revascularization was successful in 54 of 71 occlusions approached. Although 68% of those successfully treated showed sustained clinical improvement at 6-month follow-up, more experience is needed before deliberate subintimal passage can be recommended.

If the guidewire or catheter perforates the vessel, the procedure must be terminated. In such cases, it is best to stop and try at another date, if indicated. Small catheter or wire perforations in arteries of an extremity are rarely of clinical consequence as long as any anticoagulation is promptly reversed. Patients with perforations involving central vessels (renal, iliac, subclavian) must be closely monitored for bleeding. Because of the possibility of perforation, it is best to employ a 5 Fr catheter dur-ing initial manipulations until the guidewire is securely placed beyond the obstruction.

Use of Medications

As previously noted, patients should be given platelet aggregation inhibitors prior to PTA. Once the lesion has been successfully crossed, heparin should be administered (generally 5000 units, intravenously or intraarterially; the heparin effect can be monitored by activated coagula-tion time, if a coagulation monitoring machine is immediately available). Heparin need not be continued after a successful procedure, but long-term use of aspirin is strongly recommended.

In vessels prone to spasm, such as distal popliteal, tibial, and renal arter-ies, direct arterial injection of nitroglycerin (50 to 100 μg) after wire pas-sage and intermittently during subsequent manipulations is advisable. Sublingual nifedipine (10 to 20 mg) may be given before or during PTA, and its combination with injected nitroglycerin may have an additive effect, countering spasm.[54] In any case, vascular spasm can be more easi-ly prevented than treated, once present. If acute thrombosis occurs during the procedure, a thrombolytic agent infused locally often restores flow.

Choosing a Balloon

The appropriate size of balloon can be gauged by the diameter of the relatively normal artery adjacent to the lesion being treated. Conventional film angiography provides for direct measurement of a slightly magnified vessel (approximately 120% the true diameter of the lumen). Alternatively, the size of the vessel may be compared with the diameter of the catheter (or calibration markers on some catheters), if both are included on the same digital subtraction frame or 100-mm spot film.

Most angiographers choose a balloon that matches the diameter of the slightly magnified image; some prefer a balloon 1 to 2 mm larger.[54] In experimental models, a dilated artery is unlikely to rupture unless the balloon diameter exceeds 150% of the normal true diameter of the vessel.[55] Although it has been asserted that deliberate overdilatation improves results, a prospective randomized study conducted by Roubin and associates found no significant difference in restenosis rates between moderate overdilatation and underdilatation of coronary artery lesions.[56] The length of the balloon should not greatly exceed the length of the lesion; otherwise, endothelial trauma unnecessarily extends into nonstenosed portions of the vessel. Excessive balloon length increases the surface area denuded of endothelium and the risk of acute thrombosis after PTA.

Balloon technology has improved greatly since Grüntzig's first catheters. High-pressure polyethylene balloons have enhanced the effectiveness of PTA in tough, calcified lesions. Low-profile balloons are more easily positioned into tight stenoses. Catheters with short, soft tips are less likely to traumatize vessels when balloon inflation straightens the curve of a vessel. Many balloons are now available on 5 Fr catheter shafts (rather than 7 Fr), diminishing the likelihood of puncture site bleeding. Balloons have even been manufactured directly on standard-sized angiographic guidewires.[57]

Balloon Inflation, End Points, and Predictors of Success

If a high-pressure balloon is used, a balloon pressure gauge is not required, as long as hand inflation is performed with a syringe of 10 ml or greater volume. Smaller syringes can be used to generate higher pressures, and such inflations are best monitored by one of the various gauges available. The same holds true for balloons or other PTA catheters not designed to tolerate more than 7 to 8 atmospheres of pressure. When high inflation pressure is desired, the LaVeen syringe (a device with a threaded screw attached to the plunger) is useful. The manufacturer's recommended pressure limits should not be exceeded. Balloon rupture (ideally a longitudinal tear) generally does not cause arterial injury but can make catheter removal quite difficult, and cases of separation and embolization of balloon material have occurred.

Inflation proceeds with injection of 30% contrast material monitored fluoroscopically. More concentrated contrast material is viscous and slows the inflation-deflation process. A balloon should not be test-inflated prior to insertion into the patient. The profile of the device is disturbed by such a test, and introduction can be made quite difficult. As the balloon is inflated, the indentation or "waist" formed by the stenosis is noted. If it remains evident during deflation, the balloon is reexpanded until residual stenosis disappears. If a lesion is refractory to initial dilatation, a larger balloon may be tried. In selected cases, a vascular stent or atherectomy catheter may be employed.

Balloon angioplasty produces controlled injury, irreversibly stretching the vessel wall and cracking plaque, intima, and media.[58] Successful angioplasty produces intimal clefts normally, and these become endothelialized and remodeled to some extent by healing over 4 to 6 weeks. Only if clefts are seen to extend substantially beyond the PTA site should dissection be considered a complication. Because of the splits produced, a guidewire must be maintained through the lesion at all times after initial inflation until the decision is made to terminate the procedure. Otherwise, there is risk of producing an occluding dissection if a guidewire is reintroduced into the lesion. Also, should vessel rupture occur (a rare, but potentially fatal complication), an occlusion balloon can be introduced to tamponade hemorrhage while the patient is taken to surgery.

The duration of balloon inflation optimal for PTA has not been well established. Outside the coronary and brachiocephalic circulations, duration of inflation is rather arbitrary, and the balloon may be left expanded for more than 60 seconds at a time. An inflation of 20 to 40 seconds is commonly used, and multiple intermittent inflations are the rule. If there is a persistent "waist" to the balloon at the stenosis, longer inflations may result in more irreversible stretching of fibrous and elastic elements in the vessel

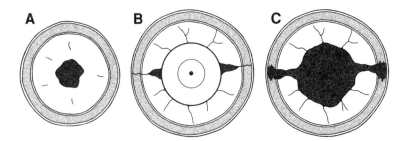

Fig. 10-1   A, Cross-section of concentric arterial stenosis. **B,** Balloon inflation produces cracking and splitting of plaque, intima, and media. **C,** Irreversibly stretched plaque and vessel maintain larger lumen diameter.

wall. If the lesion is seen to "pop" open to full vessel diameter on the initial balloon dilatation, however, multiple inflations may be superfluous.

By the nature of the angioplasty mechanism, concentric stenoses are more likely to respond than very eccentric lesions (Figs. 10-1 and 10-2). In the latter, the plaque itself may not be disrupted, and pressure simply expands the relatively normal elastic wall of the vessel. Vascular stents are well suited to treating eccentric plaques with suboptimal response to simple balloon angioplasty. Heavily calcified lesions or fibrous stenoses (such as anastomoses) can be difficult to open.

A technically successful PTA is measured by absence of residual stenosis greater than 30%, no residual systolic pressure gradient above 10 mm Hg, and good blood flow through the vessel. Additional lesions not likely to be obstructing blood flow are left alone in order to minimize the extent of endothelial trauma. Pressure measurements made before and after angioplasty are often helpful in assessing the results of treatment in iliac and renal artery lesions. Direct measurements are rarely obtained in vessels distal to the inguinal ligament. Intravascular ultrasound and duplex ultrasound have been used for early assessment of PTA effects, and they have shown that angiography often underestimates the degree of residual stenosis.[59–61] Nevertheless, the clinical utility of ultrasound in this context is dubious.[61] Angioscopy is another potential adjunct to PTA without a well-established role.[62] Turning to more mundane objective measures in

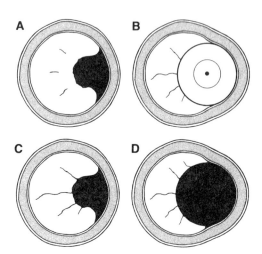

Fig. 10-2 **A,** Cross-section of eccentric arterial stenosis. **B,** Balloon inflation stretches the relatively normal portion of arterial wall preferentially. **C,** After the balloon is removed, the artery returns to pre-balloon angioplasty configuration. **D,** Stent counters the elasticity of the arterial wall and maintains luminal diameter.

the lower extremity, an increase in the ankle-brachial pressure index by at least 0.1 and/or restoration of palpable pedal pulses after PTA correlate with symptomatic improvement.

Restenosis

Postangioplasty restenosis has been a particular problem in the coronary vessels, with rates exceeding 40% in some series.[56] In the renal arteries, recurrence is less likely, with 13% to 16% restenosis rates described at 8 to 24 months of follow-up.[63,64] Similar figures can be expected in the peripheral circulation, and most recurrences are evident within 1 year.[65,66] If a patient develops new symptoms after 2 years, a new lesion at a separate site is usually responsible.[67] Despite the nonnegligible rates of recurrence, PTA remains a valuable option, particularly because most recurrent lesions can be successfully dilated a second time without any increased likelihood of subsequent recurrence.[29,40,48,68–70] It should also be noted that previous surgical endarterectomy does not present a contraindication to balloon angioplasty.[71] As noted earlier, prevention of restenosis and intimal hyperplasia is an area of intense research. Intraluminal administration of local radiation after stent placement has been reported effective in patients presenting with recurrent stenoses, but such treatment is unlikely to attain wider acceptance.[72]

LOWER EXTREMITY ANGIOPLASTY

In selecting patients for PTA in a lower extremity, it is important to correlate the location, extent, and morphology of lesions with the patient's symptoms. For limiting claudication, PTA produces good results in those with focal, isolated lesions and intact distal vessels. It is not good practice to dilate more than five discrete lesions in an extremity; surgery is a better choice. However, if a patient is suffering tissue necrosis or pain while at rest, balloon angioplasty can be applied to more extensive lesions or in the face of diffuse disease, for such patients tend to do poorly with surgery.[18]

Diagnostic arteriography is best done from the side opposite the major symptoms. If PTA is to follow immediately, many lesions in the iliac, common femoral, or proximal superficial femoral arteries can be catheterized antegrade by way of the aortic bifurcation. Should this fail, the retrograde approach can be used for pelvic lesions, or antegrade puncture employed to reach femoral or more distal obstructions. Whether the artery is entered in an antegrade or retrograde fashion, special care must be taken to avoid arterial entry above the inguinal ligament, for massive bleeding can result. Infrainguinal entry is perhaps best guaranteed by use of fluoroscopy to plan and guide puncture, with the desired site of arterial entry at or below the mid-femoral head.[73]

Gross obesity is a relative contraindication to femoropopliteal PTA because adequate postprocedural compression of the puncture site is difficult, and such patients are prone to developing large hematomas. Introducing wires, catheters, and sheaths through a deep layer of fat can also be quite problematic. If safe vascular access is unavailable, surgical arteriotomy must be considered.[74]

Aortic Procedures

Most focal occlusive disease of the abdominal aorta involves the bifurcation. However, purely aortic stenoses may arise in women with a history of smoking. These lesions are quite amenable to transluminal angioplasty, often with a single balloon, because of the small size of the aorta (less than 12 mm diameter) in most patients. Results are comparable to those of surgical bypass.[75,76] However, because of the greater stress placed on the walls of larger vessels, the aorta can rupture after PTA, particularly if heavy calcification is present.[77]

Aortic bifurcation lesions are best treated by placement of balloons from each femoral artery with simultaneous inflation ("kissing balloon" technique; Fig. 10-3). This maneuver prevents embolization to or occlusion of the contralateral iliac artery. Bifurcation stenoses can be opened in more than 90% of cases, with 90% patency at 1 year.[78,79]

Iliac Procedures

If only technically successful PTA procedures are considered, the only large-scale prospective randomized study available indicates no difference in 3-year cumulative patency between patients treated with balloon angioplasty and those who underwent surgical bypass.[3] For stenotic lesions,

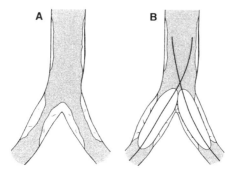

Fig. 10-3 **A,** Common iliac artery stenoses (right greater than left) from atherosclerotic plaques at the aortic bifurcation. **B,** Simultaneous balloon inflation ("kissing balloons"), with each balloon protecting its artery from possible plaque embolization or arterial occlusion caused by the balloon in the contralateral vessel.

immediate success can be expected in more than 90%, and 5-year patency rates between 63% and 90% have been recorded.[40,48,65,80]

There was early hesitancy to refer patients to transluminal angioplasty for iliac occlusion because of fears of vessel perforation or embolization. Still, some investigators have shown that recanalization can be performed safely and effectively, especially if a lesion is not longer than 5 cm.[81,82] Although a straight wire and catheter can be used, Colapinto and colleagues prefer to advance a catheter shaped like a hockey stick into the thrombus and inject small amounts of contrast material; they find that the lumen is often defined in this manner.[82] Technical success can be expected in 67% to 78% of patients, but the percentage is lower for long occlusions. However, long-term patency is good for long occlusions if they are successfully reopened.[82] Acute occlusions should not be treated by angioplasty alone, but PTA can follow successful thrombolysis (see Chapter 11 entitled Local Thrombolytic Infusion).

An advantage of aortoiliac balloon angioplasty vis-à-vis surgical bypass in men is that sexual potency may be preserved or improved.[79] In fact, PTA has been used specifically in the treatment of vasogenic impotence in isolated cases.[83] Aortoiliac PTA can provide reliable arterial inflow for infrainguinal grafts where multilevel disease is present.[84]

Femoropopliteal Procedures
Long-term results of PTA in the superficial femoral or popliteal arteries are comparable to those of surgical bypass if one acknowledges the lower initial technical success rate of PTA.[3,48] Effective dilation of stenoses can be expected in 85% to 99% of cases, but recanalization of occlusions is considerably less successful, depending on the length of the lesion.[3,46,66,68,70] Still, occlusions up to 3 cm in length can be opened as readily as focal stenoses.[66]

If one includes all procedures as a base (including unsuccessful PTAs), long-term (2- to 5-year) patency rates in patients treated for claudication are on the order of 43% to 58%.* Intact runoff vessels correlate with good long-term patency.[86] Those treated for limb salvage have a somewhat worse prognosis (see the section on Limb Salvage later in this chapter). Lesions longer than 3 to 7 cm are clearly more difficult to recanalize, and they have higher reocclusion rates.[66,68,85]

Procedures below the Knee
The use of coronary-type 0.016- and 0.018-inch guidewires, small-shaft (4.5 Fr) balloon catheters, and drugs such as nifedipine, nitroglycerin, and

---

*References 40, 46, 48, 70, 85, 86.

verapamil has greatly improved the results of balloon angioplasty in the distal popliteal artery and trifurcation vessels. In small-vessel PTA, it is reasonable to continue heparin use for several days after intervention. Schwarten and Cutcliff have achieved a remarkable 97% technical success rate in 98 patients, with limb salvage at 2 years in 86%.[19] Others have reported initial technical success of 95% or better, but primary patency as measured by sustained clinical improvement has been only 42% to 60% at 1 to 2 years follow-up.[20,21] Because many patients in these reports had concomitant PTA of more proximal lesions or proximal bypass grafts in place, one must take into account the disseminated nature of the disease treated. Surgical bypass (in situ or reversed saphenous vein grafts) in patients with distal lower extremity vascular disease has a 2-year patency of 73%; if prosthetic material must be used, however, only 30% of grafts remain open for that period.[47] If a vein is not available for graft placement, PTA should be attempted in patients with disease in the calf arteries, and it may be pursued in others with limited tibial-peroneal lesions in order to preserve the saphenous vein for later cardiac or other revascularization surgery.

Limb Salvage

When a patient is treated for rest pain or gangrene, results of revascularization, whether surgical or by balloon angioplasty, are predictably worse than for other indications for PTA. Complications of the procedure are twice as common in such patients as in those treated for claudication only.[80] Even so, it is difficult to predict who will have a good long-term outcome, and late occlusion does not necessarily mean clinical failure because many ischemic ulcers may be healed and do not recur.[18] The presence of occlusion, long-segment disease, or poor distal runoff does not necessarily preclude a good clinical result. Therefore, because many patients with rest pain or tissue loss have multiple medical problems increasing surgical risk, and many do not have donor veins for grafting, PTA can be considered a first-line treatment for limb salvage in such patients. Those who are good operative candidates should undergo surgical revascularization.

Patency at hospital discharge can be expected in about 70% of all patients treated by PTA, with long-term patency of approximately 40% at 2 to 5 years.[18,48,80] Limb salvage rates exceed long-term patency, about 50% at 3 years in those treated by a single PTA procedure without further intervention.[87,88] If a dilatation is initially successful, clinical benefit is as likely to be durable as that provided by bypass, and failed PTA is unlikely to worsen the patient's clinical status or operative risk.[18,89] Nevertheless, failure of a femoropopliteal graft in a patient treated for threatened lower extremity is more likely to result in major amputation than a failed PTA.[90]

Bypass Grafts

Regular duplex or color-flow ultrasound surveillance after vascular surgery has allowed the early recognition and treatment of failing lower extremity bypass grafts. Until recently, the most common presentation of a failing graft was acute thrombosis, a situation requiring thrombolysis followed by PTA or graft revision or by surgical thrombectomy with revision (see Chapter 11 entitled Local Thrombolytic Infusion). More than 10% of femoropopliteal or femorodistal saphenous vein grafts develop flow-limiting lesions, usually within 1 to 2 years of surgery.[91–93]

Balloon angioplasty has proved to be a valuable alternative for prolonging vein graft function (PTA of threatened synthetic grafts has not been reported to any great extent). In one series of 112 grafts, the 3-year graft primary patency rate of 40% improved to 65% assisted primary patency by early intervention with PTA.[92] Whittemore and associates described much worse results, but patients needing preliminary thrombolysis were included, and all their patients presented with ischemic symptoms, implying treatment at a later, more advanced stage of disease.[94] The best results of PTA for graft salvage are in patients with single, nonrecurrent, short (less than 15 mm long) stenoses in grafts at least 3 mm in diameter. Primary patency of 66% has been reported 2 years after PTA in such cases.[93] Berkowitz and colleagues had similar long-term success but found that mid-graft and distal anastomotic strictures were less likely to stay open in the reversed vein bypasses they treated.[91] However, even the best results of PTA for failing grafts do not surpass those of surgical revision. Choice of therapy depends on the accessibility of the lesion, the patient's surgical risk, and the preferences of the patient and referring physician.

Blue Toe Syndrome and Balloon Angioplasty

The blue toe syndrome is the sudden unilateral or bilateral appearance of digital ulcerations and severe pain, arising from a shower of emboli from a proximal source. Most are due to platelet thrombi, and treatment is needed to prevent recurrence and possible amputation.[23] Anticoagulation may not be an adequate measure, and two reports have stressed the usefulness of PTA if an iliac or femoropopliteal lesion is felt to be the source of unilateral emboli.[22,23] Brewer and associates have advocated 6 to 12 weeks of anticoagulation prior to elective angioplasty,[23] whereas Kumpe and colleagues have dilated lesions immediately at the time of discovery.[22] More experience is needed to determine the role of PTA in this clinical setting.

RENAL ARTERY ANGIOPLASTY

Renal PTA has allowed control or resolution of renovascular hypertension in many patients, who thus avoid the higher mortality and morbidity of surgical revascularization or nephrectomy. Lateralization of renin values in selectively obtained samples helps predict a beneficial result, but absence of lateralization should not be seen as a contraindication because about 50% of such patients still improve following PTA. Arguments may be made that PTA should be used to prevent renal artery occlusion whether or not hypertension responds to the procedure. Without treatment, renal artery stenosis may progress to occlusion within 2 years in 11%.[95] Particularly vulnerable to occlusion are patients with unilateral renal artery stenosis being treated with angiotensin-converting enzyme (ACE) inhibitors; more than a quarter may suffer renal artery thrombosis within 6 months.[96] Balloon angioplasty has demonstrated value in selected patients with severe renal vascular disease and renal insufficiency, including individuals with renal transplants and others with solitary functioning kidneys. It has also been used to open the lesions of Takayasu's arteritis.[97]

Patients undergoing renal artery angioplasty should have continual monitoring afterward, preferably in an intensive care unit, because blood pressure can change rapidly. If blood pressure drops, it is likely to do so in the first 1 to 2 days after PTA. However, transient early hypertension can be noted in 30% of patients within 2 hours of the procedure and may persist up to 24 hours, presumably a renin wash-out phenomenon.[98] It is advisable not to discontinue antihypertensive medications prior to PTA, and ACE inhibitors help prevent a sudden drop of blood pressure after dilation.[54]

Patients with extremely atherosclerotic "shaggy" aortas should have PTA only after very careful deliberation, for they are more likely to experience cholesterol embolization, a cause of renal loss or death in isolated cases.[25,99] Simmons catheters are effective in catheterizing most renal arteries, but difficult stenoses may require changing the degree of inspiration or injection of contrast material during catheter advancement.[54] In some cases a coaxial catheter balloon system is useful in catheterizing stenoses, particularly in branch renal vessels.

The guidewire placed after initial catheterization of the lesion must be long enough to allow exchange for the dilating catheter. In practice, a Rosen 1.5-mm J-tip wire (180 cm long) is a good choice for most exchanges. However, care must be taken to prevent traumatization of small branch vessels; otherwise, use of a straight-tip exchange wire is advised. During balloon catheter introduction, the position of the wire must be followed carefully by fluoroscopy to prevent accidental withdrawal or excessive advancement of wire. Spasm can be a difficult problem in renal angioplasty; premedication with nifedipine and frequent intraarterial injections of nitroglycerin (100 to 200 µg) are strongly recommended.

Hydration is particularly important because many patients already have functional impairment of the kidneys prior to PTA. Martin and associates have found that administration of mannitol (25%) over 8 hours at 50 ml/hour in those deemed to be at high risk for contrast material–related renal failure has dropped the incidence of this complication from 11% to 5%.[51]

In order to put renal PTA into context, one must be aware of the results of surgery. One recent series of 285 patients who underwent bypass or endarterectomy produced 5.6% operative mortality and a 5-year cumulative patency rate of 75%.[100] Overall, surgery may provide more consistent long-term clinical results but at the cost of higher early mortality.

Hypertension
Technical success for renal artery balloon angioplasty has been reported between 81% and 97%.* Major complications are seen in 11% to 13%, and risks of permanent impairment of renal function, nephrectomy, and death are each under 1%.[99,101] Use of undersized balloons and residual stenosis greater than 30% are factors associated with increased recurrence.[54] Bilateral lesions can be treated during one session without any increase in morbidity. However, if any difficulty is encountered in the treatment of one kidney, deferring dilation of the opposite side is prudent.

Fibromuscular Dysplasia
Clinical results in hypertension (cure regarded as diastolic blood pressure less than 90 mm Hg without medications; improvement regarded as diastolic pressure that significantly drops on the same or fewer medications) are best for patients with fibromuscular dysplasia (FMD). At 6-month to 2-year follow-up, 81% to 100% of those with successful dilations show clinical benefit.[24,63,99,101 103] Cumulative 5-year patency in FMD among those with initial response has been 89%, underscoring the durability of results.[99] Restenosis rates for FMD are low. Technical failure to dilate is more common in the very tough lesions of adventitial fibroplasia.[27] Still, atypical fibromuscular lesions unlikely to represent medial fibroplasia are worth attempting, for many *can* be effectively dilated.[104]

Atherosclerosis
Renovascular hypertension from atherosclerotic disease responds to PTA in a less predictable manner, and few patients are likely to be cured of their high blood pressure. Whereas 47% to 65% of patients have at least some improvement 6 to 16 months after dilatation of unilateral renal artery lesions, only 14% to 46% of those treated for bilateral lesions have had the benefit persist for that long a time.[101,103] Sos and colleagues

---

*References 27, 51, 54, 63, 64, 99, 101.

attributed their very poor clinical results in bilateral atheromatous disease to an inability to achieve a satisfactory technical result.[103] Klinge and colleagues, however, reported treatment of 42 patients with bilateral lesions, with good initial clinical response in 38 (90%).[99] In the same study, of all 133 patients in whom dilatation of atherosclerotic lesions was attempted, 77% had cure or improvement in their hypertension at 6 months, and the cumulative 5-year response stayed high. A more recent report confirmed the durability of results, with deterioration of blood pressure control in only 21% at 5 years.[27] The difference in these reports might be explained by improvement in technique, equipment, and patient selection with time.

Dilatation of Ostial Stenoses
Many atherosclerotic lesions are ostial; that is, the stenosis involves the main renal artery near its origin. Ostial stenosis dilatation procedures have generally had poor technical and clinical results, ostensibly because it is aortic plaque that is actually subjected to longitudinal displacement, rather than renal plaque undergoing the desired radial disruption (Fig. 10-4). Which particular lesion actually is ostial depends on the thickness of plaques involving the aorta. In practice, this can only be estimated, but narrowings in the first 5 to 10 mm of the renal artery probably involve its origin. In addition, tight ostial stenoses are more difficult to catheterize than more distal lesions. Although success is not as good as for nonostial stenoses, PTA is still worth pursuing in selected patients. Klinge and colleagues achieved a satisfactory technical result in 82% of their ostial stenosis patients, with subsequent recurrent hypertension in 18%.[99] By contrast, Losinno and colleagues found that although 88% with nonostial atherosclerotic stenoses had their hyper-

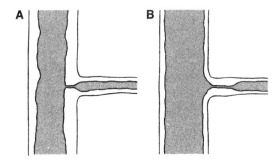

Fig. 10-4 Two renal artery stenoses. **A,** The narrowing is caused by plaque within the aorta and would not likely respond to balloon angioplasty; **B,** the stenosis is truly within the renal artery. On angiography such stenoses may be very difficult to distinguish.

tension cured or improved, only 39% with ostial lesions had a positive response.[27] Martin and associates have found that response to PTA performed to improve renal function did not depend on the ostial versus nonostial location of stenosis.[25]

Special Situations in Renal Angioplasty

Renal Transplants

The incidence of renal artery stenosis after transplantation varies widely but can be as high as 16%.[105] End-to-end anastomoses to the internal iliac artery are best approached by catheterization from the contralateral femoral artery; end-to-side anastomoses to the external iliac should be catheterized from the ipsilateral approach. Most stenoses involve the anastomosis or the main renal artery, and balloon dilatation can be performed with at least 69% technical success.[105-107] Improvement in function and hypertension is maintained in 50% to 63% at 1 year or more.[24,105,106,108] Restenosis rates can be high, but recurrent lesions usually respond to a second dilatation procedure.[107]

Azotemia

Patients with azotemia and renal vascular disease may have a single functioning kidney, two kidneys with bilateral lesions, or two kidneys with only unilateral arterial obstruction. Hypertension is a common accompanying problem. Persons suffering severe and long-standing renal insufficiency are not likely to benefit from an attempted balloon angioplasty; in particular, those with unilateral stenosis (as opposed to bilateral stenosis or stenosis in the vessel supplying a single functioning kidney) rarely show any improvement.[27] Even so, in larger series roughly half of those not yet on dialysis have improved or (more commonly) stabilized function at 1 year of follow-up.[25,28,109-111] Balanced against this potential benefit is the possibility of at least transient deterioration of renal status in about one in four of such patients.[24,111] Diabetics are less likely than nondiabetics to maintain stable renal function at 1 year.[111] Treatment can be justified by the high mortality and cost of chronic hemodialysis in patients who are not candidates for transplantation.

Recanalization of Occlusions

Kadir and colleagues have used angioplasty to treat acute arterial occlusion in five patients with solitary kidneys, achieving return of function in three.[26] In another report, 6 of 10 subacute occlusions were reopened, with significant improvement in renal function in all 6 patients, including 3 who discontinued hemodialysis.[112] Others have approached chronically occluded vessels with balloons and have produced mixed results.[54,99] Such attempts are best reserved for extraordinary situations.

Surgery for Failure or Complication of Balloon Angioplasty

Although balloon angioplasty may fail or be responsible for acute arterial occlusion or rupture in a small number of cases, prompt surgical intervention can usually salvage the kidney. Beebe and associates found that their surgical approach was altered by attempted PTA in only one of nine patients, and all but one have a good result at a mean of 3 years of follow-up.[24] Revascularization was successful in 10 of 13 kidneys treated by McCann and colleagues, including 4 of 5 experiencing a complication of angioplasty.[4]

SUBCLAVIAN BALLOON ANGIOPLASTY

Despite initial fears that balloon angioplasty in the brachiocephalic vessels would be complicated by stroke, subclavian PTA has proved quite safe, even with antegrade flow in a vertebral artery originating distal to the treated lesion.[113] Balloon angioplasty has been used effectively at a number of centers in patients suffering subclavian steal syndrome.[29,113,114] In one series of 50 patients, 90% technical success was achieved, and 37 of 44 successfully treated patients had sustained clinical improvement at a mean follow-up interval of more than 3 years.[115] Similar durable results have been reported from Nuremberg, but in that study only two thirds of 125 patients treated were available for late follow-up.[116] Balloon angioplasty has also been successful in the treatment of five of six patients with brachiocephalic lesions of Takayasu's arteritis.[97]

Subclavian arteries have been recanalized in a small number of cases, but results have been generally poor for occlusions.[29,114,116,117] Düber and associates reopened seven of eight subclavian occlusions (all in patients with absent or reversed vertebral artery flow), but obstruction recurred in four cases.[117] Of note, they also placed a Strecker stent in one patient who later developed an episode of cerebellar ischemia. Lesions involving the segment from which a patent vertebral artery arises are best not dilated. If a stenosis is near (but not involving) the vertebral artery, a balloon can be inflated across the vertebral artery origin with little danger of adverse consequences.[113]

In all cases of subclavian angioplasty, it is strongly suggested that a full four-vessel cerebral study be obtained to assess the pattern of intracranial circulation before an intervention is attempted. Although the retrograde brachial or axillary approach has been employed, it is not as likely to be successful as a femoral approach. Upper extremity arterial access is also more prone to complicating hematoma or puncture site occlusion.

OTHER APPLICATIONS

Aside from its application in coronary artery disease and in instances of cerebrovascular disease, transluminal angioplasty has also been applied to mesenteric ischemia. With the exception of ostial stenosis and median arcuate ligament compression of the celiac axis, mesenteric PTA has had good technical success but a high incidence of restenosis.[31] Long-term results with central venous and dialysis access stenosis PTA have been disappointing. Still, the relatively short life of a dialysis shunt and the difficulty of treating central venous strictures by other means, as well as the low morbidity of a second PTA procedure, support the use of transluminal dilatation for these clinical problems.[30,118] Vascular stents are being applied with greater frequency for the alleviation of central venous obstructions, but wide experience and long-term follow-up are still lacking (see Chapter 9 entitled Dialysis Access, Central Venous Catheters, and Other Central Venous Problems).

SALVAGE OF PROCEDURES COMPLICATED BY THROMBOSIS OR EMBOLISM

If catheterization or dilatation of a lesion results in acute arterial thrombosis, all is not necessarily lost. Immediate local infusion of urokinase or other thrombolytic agent can reestablish flow in the great majority of cases[119] (see Chapter 11 entitled Local Thrombolytic Infusion). However, distal embolization of plaque fragments causes occlusion unresponsive to thrombolysis.

Distal embolization (as well as thrombotic occlusion) can be treated by passage of a Fogarty embolectomy catheter into the affected vessel by way of a sheath.[120] If this maneuver is chosen, the sheath should be cut or the cap of the sheath removed after the Fogarty catheter is withdrawn, in order to allow any retained clot or debris to be flushed out of the sheath by backbleeding.

Starck and associates have used percutaneous aspiration thromboembolectomy (PAT) in similar situations.[121] The PAT procedure involves use of a special long 8 Fr sheath with a removable hemostasis valve. A minimally tapered, thin-wall catheter is passed to the clot or obstruction, and strong suction is applied with a large syringe. The catheter is removed, the debris expelled, and the procedure repeated until distal runoff is reestablished.

COST-EFFECTIVENESS OF PERCUTANEOUS ANGIOPLASTY

Up to 40% of patients presenting with lesions amenable to surgical revascularization are candidates for balloon angioplasty.[122] Hospital stays and treatment charges may be less than one third those of surgically treated patients.[122] Although no large prospective cost-comparison studies are at hand, it is reasonable to assume that even if the costs of complications and technical failures are factored in, PTA remains clearly less expensive than surgical bypass. Average hospital stay is but a fraction of that for surgical patients.[48] Nevertheless, recent epidemiologic studies have indicated that use of balloon angioplasty in the lower extremities has neither decreased the number of vascular surgical procedures (particularly for critical ischemia) nor decreased the amputation rate.[123,124] The reasons for the increase in vascular procedures are no doubt complex, including use of PTA as an adjunct to surgery, failed PTA resulting in surgery, and application of PTA to patients with milder symptoms, whereas the rise in amputation rate may simply reflect an aging population.[124] In any case, widespread use of PTA for peripheral vascular disease may not result in the large cost savings envisioned by early proponents. Much research remains to be done to determine the optimal indications for endovascular procedures.

NEW DIRECTIONS

Because of the lower success rates of PTA in recanalization of long occlusions and in patients with diffuse disease, and because of continuing problems with restenosis, a number of novel interventions and devices have been developed and are being tested.

Enclosed Thrombolysis as an Adjunct to PTA

Recanalization of femoropopliteal occlusions longer than 5 cm resulted in reocclusion within 6 months in 22 of 23 lesions treated in one recent study.[125] Because Jørgensen and colleagues had similarly dismal results for long occlusions,[87] they created a double-balloon catheter system for bathing a recanalized segment with thrombolytic enzymes. By removing residual thrombus in the 10- to 25-cm segment enclosed by two balloons inflated for 30 minutes, they reduced early rethrombosis from 41% in those treated with PTA alone to 9%.[126] One-year cumulative patency rose to 80% in the same report. This work remains to be duplicated by others.

Mechanical and Other Atherectomy Devices

Transluminal systems for mechanical removal or disruption of plaque have already entered clinical use. The Simpson atherectomy catheter, 7 Fr or 9 Fr in diameter, can be inserted through a percutaneous sheath. A motor-driven cutting blade is housed in a cylindrical metal capsule. The aperture of the capsule is forced against a plaque by a low-pressure balloon inflated on the side of the capsule opposite the cutting aperture. Although a small wire is appended to the leading end of the capsule, the catheter is not guided *over* a wire. The Simpson catheter must work through an established lumen; an occluded vessel must be partially reopened to allow its introduction. Also, because only a finite amount of material can be held by the capsule, the catheter must be repeatedly removed and emptied for extensive atherectomy procedures. In one randomized study of 30 patients with angiographic follow-up, 1-year patency (as defined by absence of stenosis of 50% or more in the treated segment) was 77% in those treated by conventional PTA versus only 25% in those treated by Simpson catheter atherectomy.[10] Other series of 46 and 94 patients have found 18- and 24-month patency rates of under 50%.[11,12] Because these results are no better than those obtained by balloon angioplasty, directional atherectomy is best limited to resection of intimal flaps obstructing flow or possibly eccentric plaques not responding to simple PTA.

The Kensey catheter uses a rotating cam to bore through and pulverize occlusive lesions. Embolic particles from fragmented plaque have produced small cerebral and renal infarcts in animal models, but peripheral embolization has not been a clinical problem in the lower extremities.[127,128] Because the catheter creates only a small lumen, balloon dilatation must be performed at the conclusion of most recanalizations. A high rate of vascular perforation with this device[127] has precluded larger trials.

The Auth burr is a rotating, football-shaped, brass device containing embedded diamond chips. Due to its relative lack of compliance, calcified plaque is abraded preferentially by the burr, most particles resulting being less than 10 micrometers in diameter.[129] Because of their size (up to 4.5 mm in diameter), larger burrs must be introduced through a surgical arteriotomy. The recanalization of occlusions is limited to lesions that can be traversed prior to atherectomy, for the Auth device is advanced over a guidewire. Although early recanalization rates were promising in a multicenter trial, there was a high incidence of thromboembolic complications and vessel perforations, and the 2-year patency rate was only 19%.[9]

As in the case of laser-assisted angioplasty, atherectomy catheters of these and other designs have been more of a disappointment than a panacea. All devices tested to date have been more expensive than conventional balloon catheters. At the same time, they have generally demonstrated inferior performance in routine application. If safe and effective measures for maintaining patency and preventing restenosis are found (presumably on a pharmacologic or immunologic basis, the discoverer no doubt winning a Nobel prize), recanalization catheters may experience a renaissance.

Endovascular Stents

Vascular stents are metallic meshes of stainless steel, tantalum, or titanium alloys that are introduced by means of sheaths and fixed into place by inflation of a balloon carrier-catheter or by properties of self-expansion.[130–132] Stents are meant to improve the results of PTA by resisting any elastic elements in vascular segments not opened completely by balloon alone and to tack down intimal flaps. At present, the Palmaz stent is the only one approved by the FDA for intravascular use in the United States, and it has been released for use in iliac artery lesions. The Palmaz stent is deployed after a sheath is first advanced through the obstruction. When the balloon carrying the stent is properly positioned, the sheath is withdrawn and the balloon inflated. The balloon used should be slightly larger than the desired lumen size to allow the stent to embed itself within the arterial wall.[130] The Palmaz stent is easily introduced and readily visible on fluoroscopic monitoring. Another advantage to this stent is the ability to increase its diameter after placement by using a larger balloon. However, the device is not flexible and is poorly suited for tortuous vessels. Two-year patency of Palmaz stents used to treat iliac artery stenoses or occlusions has been reported at 65%.[15]

Wallstents are self-expanding upon release from the specially designed introducing catheter. They exert continuous radial pressure until the manufactured diameter is attained. They are quite flexible and may be deployed in curved vessels or from a contralateral femoral approach. Wallstents may also be withdrawn or removed, if positioning is deemed unsatisfactory (as long as they are not fully released). Disadvantages include poor radiopacity, and relatively greater stent shortening with expansion. The latter feature may make proper positioning somewhat tricky. Long-term results in treating iliac lesions have been comparable to those of Palmaz stents.[13,15]

In renal arteries, stents have been used to treat ostial lesions, recurrent stenoses, and stenoses refractory to balloon dilatation. Hennequin and colleagues found a 20% rate of significant (at least 50%) narrowing at 1 to 2 years in 20 patients with renal Wallstents.[16] All angiograms showed some intimal thickening within the stents, but this lining stabilized in appearance after 6 months in most cases. Even when placed for ostial lesions, stents should not project into the aorta more than 1 or 2 mm.

Results of stenting smaller vessels have been rather disappointing. One-year primary patency of self-expanding stents in femoropopliteal lesions has been less than 50%.[14] At present, it is wise to limit application of these expensive devices to large or medium-sized arteries obstructed by post-PTA dissections or to elastic or eccentric lesions producing unsatisfactory PTA results. Recurrent stenoses in larger, high-flow arteries may be stented. Potential future applications for covered or uncovered stents may include treatment of spontaneous aortic dissection, aneurysms, or post-traumatic pseudoaneurysms.[133]

During stent placement, overlapping major branch or collateral vessels is best avoided, even though flow may be preserved early on. We have noted occlusion of a previously normal internal iliac artery 1 year after a stent was placed across its origin. Placement in vessels at areas of flexion, such as the common femoral artery or popliteal artery, should also be avoided. Finally, great care must be taken to maintain sterile technique during insertion. As implanted foreign bodies, stents are susceptible to bacterial contamination. Stent infection can be disastrous.[45]

REFERENCES

1. Dotter C, Judkins MP: Transluminal treatment of arteriosclerotic obstruction: Description of a new technique and preliminary report of its application. *Circulation* 1964; 30:654–670.
2. Grüntzig A, Hopff H: Perkutane rekanalisation chronischer arterieller verschlüsse mit einem neuen dilatationskatheter: Modifikation der Dotter-technik. *Dtsch Med Wochenschr* 1974; 99:2502–2505.
3. Wilson SE, Wolf GL, Cross AP, et al: Percutaneous transluminal angioplasty versus operation for peripheral arteriosclerosis. *J Vasc Surg* 1989; 9:1–9.
4. McCann RL, Bollinger RR, Newman GE: Surgical renal artery reconstruction after percutaneous transluminal angioplasty. *J Vasc Surg* 1988; 8:389–394.
5. Rutherford RB, Becker GJ: Standards for evaluating and reporting the results of surgical and percutaneous therapy for peripheral vascular disease. *J Vasc Interv Radiol* 1991; 2:169–174.
6. Douek PC, Leon MB, Geschwind H, et al: Occlusive peripheral vascular disease: A multicenter trial of fluorescence-guided pulsed dye laser-assisted balloon angioplasty. *Radiology* 1991; 180:127–133.
7. Miller BV, Sharp WJ, Shamma AR, et al: Surveillance for recurrent stenosis after endovascular procedures: A prospective study. *Arch Surg* 1991; 126:867–872.
8. Siegel RJ, Fishbein MC, Forrester J, et al: Ultrasonic plaque ablation: A new method for recanalization of partially or totally occluded arteries. *Circulation* 1988; 78:1443–1448.
9. Ahn SS, Yeatman LA, Deutsch LS, et al: Peripheral atherectomy with the Rotablator: A multicenter report. *J Vasc Surg* 1994; 19:509–515.
10. Vroegindeweij D, Kemper FJM, Tielbeek AV, et al: Recurrence of stenoses following balloon angioplasty and Simpson atherectomy of the femoro-popliteal segment: A randomised comparative 1-year follow-up study using colour flow duplex. *Eur J Vasc Surg* 1992; 6:164–171.
11. Lugmayr H, Pachinger O, Deutsch M: Langzeitresultate der perkutanen Atherektomie bei peripherer arterieller Verschlußkrankheit. *Rofo* 1993; 158:532–535.
12. Cavallari N, Feldhaus RJ, McGill JE, et al: Peripheral directional atherectomy: Arteriographic vs hemodynamic assessment of cumulative patency. *Vasc Surg* 1993; 27:329–336.
13. Long AL, Page PE, Raynaud AC, et al: Percutaneous iliac artery stent: Angiographic long-term follow-up. *Radiology* 1991; 180:771–778.
14. Sapoval MR, Long AL, Raynaud AC, et al: Femoropopliteal stent placement: Long-term results. *Radiology* 1992; 184:833–839.
15. Strunk HM, Schild HH, Düber C, et al: Ergebnisse angiographischer Verlaufskontrollen nach perkutaner Stentimplantation in Beckenarterien mit Vergleich zwischen Wall- und Palmaz-Stent. *Rofo* 1993; 159:251–257.

16. Hennequin LM, Joffre FG, Rousseau HP, et al: Renal artery stent placement: Long-term results with the Wallstent endoprosthesis. *Radiology* 1994; 191:713–719.
17. Cragg AH, Dake MD: Percutaneous femoropopliteal graft placement. *Radiology* 1993; 187:643–648.
18. Milford MA, Weaver FA, Lundell CJ, Yellin AE: Femoropopliteal percutaneous transluminal angioplasty for limb salvage. *J Vasc Surg* 1988; 8:292–299.
19. Schwarten DE, Cutcliff WB: Arterial occlusive disease below the knee: Treatment with percutaneous transluminal angioplasty performed with low-profile catheters and steerable guide wires. *Radiology* 1988; 169:71–74.
20. Brown KT, Moore ED, Getrajdman GI, Saddekni S: Infrapopliteal angioplasty: Long-term follow-up. *J Vasc Interv Radiol* 1993; 4:139–144.
21. Sivananthan UM, Browne TF, Thorley PJ, Rees MR: Percutaneous transluminal angioplasty of the tibial arteries. *Br J Surg* 1994; 81:1282–1285.
22. Kumpe DA, Zwerdlinger S, Griffin DJ: Blue digit syndrome: Treatment with percutaneous transluminal angioplasty. *Radiology* 1988; 166:37–44.
23. Brewer ML, Kinnison ML, Perler BA, White RI, Jr: Blue toe syndrome: Treatment with anticoagulants and delayed percutaneous transluminal angioplasty. *Radiology* 1988; 166:31–36.
24. Beebe HG, Chesebro K, Merchant F, Bush W: Results of renal artery balloon angioplasty limit its indications. *J Vasc Surg* 1988; 8:300–306.
25. Martin LG, Casarella WJ, Gaylord GM: Azotemia caused by renal artery stenosis: Treatment by percutaneous angioplasty. *Am J Roentgenol* 1988; 150:839–844.
26. Kadir S, Watson A, Burrow C: Percutaneous transcatheter recanalization in the management of acute renal failure due to sudden occlusion of the renal artery to a solitary kidney. *Am J Nephrol* 1987; 7:445–449.
27. Losinno F, Zuccala A, Busato F, Zucchelli P: Renal artery angioplasty for renovascular hypertension and preservation of renal function: Long-term angiographic and clinical follow-up. *Am J Roentgenol* 1994; 162:853–857.
28. Pattynama PMT, Becker GJ, Brown J, et al: Percutaneous angioplasty for atherosclerotic renal artery disease: Effect on renal function in azotemic patients. *Cardiovasc Intervent Radiol* 1994; 17:143–146.
29. Erbstein RA, Wholey MH, Smoot S: Subclavian artery steal syndrome: Treatment by percutaneous transluminal angioplasty. *Am J Roentgenol* 1988; 151:291–294.
30. Glanz S, Gordon DH, Lipkowitz GS, et al: Axillary and subclavian vein stenoses: Percutaneous angioplasty. *Radiology* 1988; 168:371–373.
31. Odurny A, Sniderman KW, Colapinto RF: Intestinal angina: Percutaneous transluminal angioplasty of the celiac and superior mesenteric arteries. *Radiology* 1988; 167:59–62.
32. Ali MK, Ewer MS, Balakrishnan PV, et al: Balloon angioplasty for superior vena cava obstruction. *Ann Intern Med* 1987; 107:856–857.
33. Lemarbre L, Hudon G, Coche G, Bourassa MG: Outpatient peripheral angioplasty: Survey of complications and patients' perceptions. *Am J Roentgenol* 1987; 148:1239–1240.
34. Struk DW, Rankin RN, Eliasziw M, Vellet AD: Safety of outpatient peripheral angioplasty. *Radiology* 1993; 189:193–196.

35. Richter E-I, Zeitler E: *Percutaneous transluminal angioplasty: Adjunct drug therapy*. In Dotter CT, Grüntzig AR, Schoop AW, editors: *Percutaneous Transluminal Angioplasty: Technique, Early and Late Results*. 1983, Berlin: Springer-Verlag. pp 84–90.

36. Cunningham D, Kumar B, Siegal BA, et al: Aspirin inhibition of platelet deposition at angioplasty sites: Demonstration by platelet scintigraphy. *Radiology* 1984; 151:487–490.

37. Fellmeth BD, Bookstein JJ, Lurie AL, Dillard JP: Rapid progression of peripheral vascular disease after diagnostic angiography. *Radiology* 1990; 175:71–74.

38. Gardiner GA, Jr, Meyerovitz MF, Stokes KR, et al: Complications of transluminal angioplasty. *Radiology* 1986; 159:201–208.

39. Jensen SR, Voegeli DR, Crummy AB, et al: Iliac artery rupture during transluminal angioplasty: Treatment by embolization and surgical bypass. *Am J Roentgenol* 1985; 145:381–382.

40. Johnston KW, Rae M, Hogg-Johnston SA, et al: 5-year results of a prospective study of percutaneous transluminal angioplasty. *Ann Surg* 1987; 206:403–413.

41. Fraedrich G, Beck A, Bonzel T, Schlosser V: Acute surgical intervention for complications of percutaneous transluminal angioplasty. *Eur J Vasc Surg* 1987; 1:197–203.

42. Belli AM, Cumberland DC, Knox AM, et al: The complication rate of percutaneous peripheral balloon angioplasty. *Clin Radiol* 1990; 41:380–383.

43. Schräder R, Steinbacher S, Burger W, et al: Collagen application for sealing of arterial puncture sites in comparison to pressure dressing: A randomized trial. *Cathet Cardiovasc Diagn* 1992; 27:298–302.

44. McCready RA, Siderys H, Pittman JN, et al: Septic complications after cardiac catheterization and percutaneous transluminal coronary angioplasty. *J Vasc Surg* 1991; 14:170–174.

45. Therasse E, Soulez G, Cartier P, et al: Infection with fatal outcome after endovascular metallic stent placement. *Radiology* 1994; 192:363–365.

46. Hunink MGM, Donaldson MC, Meyerovitz MF, et al: Risks and benefits of femoropopliteal percutaneous balloon angioplasty. *J Vasc Surg* 1993; 17:183–192.

47. Veterans Administration Cooperative Study Group 141: Comparative evaluation of prosthetic, reversed, and in situ vein bypass grafts in distal popliteal and tibial-peroneal revascularization. *Arch Surg* 1988; 123:434–438.

48. Cole SEA, Baird RN, Horrocks M, Jeans WD: The role of balloon angioplasty in the management of lower limb ischemia. *Eur J Vasc Surg* 1987; 1:61–65.

49. Taylor LM, Jr, Hamre D, Dalman RL, Porter JM: Limb salvage vs amputation for critical ischemia: The role of vascular surgery. *Arch Surg* 1991; 126:1251–1258.

50. Cronin TG, Calandra JD, Sheridan PH, et al: Retrograde puncture of popliteal artery for access to peripheral arteries for laser angioplasty. *Semin Intervent Radiol* 1988; 5:281–282.

51. Martin LG, Casarella WJ, Alspaugh JP, Chuang VP: Renal artery angioplasty: Increased technical success and decreased complications in the second 100 patients. *Radiology* 1986; 159:631–634.

52. McDermott JC, Babel SG, Crummy AB, et al: Review of the uses of digital "road map" techniques in interventional radiology. *Ann Radiol (Paris)* 1989; 32:11–13.

53. Bolia A, Miles KA, Brennan J, Bell PRF: Percutaneous transluminal angio-plasty of occlusions of the femoral and popliteal arteries by subintimal dissection. *Cardiovasc Intervent Radiol* 1990; 13:357–363.
54. Tegtmeyer CJ, Sos TA: Techniques of renal artery angioplasty. *Radiology* 1986; 161:577–586.
55. Zollikofer CL, Salomonowitz E, Castañeda-Zuñiga WR, et al: The relationship between arterial and balloon rupture in experimental angioplasty. *Am J Roentgenol* 1985; 144:777–779.
56. Roubin GS, Douglas JS, Jr, King SB, et al: Influence of balloon size on initial success, acute complications, and restenosis after percutaneous transluminal coronary angioplasty: A prospective randomized study. *Circulation* 1988; 78:557–565.
57. Tegtmeyer CJ: Guide wire angioplasty balloon catheter: Preliminary report. *Radiology* 1988; 169:253–254.
58. Wolf GL, LeVeen RF, Ring EJ: Potential mechanisms of angioplasty. *Cardiovasc Intervent Radiol* 1984; 7:11–17.
59. Engeler CE, Yedlicka JW, Letourneau JG, et al: Intravascular sonography in the detection of arteriosclerosis and evaluation of vascular interventional procedures. *Am J Roentgenol* 1991; 156:1087–1090.
60. Kinney EV, Bandyk DF, Mewissen MW, et al: Monitoring functional patency of percutaneous transluminal angioplasty. *Arch Surg* 1991; 126:743–747.
61. Sacks D, Robinson ML, Summers TA, Marinelli DL: The value of duplex sonography after peripheral artery angioplasty in predicting subacute restenosis. *Am J Roentgenol* 1994; 162:179–183.
62. Winkelbauer F, Holzenbein T, Ammann ME, et al: Percutaneous angioscopy: Improved technique. *Cardiovasc Intervent Radiol* 1993; 16:374–376.
63. Tegtmeyer CJ, Kellum CD, Ayers C: Percutaneous transluminal angioplasty of the renal artery. *Radiology* 1984; 153:77–84.
64. Plouin PF, Darné B, Chatellier G, et al: Restenosis after a first percutaneous transluminal renal angioplasty. *Hypertension* 1993; 21:89–96.
65. Van Andel GJ, van Erp WFM, Krepel VM, Breslau PJ: Percutaneous transluminal dilatation of the iliac artery: Long-term results. *Radiology* 1985; 156:321–323.
66. Krepel VM, van Andel GJ, van Erp WFM, Breslau PJ: Percutaneous transluminal angioplasty of the femoro-popliteal artery: Initial and long-term results. *Radiology* 1985; 156:325–328.
67. Thorvinger B, Norgren L, Albrechtsson U: Patency after iliac and femoro-popliteal angioplasty: Difference between angiographic and clinical results. *Acta Radiol* 1992; 33:29–30.
68. Murray RR, Jr, Hewes RC, White RI, Jr, et al: Long-segment femoropopliteal stenoses: Is angioplasty a boon or a bust? *Radiology* 1987; 162:473–476.
69. Greminger P, Schneider E, Siegenthaler W, Vetter W: Renovaskuläre hypertonie. *Internist (Berl)*1988; 29:246–251.
70. Matsi PJ, Manninen HI, Vanninen RL, et al: Femoropopliteal angioplasty in patients with claudication: Primary and secondary patency in 140 limbs with 1–3-year follow-up. *Radiology* 1994; 191:727–733.
71. Tisnado J, Vines FS, Barnes RW, et al: Percutaneous transluminal angioplasty following endarterectomy. *Radiology* 1984; 152:361–364.

72. Lierman D, Bottcher HD, Kollath J, et al: Prophylactic endovascular radiotherapy to prevent intimal hyperplasia after stent implantation in femoropopliteal arteries. *Cardiovasc Intervent Radiol* 1994; 17:12–16.

73. Rupp SB, Vogelzang RL, Nemcek AA, Jr, Yungbluth MM: Relationship of the inguinal ligament to pelvic radiographic landmarks: Anatomic correlation and its role in femoral arteriography. *J Vasc Interv Radiol* 1993; 4:409–413.

74. Wilms G, Nevelsteen A, Baert A, Suy R: Intraoperative angioplasty. *Cardiovasc Intervent Radiol* 1987; 10:8–12.

75. Charlebois N, Saint-Georges G, Hudon G: Percutaneous transluminal angioplasty of the lower abdominal aorta. *Am J Roentgenol* 1986; 146:369–371.

76. Odurny A, Colapinto RF, Sniderman KW, Johnston KW: Percutaneous transluminal angioplasty of abdominal aortic stenoses. *Cardiovasc Intervent Radiol* 1989; 12:1–6.

77. Berger T, Sörenson R, Konrad J: Aortic rupture: A complication of transluminal angioplasty. *Am J Roentgenol* 1986; 146:373–374.

78. Tegtmeyer CJ, Kellum CD, Kron IL, Mentzer RM, Jr: Percutaneous transluminal angioplasty in the region of the aortic bifurcation. *Radiology* 1985; 157:661–665.

79. Ravimandalam K, Rao VRK, Kumar S, et al: Obstruction of the infrarenal portion of the abdominal aorta: Results of treatment with balloon angioplasty. *Am J Roentgenol* 1991; 156:1257–1260.

80. Zeitler E, Richter EI, Roth FJ, Schoop W: Results of percutaneous transluminal angioplasty. *Radiology* 1983; 146:57–60.

81. Rubinstein AJ, Morag B, Peer A, et al: Percutaneous transluminal recanalization of common iliac artery occlusions. *Cardiovasc Intervent Radiol* 1987; 10:16–20.

82. Colapinto RF, Stronell RD, Johnston WK: Transluminal angioplasty of complete iliac obstructions. *Am J Roentgenol* 1986; 146:859–862.

83. Castañeda-Zuñiga WR, Smith A, Kaye K, et al: Transluminal angioplasty for treatment of vasculogenic impotence. *Am J Roentgenol* 1982; 139:371–373.

84. Wilson SE, White GH, Wolf G, et al: Proximal percutaneous balloon angioplasty and distal bypass for multilevel arterial occlusion. *Ann Vasc Surg* 1990; 4:351–355.

85. Henricksen LO, Jørgensen B, Holstein PE, et al: Percutaneous transluminal angioplasty of infrarenal arteries in intermittent claudication. *Acta Chir Scand* 1988; 154:573–576.

86. Johnston KW: Femoral and popliteal arteries: Reanalysis of results of balloon angioplasty. *Radiology* 1992; 183:767–771.

87. Jørgensen B, Tønnesen KH, Holstein P: Late hemodynamic failure following percutaneous transluminal angioplasty for long and multifocal femoropopliteal stenoses. *Cardiovasc Intervent Radiol* 1991; 14:290–292.

88. Matsi PJ, Manninen HI, Suhonen MT, et al: Chronic critical lower-limb ischemia: Prospective trial of angioplasty with 1–36 months follow-up. *Radiology* 1993; 188:381–387.

89. Blair JM, Gewertz BL, Moosa H, et al: Percutaneous transluminal angioplasty versus surgery for limb-threatening ischemia. *J Vasc Surg* 1989; 9:698–703.

90. Fletcher JP, Fermanis G, Little JM, Kershaw LZ: The role of percutaneous transluminal angioplasty and femoropopliteal bypass in patients with threatened limb. *Vasc Surg* 1988; 22:226–230.
91. Berkowitz HD, Fox AD, Deaton DH: Reversed vein graft stenosis: Early diagnosis and management. *J Vasc Surg* 1992; 15:130–142.
92. London NJM, Sayers RD, Thompson M, et al: Interventional radiology in the maintenance of infrainguinal vein graft patency. *Br J Surg* 1993; 80:187–193.
93. Sanchez LA, Suggs WD, Marin ML, et al: Is percutaneous balloon angioplasty appropriate in the treatment of graft and anastomotic lesions responsible for failing vein bypasses? *Am J Surg* 1994; 168:97–101.
94. Whittemore AD, Donaldson MC, Polak JF, Mannick JA: Limitations of balloon angioplasty for vein graft stenosis. *J Vasc Surg* 1991; 14:340–345.
95. Zierler RE, Bergelin RO, Isaacson JA, Strandness DE: Natural history of atherosclerotic renal artery stenosis: A prospective study with duplex ultrasonography. *J Vasc Surg* 1994; 19:250–258.
96. Postma CT, Hoefnagels WHL, Barentsz JO, et al: Occlusion of unilateral stenosed renal arteries: Relation to medical treatment. *J Hum Hypertens* 1989; 3:185–190.
97. Kumar S, Mandalam R, Rao VRK, et al: Percutaneous transluminal angioplasty in nonspecific aortoarteritis (Takayasu's disease): Experience of 16 cases. *Cardiovasc Intervent Radiol* 1990; 12:321–325.
98. Svigals PJ, McLean GK, Davis JE, et al: Transient hypertension after percutaneous transluminal renal artery angioplasty. *Radiology* 1986; 161:293–294.
99. Klinge J, Mali WPTM, Puijlaert CBAJ, et al: Percutaneous transluminal renal angioplasty: Initial and long-term results. *Radiology* 1989; 171:501–506.
100. Cambria RP, Brewster DC, Litalien GJ, et al: The durability of different reconstructive techniques for atherosclerotic renal artery disease. *J Vasc Surg* 1994; 20:76–87.
101. Martin LG, Price RB, Casarella WJ, et al: Percutaneous angioplasty in clinical management of renovascular hypertension: Initial and long-term results. *Radiology* 1985; 155:629–633.
102. Miller GA, Ford KK, Braun SD, et al: Percutaneous transluminal angioplasty vs surgery for renovascular hypertension. *Am J Roentgenol* 1985; 144:447–450.
103. Sos TA, Pickering TG, Sniderman K, et al: Percutaneous transluminal renal angioplasty in renovascular hypertension due to atheroma or fibromuscular dysplasia. *N Engl J Med* 1983; 309:274–279.
104. Archibald GR, Beckman CF, Libertino JA: Focal renal artery stenosis caused by fibromuscular dysplasia: Treatment by percutaneous transluminal angioplasty. *Am J Roentgenol* 1988; 151:593–596.
105. Raynaud A, Bedrossian J, Remy P, et al: Percutaneous transluminal angioplasty of renal transplant arterial stenoses. *Am J Roentgenol* 1986; 146:853–857.
106. Fauchald P, Vatne K, Paulsen D, et al: Long-term clinical results of percutaneous transluminal angioplasty in transplant renal artery stenosis. *Nephrol Dial Transplant* 1992; 7:256–259.

107. Benoit G, Moukarzel M, Hiesse C, et al: Transplant renal artery stenosis: Experience and comparative results between surgery and angioplasty. *Transpl Int* 1990; 3:137–140.

108. Matalon TAS, Thompson MJ, Patel SK, et al: Percutaneous transluminal angioplasty for transplant renal artery stenosis. *J Vasc Interv Radiol* 1992; 3:55–58.

109. Madias NE, Kwon OJ, Millan VG: Percutaneous transluminal renal angioplasty: A potentially effective treatment for preservation of renal function. *Arch Intern Med* 1982; 142:693–697.

110. Courthéoux P, Mani J, Mercier V, et al: L'angioplastie endoluminale percutanée des sténoses des artères rénales sur rein considéré comme unique. *Ann Radiol (Paris)* 1988; 31:177–180.

111. Connolly JO, Higgins RM, Walters HL, et al: Presentation, clinical features and outcome in different patterns of atherosclerotic renovascular disease. *Q J Med* 1994; 87:413–421.

112. Boyer L, Ravel A, Boissier A, et al: Percutaneous recanalization of recent renal artery occlusions: Report of 10 cases. *Cardiovasc Intervent Radiol* 1994; 17:258–263.

113. Vitek JJ: Subclavian artery angioplasty and the origin of the vertebral artery. *Radiology* 1989; 170:407–409.

114. Motarjeme A, Keifer JW, Zuska AJ, Nabawi P: Percutaneous transluminal angioplasty for treatment of subclavian steal. *Radiology* 1985; 155:611–613.

115. Millaire A, Trinca M, Marache P, et al: Subclavian angioplasty: Immediate and late results in 50 patients. *Cathet Cardiovasc Diagn* 1993; 29:8–17.

116. Qi JP, Zeitler E: Katheterdilatation der arteriellen Stenosen supraaortaler Gefäße und Spätergebnisse. *Rofo* 1991; 155:357–362.

117. Düber C, Klose KJ, Kopp H, Schmiedt W: Percutaneous transluminal angioplasty for occlusion of the subclavian artery: Short- and long-term results. *Cardiovasc Intervent Radiol* 1992; 15:205–210.

118. Rodriguez-Perez JC, Maynar M, Rams A, et al: Percutaneous transluminal angioplasty as best treatment in stenosis of vascular access for hemodialysis. *Nephron* 1989; 51:192–196.

119. Katzen BT: Technique and results of "low-dose" infusion. *Cardiovasc Intervent Radiol* 1988; 11:S41–S47.

120. Zimmerman JJ, Cipriano PR, Hayden WG, Fogarty TJ: Balloon embolectomy catheter used percutaneously. *Radiology* 1986; 158:260–262.

121. Starck EE, McDermott JC, Crummy AB, et al: Percutaneous aspiration thromboembolectomy. *Radiology* 1985; 156:61–66.

122. Kinnison ML, White RI, Jr, Bowers WP, Dunlap ED: Cost incentives for peripheral angioplasty. *Am J Roentgenol* 1985; 145:1241–1244.

123. Tunis SR, Bass EB, Steinberg EP: The use of angioplasty, bypass surgery, and amputation in the management of peripheral vascular disease. *N Engl J Med* 1991; 325:556–562.

124. Pell JP, Whyman MR, Fowkes FGR, et al: Trends in vascular surgery since the introduction of percutaneous transluminal angioplasty. *Br J Surg* 1994; 81:832–835.

125. Currie IC, Wakeley CJ, Cole SEA, et al: Femoropopliteal angioplasty for severe limb ischaemia. *Br J Surg* 1994; 81:191–193.

126. Jørgensen B, Tønnesen KH, Nielsen JD, et al: Segmentally enclosed thrombolysis in percutaneous transluminal angioplasty for femoropopliteal occlusions: A report from a pilot study. *Cardiovasc Intervent Radiol* 1991; 14:293–298.
127. Snyder SO, Jr, Wheeler JR, Gregory RT, et al: The Kensey catheter: Preliminary results with a transluminal atherectomy tool. *J Vasc Surg* 1988; 8:541–543.
128. Kensey KR, Nash JE, Abrahams C, Zarins CK: Recanalization of obstructed arteries with a flexible, rotating tip catheter. *Radiology* 1987; 165:387–389.
129. Ahn SS, Auth D, Marcus DR, Moore WS: Removal of focal atheromatous lesions by angioscopically guided high-speed atherectomy: Preliminary experimental observations. *J Vasc Surg* 1988; 7:292–300.
130. Palmaz JC: Intravascular stents: Tissue-stent interactions and design considerations. *Am J Roentgenol* 1993; 160:613–618.
131. Strecker EP, Romaniuk P, Schneider B, et al: Perkutan implantierbare, durch ballon aufdehnbare gefäßprothese: Erste klinische ergebnisse. *Dtsch Med Wochenschr* 1988; 113:538–542.
132. Günther RW, Vorwerk D, Bohndorf K, et al: Venous stenoses in dialysis shunts: Treatment with self-expanding metallic stents. *Radiology* 1989; 170:401–405.
133. Marin ML, Veith FJ, Panetta TF, et al: Transluminally placed endovascular stented graft repair for arterial trauma. *J Vasc Surg* 1994; 20:466–473.

11

Local Thrombolytic Infusion

KEY CONCEPTS

1. Local thrombolytic infusion may be equivalent to surgical thrombectomy in many cases of acute embolization or thrombosis, but it has lower mortality and lower serious morbidity.
2. Thrombolysis, combined with balloon angioplasty or surgical revision, can salvage bypass grafts, but long-term results are inferior to those of treated native vessel occlusions, particularly for saphenous vein grafts.
3. Results are best for occlusions shorter than 15 to 25 cm, with a duration of less than 1 week, and with intact runoff.
4. Urokinase has a more predictable effect, higher rates of lysis, and fewer complications than streptokinase.
5. Recombinant-type tissue plasminogen activator (rt-PA) is a powerful lytic agent, effective but also more prone to produce serious bleeding.
6. Whatever the agent used, pulse-spray or higher-rate infusions with rapid catheter advancement can decrease total dose, cost, and sometimes infusion duration.

INTRODUCTION AND INDICATIONS

Acute arterial occlusion from embolization or thrombosis can be approached surgically by thrombectomy or bypass graft placement. When possible, thrombectomy is desirable because the patient's native artery and collateral vessels may be preserved. Thrombectomy, however, is quite dependent on how rapidly the patient reaches the surgeon. Early operation can lead to amputation rates below 5%, but delay of as little as 12 hours increases risk of limb loss to 32%.[1] Use of a Fogarty catheter has produced limb salvage in 62% to 96% of patients, but may be associated with surgical mortality of 17% and complications in 44%.[1,2] Surgery for occluded arterial grafts has an even more dismal prognosis. Thrombectomy and graft revision may have a 6-month limb preservation rate of only 23%.[3]

For these reasons, an effective adjunct or alternative to surgery has been sought. Although systemic administration of thrombolytic (fibrinolytic) drugs has shown benefit in the treatment of severe pulmonary embolism, central venous thrombosis, and acute myocardial infarction, results in the treatment of peripheral arterial occlusion have been disappointing.[4] Moreover, systemic lysis can result in severe bleeding complications.

In 1974, Dotter and colleagues[5] reported the first local arterial infusion of streptokinase. The rationale for the procedure was to deliver a concentrated dose of enzyme to the occlusion while avoiding the hazards of a systemic lytic state. Initial success was low and complications quite frequent, limiting the general acceptance of local thrombolytic infusion. However, refinements in technique of administration, patient selection, and the availability of the newer agents, urokinase and recombinant tissue-type plasminogen activator (rt-PA), have improved clinical results.

Local streptokinase infusion for embolic arterial occlusion is now associated with a 3% amputation rate and 3.5% hospital mortality.[6] In some studies successful lysis combined with surgical revision in graft occlusion has doubled graft patency and limb salvage rates in comparison to surgical treatment alone.[3,7] The experiences of other investigators with longer-term follow-up, however, have not been so positive.[8–10] The only published large-scale randomized study comparing local infusion of urokinase and surgical treatment of acute (less than 1 week in duration) peripheral vascular occlusions has produced some unexpected results. Ouriel and associates found comparable 1-year limb salvage rates and costs of treatment in the 114 patients randomized, but cumulative survival at 1 year was significantly better in the group treated with urokinase— 84% versus 58% in the surgical group.[11] The difference in survival was attributed in large measure to increased cardiopulmonary complications in the operative treatment group.

Thrombolysis is thus an established alternative therapy for acute arterial occlusions of more than just a few hours' duration in patients without immediate danger of limb loss. It is more likely to provide sustained benefit in native vessel occlusions than in thrombosed bypass grafts. Local infusion may also be advised for those with more chronic occlusion who present a high surgical risk. Although the greatest experience with thrombolytic infusion has been in the arteries of the lower extremity, it has also been used for central venous occlusion, hemodialysis access clots, acute upper extremity ischemia, and, in exceptional circumstances, for renal and visceral artery occlusions.[12–23] When necessary, surgery can be safely performed shortly after cessation of infusion of any of the available drugs.

PATIENT SELECTION AND PRECAUTIONS

Contraindications to the use of thrombolytics include active hemorrhage, presence of a bleeding diathesis, recent cerebrovascular accident, craniotomy within the previous 2 months, intracranial tumor, tissue necrosis, and life-threatening ischemia. Patients with motor and sensory paresis are at risk for the revascularization syndrome, which may be fatal.[24] Patients with a compartment syndrome are prone to massive myoglobinuria and should have surgical fasciotomy.[25]

Recent noncranial surgery is only a relative contraindication. Streptokinase has been used less than 3 days after surgery with no wound bleeding.[26] Cardiac or valve thrombi have caused serious complications in isolated cases,[27,28] but in general they have been associated with a surprisingly low incidence of new emboli during thrombolytic therapy.[4]

Prognostic Factors

Older clots are less susceptible to lysis because of the cross-linking of fibrin chains that occurs with time.[29] Data on the dependence of successful lysis with time are conflicting, but there are strong indications that clots or emboli less than 6 weeks old are twice as likely to lyse with directed infusion as older lesions.[6,26,30] Browse and colleagues found that not only were clots less than 1 week old twice as likely to lyse completely as those older than 1 month but also long-term patency of the successfully reopened vessels was substantially better in the group with short-duration occlusions.[31] Others have had a positive response in many chronic occlusions and suggest that thrombolysis be tried in clots up to 6 months of age.[32]

Length of occlusion also has a bearing on response. Recanalization is twice as likely to succeed if an occlusion is less than 10 cm long.[33] A similar effect was noted by Hess and associates[6] in their series of more than 500 patients treated with streptokinase, but better success was noted in lesions up to 25 cm. With the use of rt-PA, length of the occluded segment may have less of an effect on recanalization success.[34] Absence of any visible runoff on initial arteriography makes successful treatment unlikely, but some patients may still benefit from infusion.[35,36]

Monitoring and Patient Care

All persons submitting to thrombolytic infusion should be placed in an intensive care unit for the duration of treatment. Intramuscular injections and arterial punctures must be avoided, and venipunctures kept to a minimum. Patients should be closely watched for signs of fluid overload or renal failure, in addition to bleeding. If streptokinase is used, low-grade fever may be expected.

Laboratory studies to be obtained before onset of therapy include hematocrit, thrombin time (TT), and fibrinogen levels. If heparin is given as a simultaneous infusion, activated partial thromboplastin time (PTT) should also be followed. Fibrinogen and TT are checked at 4 hours and then every 12 hours afterward. A blood sample should be drawn every 4 hours for PTT to allow dosage adjustment of heparin. Changes in fibrinogen and TT indicate a systemic lytic effect. A TT two or three times that of control is considered to be therapeutic, and virtually all patients with local streptokinase infusion have such prolongation by 48 hours of infusion.[26] Lytic therapy should be adjusted if serum fibrinogen falls below 150 mg/dl and stopped if it drops below 100 mg/dl. The need to monitor serum fibrinogen has been controversial.[37] In some reports major hemorrhages and fatalities have occurred without depression of fibrinogen.[9,38] However, significant bleeding complications have tended to arise in those with levels under 150 mg/dl in the experience of others.[11]

AGENTS AND PHARMACOLOGY

One point to be remembered about fibrinolytic agents is that, although they can produce systemic changes in blood coagulation, uninjured vessels do not bleed spontaneously.[29] Thrombolytics drugs attack fibrin plugs, and sites of vascular injury are prone to hemorrhage. All thrombolytic drugs available work by activating the body's endogenous lytic enzyme, plasmin. A systemic lytic state can be reversed by stopping infusion and administering plasma or cryoprecipitate. ε-Aminocaproic acid (Amicar) is a plasmin inhibitor that can also reverse the effects of thrombolysis, but it is potentially dangerous and rarely, if ever, indicated.[39]

Streptokinase

Streptokinase is an indirect plasminogen activator that also has the effect of depleting plasminogen. Because of this plasminogen depression, systemic heparinization is recommended for several days after successful lysis to prevent reocclusion.[39] In systemic doses, streptokinase also depletes fibrinogen and clotting factors V and VIII. Streptokinase has a higher affinity for circulating plasminogen than urokinase or rt-PA and is thus more likely to produce a systemic lytic state.[29] The production of fibrin degradation products (or fibrin split products) is common to all fibrinolytics and can competitively inhibit fibrin polymerization. The plasma half-life of streptokinase is 23 minutes.

Derived from group C β-hemolytic streptococci, streptokinase is antigenic and has been associated with anaphylaxis on rare occasions. Antibodies to streptokinase begin rising several days after exposure, and elevation may persist up to 6 months.[29] Virtually everyone has some antibodies to streptococci, and much of the irregular dose response to systemic streptokinase therapy can be traced to neutralizing antibodies.

Urokinase

Urokinase, unlike streptokinase, is a direct plasminogen activator that allows more predictability of dose response.[40] It depletes the same factors that streptokinase does, although it is more clot-specific and less likely to produce a lytic state. It has a plasma half-life of 16 minutes and, being an endogenous human protein, elicits no immune response.[29] Nevertheless, in the past several years we and many others have observed patients who develop rigors, usually within an hour of bolus administration. No underlying contaminant has been established as the cause of this phenomenon.[41] Fortunately, urokinase-associated rigors, although disconcerting, are limited and generally of no great consequence. When this side effect is encountered, it readily responds to intravenous meperidine.

Lysyl-Plasminogen

Lysyl-plasminogen has been used by French investigators to potentiate the effects of urokinase.[42] It is produced by the proteolysis of native plasminogen, and the resulting enzyme has a higher affinity for fibrin.

Recombinant Tissue-Type Plasminogen Activator

Another endogenous human protein, rt-PA activator is a serine protease produced in quantity by recombinant gene technology.[43] It has very high affinity for fibrin and low affinity for circulating plasminogen. The plasma half-life of this agent is 5 to 8 minutes.[29]

STREPTOKINASE VERSUS UROKINASE

In choosing between these two most commonly employed fibrinolytic agents, one must balance considerations of efficacy, complication rates, previous exposure to streptokinase or high circulating antibodies, and cost. Mean infusion time has been long with successful lysis by streptokinase, up to 120 hours, but urokinase in equivalent low-dose infusions can take nearly as long to produce the desired effect.[40] However, at doses of similar efficacy, streptokinase causes more bleeding and other complications.[30,37,40,44,45] Streptokinase affects fibrinogen levels in most people after just 12 hours of infusion, whereas urokinase does not.

Even so, streptokinase has been used successfully in many cases, and the higher-dose, rapid catheter advancement techniques popular in Europe decrease treatment time considerably.[6,32] Urokinase costs about six times as much as streptokinase.[40]

MODES OF INFUSION

In general, the smallest possible catheter should be used to enter the clot. Katzen prefers an infusable guidewire because it is more readily visible with fluoroscopy and less likely to be coated with thrombus.[18] When possible, placement through an area of reduced flow should be avoided. A sheath or coaxial system can administer a portion of the dose proximally, decreasing the possibility of clot formation on the infusing catheter.

The catheter or guidewire delivering the thrombolytic agent should be embedded in thrombus.[46] Placement in a patent vessel above the occlusion may result in loss of infusate into collateral vessels.

Original Low-Dose Protocols

The first doses tried for local therapy were rather arbitrarily set as 5% to 10% of systemic. For streptokinase, with a systemic loading dose of 250,000 units administered over 30 minutes and infusion at 100,000 units/hour, this dose meant intraarterial infusion at 5000 units/hour in a concentration of 100 units/ml.

Systemic urokinase is given at 4400 units/kg/hour after a bolus of 4400 units/kg (or 308,000 units for the proverbial 70-kg man). The local dose commonly used for low-dose infusion is 20,000 units/hour.

No loading dose is usually given for local lysis because it defeats the purpose of avoiding systemic lytic effects. A loading dose is sometimes given for streptokinase infusions in order to overcome circulating antibodies. With both urokinase and streptokinase, lower-dose infusions often take up to 5 days, and angiography must be repeated every 8 to 12 hours to assess progress and to reposition the catheter. With these protocols not only is hospitalization (especially intensive care monitoring) prolonged but also bleeding complications may be more likely to arise.

Higher-Dose Local Streptokinase

In the protocol used by Hess and colleagues,[6] the infusing catheter is placed immediately above the clot, and three separate doses of 1000 units of streptokinase (dissolved in 2 ml of normal saline) are given at 3-minute intervals. The catheter is then advanced into clot, followed by similar repeated injections and intermittent 1-cm advancement. The final 2 to 3 cm of the occlusion need not be traversed. Any residual nonobstructing thrombus may resolve with the "afterlysis" effect of continued fibrinolysis for some time after infusion ceases. This method may reduce total dose to 20,000 to 30,000 units and keep procedure time under 90 minutes![6] The entire recanalization can be performed without removing the patient from the angiography suite. Local bleeding can be detected and controlled immediately. Such aggressive efforts at fibrinolysis can quickly reveal lesions amenable to balloon angioplasty.[33] Most failures with this protocol are the result of vessel dissection from guidewire and/or catheter manipulation. Such a complication must be addressed by stopping local infusion.

Many Europeans favor the use of streptokinase with this or similar techniques.[35] Urokinase is reserved for those patients with exposure to streptokinase within the previous several months or who otherwise have high antibody levels.

Higher-Dose Local Urokinase

The method of higher-dose urokinase infusion described by McNamara and Fischer in 1985[24] has been widely applied in the United States. The infusing catheter is placed near the obstructing clot, and a straight guidewire is passed as far as possible into the thrombus. Chances for successful lysis are high if a small channel passing completely through the obstruction can be created.[46] Urokinase (500,000 units in 200 ml of saline) is infused directly into the proximal clot at 4000 units/min. Response is checked by arteriography every 2 to 4 hours, with repeat passage of guidewire and further advancement of the catheter as lysis proceeds. With recanalization and restoration of antegrade flow, infusion is slowed to 1000 units/min. For practical considerations, infusions begun late in the day or at night are started at this lower rate, and follow-up arteriography is done the next morning.[47] Infusion is stopped when all clot lyses (an average of 18 hours in their series), and the catheter is removed 1 hour after heparin and urokinase are discontinued.[24] Any necessary anticoagulation can be resumed 12 hours afterward.

If there is distal embolization of clot, the catheter should be advanced to the level undergoing embolization and infusion continued at 4000 units/min. This maximum rate of infusion should not be exceeded because systemic effects of urokinase rapidly become evident.[48] Some have recommended that the catheter be placed through thrombus at the onset and 30,000 to 60,000 units of urokinase injected as a bolus during withdrawal before local infusion into proximal clot is started (Fig. 11-1).[3] Failure to

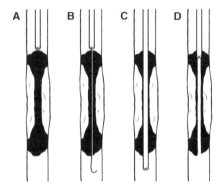

Fig. 11-1 Steps in conventional clot lysis with an endhole catheter. **A,** The catheter is advanced to the level of occlusion. **B,** A guidewire is passed through the clot. **C,** The catheter has been advanced into the vessel lumen distal to the occlusion. Injection of contrast medium at this point confirms position and allows examination of the distal vessels. **D,** The catheter is withdrawn to a position where the tip is just within the thrombus. Local infusion of fibrinolytic enzyme is begun.

see at least 10% lysis of the occluded segment after 500,000 units is an indication to discontinue lytic therapy.

Heparin helps prevent the formation of clot on the infusing catheter (dropping the incidence of this problem from 29% to 4%), but it must be given in doses high enough to cause threefold to fivefold prolongation of the PTT.[24] McNamara and Fischer have not found an increase in bleeding complications from such anticoagulation, although they caution against treating patients on warfarin or through an aortofemoral graft. Doses of heparin that produce a lesser degree of PTT prolongation are not uniformly effective.[44,49] Splitting the infusion between the sideport of a proximal sheath and the distal catheter or open-ended guidewire may also counter clot build-up.[47]

Pulse-Spray Thrombolysis
Tip-occluded multi-sidehole or multislit catheters allow the forceful injection of fibrinolytic agent around the tip-occluding wire by means of a Touhy-Borst adapter (Fig. 11-2). In the pulse-spray technique described by Valji and associates, highly concentrated urokinase (25,000 units/ml) is injected in 0.2-ml aliquots by a tuberculin syringe.[50] The guidewire and catheter are initially passed through the occlusion, and an angiogram is performed to outline the distal vessels. Aliquots are then administered at about 30-second intervals for the first 15 to 20 minutes and then every minute thereafter. Early in the treatment, injection into the most distal 1 cm of thrombus is avoided in order to minimize the risk of distal embolization.

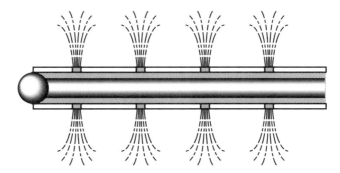

Fig. 11-2 Longitudinal section of tip-occluded pulse-spray catheter. The occluding wire tip prevents injection through the catheter endhole and forces the fluid to spray through the sideholes.

Flow is usually restored in 30 to 60 minutes, and in many cases complete lysis occurs by 90 minutes. If small defects are present that do not change within an hour of further treatment ("lytic stagnation"), the procedure is terminated.[51] If more major defects remain, overnight conventional continuous urokinase infusion may be pursued. Because some investigators maintain the need to resolve all evident thrombus to prevent early reocclusion, they perform overnight infusions routinely.[52,53]

Recombinant Tissue-Type Plasminogen Activator
Recombinant tissue-type plasminogen activator is still undergoing clinical investigation in peripheral vascular occlusions, but it may be administered intraarterially at the rate of 0.05 mg/kg/hour. This dose has been reported to be as effective and as safe as infusion of 0.1 mg/kg/hour.[43] Still, rt-PA given at similar rates has been associated with more bleeding complications than urokinase treatment.[54] Because of its potency, rt-PA may be more likely to produce fatal intracranial hemorrhage, and some would caution against the concomitant use of aspirin and rt-PA.[9] In Europe, Hess's intermittent catheter-advancement technique has been adapted for rt-PA. The dose typically administered in such a regimen, 5 mg over a 2-hour period, has not produced significant bleeding.[34,55]

RESULTS

Published results of local thrombolytic infusion are difficult to compare because of differences in patient selection, agent and technique used, adjunctive surgery or percutaneous angioplasty, definitions of success, and clinical follow-up. Care must be taken to discount those reports with only short-term follow-up (such as defining clinical success by patency or relief of symptoms at 30 days). High rates of early lysis and technical success may be offset by reocclusion and possible limb loss within 6 to 12 months. Strict adherence to reporting standards in future publications may make the medical literature easier to interpret with regard to thrombolysis and other vascular procedures.[56] With these caveats, certain trends are evident.

Emboli and in situ thrombi lyse with about equal success, but if the reopened vessel stays patent for 2 weeks, 5-year patency is about 90% for emboli but only 59% for thrombosis associated with a preexisting lesion.[6] Ouriel and associates also noted better long-term outcomes in patients treated for peripheral emboli.[11] McNamara has observed that emboli may need infusion for nearly twice as long as thrombi.[48]

Surgical or endovascular correction of underlying stenosis is needed in many (if not most) who undergo successful lysis. For nonembolic occlusions, failing to find an underlying correctable lesion is actually a poor prognostic sign.[8,46] Long-term patency of a vessel and relief of symptoms without a *major* surgical intervention are reasonable outcome criteria for judging results.

Early Success
Most series with standard low-dose streptokinase treatment have reported partial or complete lysis in 50% to 56% of cases.[6,14,22,26] Others have had a greater degree of success with the low-dose streptokinase protocol, perhaps related to patient selection.[31,57,58] The more rapid infusions with streptokinase have been successful in restoring circulation in 71% to 77% of patients.[33,35,59]

The higher-dose urokinase methods of infusion have produced lysis in 70% to 95% of cases, and lysis has been complete more often than with streptokinase.* However, one investigation comparing low and high rates of urokinase infusion (50,000 units/hour versus 250,000 units/hour) found no improvement in recanalization rates with the higher doses, and complications were significantly increased.[61] Others have not had very gratifying results with higher-dose urokinase.[8] Smith and associates report a positive early clinical outcome in only 52% of the native vessels treated.[38]

Pulse-spray and rapid catheter advancement techniques using urokinase or rt-PA have achieved high degrees of early recanalization.[34,50,53,55] However, Kandarpa and colleagues compared pulse-spray and conventional infusion in 25 patients, and they found no difference in positive clinical outcome at 30 days (64% for the entire group).[52] Similar observations have been made in comparing rapid catheter advancement protocols and overnight infusions.[62]

*References 10, 11, 18, 24, 36, 42, 44, 60.

Long-Term Results

Two-year patency of reopened vessels has been reported as 64%, but the balloon dilatation treatment of suitable underlying lesions may improve long-term patency to 82%, a number comparable to that obtained with successful surgical thrombectomy.[33,35] However, when one includes the early treatment failures (analyzing on an "intent to treat" basis), the figures are not nearly so impressive. Browse and associates found a strong correlation between duration of symptoms at the time of presentation and 1-year patency; 50% of all patients treated for occlusions of 1 week's duration or less had patent vessels at 1 year versus only 15% of those treated for longer-standing occlusions.[31] Iliac arteries are more likely to stay open than more distal vessels, and the best predictor of reocclusion is the presence of a residual uncorrected flow-limiting lesion.[63]

Arterial Bypass Grafts

Technical success rates are as high for reopening occluded grafts as they are for native vessels.[8,10,31,60–62] The presence of a "stump" at the proximal end of an occluded graft may have positive prognostic significance, and it is certainly helpful in guiding catheterization of the clot.[18] No substantial differences in early response between autologous vein grafts and bypasses of synthetic material have been found by most authors.[37,64] Ouriel and colleagues, however, could recanalize only 55% of vein grafts, compared to 80% of the synthetic conduits treated.[46] Both initial lysis and long-term patency tend to be better in aortoiliac or aortofemoral grafts.[8,63,64] Faggioli and associates reported 92% patency at 18 months for suprainguinal grafts successfully lysed with subsequent PTA or surgical correction of underlying lesions, compared to 40% patency in similarly treated infrainguinal grafts.[8] Below-knee synthetic grafts have a particularly dismal outcome. The 1-year patency of less than 20%, nevertheless, is similar to that of surgical revision.[9] As in native arterial occlusions, ultimate results of thrombolysis are improved substantially if an underlying lesion responsible for graft occlusion is found and treated.[3,37]

Dialysis Access

Standard low-dose thrombolytic therapy for clotted dialysis fistulae or grafts has been disappointing.[14,65] However, Davis and colleagues[15] have developed a more intensive technique using crossed catheters "lacing" thrombus with urokinase. They have managed to lyse thrombus in 90% of the grafts treated, and 62% of their patients have avoided surgical revision for at least 6 months. Equally good results have been reported by Beathard, who used a similar pulse-spray technique with heparinized saline alone (see Chapter 9 entitled Dialysis Access, Central Venous Catheters, and Other Central Venous Problems).[66]

Venous Occlusions

Superior vena caval, subclavian, and axillary vein occlusions have been treated with varying success. Some investigators have reported good results for both primary and secondary thromboses in subclavian veins, but experience is limited (see Chapter 9 entitled Dialysis Access, Central Venous Catheters, and Other Central Venous Problems).[13,14,26,67,68] Other central venous infusions have successfully treated patients with occlusion of the iliac veins and inferior vena cava, as well as transplant renal vein occlusion.[12,20] Vascular stents have been placed after thrombolysis in some central veins.[12]

Other Vessels

Isolated cases of superior mesenteric artery embolus have been successfully treated by local infusion of streptokinase.[21,22] Thrombolytic therapy may be instituted only in the absence of bowel necrosis; otherwise, the patient should be taken immediately to surgery.

Renal artery occlusions have lysed up to 10 days after thrombosis, and 67% of patients treated have had perfusion reestablished.[18,19] Thrombolysis has produced benefit to patients with acute hand ischemia comparable to that seen in lower extremity clots.[16,17] If the infusing catheter is placed from a femoral artery, the potential for cerebral embolization from catheter-associated thrombus must be kept in mind.[17]

COMPLICATIONS

Potential complications of local thrombolytic infusion include hemorrhage, synthetic graft permeation, distal embolization, new thrombus arising on the infusion catheter, limb loss, sepsis, and death. Fortunately, most serious complications are related to hemorrhage and respond to transfusion or surgical evacuation of hematoma.

Bleeding has been more common with streptokinase in prolonged, low-dose infusions. Major hemorrhage has been described in 7% to 32% of patients, with most such series reporting in the 12% to 17% range.* Protocols using more rapid infusion of streptokinase have dropped the incidence of severe bleeding to 2% to 4%.[6,32] In comparison, transfusion or other intervention for hemorrhage has been necessary in 3% to 11% of patients treated with higher-dose local urokinase.†

Distal macroembolization or microembolization is not rare but in most cases resolves with further thrombolysis. Rates of clinical embolization cited have been fairly uniform, from 11% to 14%.[6,22,24,32,69] Severe limb

---

*References 3, 14, 22, 25, 26, 45.
†References 3, 11, 18, 24, 30, 42, 45.

deterioration has been reported in only 2% of local infusions in one multi-center review, but whenever this complication arises immediate surgery is warranted.[69]

Isolated reported deaths have been due to retroperitoneal hemorrhage or myocardial infarction.[25,30] Fatal intracranial hemorrhage does occur with urokinase protocols,[8,11] but it appears to be a greater threat with rt-PA.[9,62] Up to 15% hospital mortality may be seen, but many deaths are attributable to other concomitant severe disease.[46,49] It is rare that limb loss is directly due to choice of thrombolysis for therapy. Most of those undergoing amputation may have been expected to have the same outcome with surgical thrombectomy.

NEW DIRECTIONS AND MECHANICAL ALTERNATIVES

Despite the benefits of local thrombolytic infusion, it is clear that treatment must be made safer, more effective, less labor-intensive, and less expensive in order to gain wide acceptance in the treatment of vascular occlusion. Pulse-spray and rapid catheter advancement methods have not completely fulfilled their initial promise, although the total dose of enzyme needed to reopen a vessel may be decreased. The addition of ultrasound energy during infusion may enhance lysis.[70] A major challenge is prevention of reocclusion, for the early benefits of many thrombolytic procedures disappear within weeks to months.

There are alternatives to enzymatic clot lysis and surgical revascularization. Percutaneous aspiration embolectomy represents a reasonable alternative for acute emboli with good long-term limb salvage and low mortality.[71] Technical improvements, such as the corkscrew wire for rotational aspiration thromboembolectomy and an expanding "tulip" sheath, may enhance application of this technique.[71,72] Other lines of investigation center on percutaneous thrombectomy catheters employing saline jets or coweled "impellers."[73,74] Concerns about distal embolization and hemolysis remain to be resolved before such devices can be applied clinically. Nevertheless, such catheters have the potential to "debulk" occlusions, either replacing local catheter infusions or shortening the duration of any ancillary infusions.

REFERENCES

1. Johnson JA, Cogbill TH, Strutt PJ: Late results after femoral artery embolectomy. *Surgery* 1988; 103:289–293.
2. Genton E, Clagett GP, Salzman EW: Antithrombotic therapy in peripheral vascular disease. *Chest* 1986; 89:75–81.
3. Koltun WA, Gardiner GA, Jr, Harrington DP, et al: Thrombolysis in the treatment of peripheral arterial vascular occlusions. *Arch Surg* 1987; 122:901–905.

4. Marder VJ, Sherry S: Thrombolytic therapy: Current status (part 2). *N Engl J Med* 1988; 318:1585–1595.
5. Dotter CT, Rösch J, Seaman AJ: Selective clot lysis with low-dose streptokinase. *Radiology* 1974; 111:31–37.
6. Hess H, Mietaschk A, Brückl R: Peripheral arterial occlusions: A 6-year experience with local low-dose thrombolytic therapy. *Radiology* 1987; 163:753–758.
7. Graor RA, Risius B, Young JR, et al: Thrombolysis of peripheral arterial bypass grafts: Surgical thrombectomy compared with thrombolysis. *J Vasc Surg* 1988; 7:347–355.
8. Faggioli GL, Peer RM, Pedrini L, et al: Failure of thrombolytic therapy to improve long-term vascular patency. *J Vasc Surg* 1994; 19:289–296.
9. Lacroix H, Suy R, Verheyen L, et al: Local thrombolysis for occluded arterial grafts: Is the yield worth the effort? *J Cardiovasc Surg (Torino)* 1994; 35:187–191.
10. Parent FN, Piotrowski JJ, Bernhard VM, et al: Outcome of intraarterial urokinase for acute vascular occlusion. *J Cardiovasc Surg (Torino)* 1991; 32:680–690.
11. Ouriel K, Shortell CK, Deweese JA, et al: A comparison of thrombolytic therapy with operative revascularization in the initial treatment of acute peripheral arterial ischemia. *J Vasc Surg* 1994; 19:1021–1030.
12. Semba CP, Dake MD: Iliofemoral deep venous thrombosis: Aggressive therapy with catheter-directed thrombolysis. *Radiology* 1994; 191:487–494.
13. Druy EM, Trout HH, Giordano JM, Hix WR: Lytic therapy in the treatment of axillary and subclavian vein thrombosis. *J Vasc Surg* 1985; 2:821–827.
14. Becker GJ, Rabe FE, Richmond BD, et al: Low-dose fibrinolytic therapy: Results and new concepts. *Radiology* 1983; 148:663–670.
15. Davis GB, Dowd CF, Bookstein JJ, et al: Thrombosed dialysis grafts: Efficacy of intrathrombotic deposition of concentrated urokinase, clot maceration, and angioplasty. *Am J Roentgenol* 1987; 149:177–181.
16. Widlus DM, Venbrux AC, Benenati JF, et al: Fibrinolytic therapy for upper-extremity arterial occlusions. *Radiology* 1990; 175:393–399.
17. Coulon M, Goffette P, Dondelinger RF: Local thrombolytic infusion in arterial ischemia of the upper limb: Mid-term results. *Cardiovasc Intervent Radiol* 1994; 17:81–86.
18. Katzen BT: Technique and results of "low-dose" infusion. *Cardiovasc Intervent Radiol* 1988; 11:S41–S47.
19. Morag B, Rubinstein Z, Schneiderman J: Renal artery occlusion: Intra-arterial thrombolytic therapy. *J Intervent Radiol* 1988; 3:77–80.
20. Robinson JM, Cockrell CH, Tisnado J, et al: Selective low-dose streptokinase infusion in the treatment of acute transplant renal vein thrombosis. *Cardiovasc Intervent Radiol* 1986; 9:86–89.
21. Vujic I, Stanley J, Gobien RP: Treatment of acute embolus of the superior mesenteric artery by topical infusion of streptokinase. *Cardiovasc Intervent Radiol* 1984; 7:94–96.
22. Kakkasseril JS, Cranley JJ, Arbaugh JJ, et al: Efficacy of low-dose streptokinase in acute arterial occlusion and graft thrombosis. *Arch Surg* 1985; 120:427–429.
23. Yankes JR, Uglietta JP, Grant J, Braun SD: Percutaneous transhepatic recanalization and thrombolysis of the superior mesenteric vein. *Am J Roentgenol* 1988; 151:289–290.

24. McNamara TO, Fischer JR: Thrombolysis of peripheral arterial and graft occlusions: Improved results using high-dose urokinase. *Am J Roentgenol* 1985; 144:769–775.
25. Lang EK: Streptokinase therapy: Complications of intra-arterial use. *Radiology* 1985; 154:75–77.
26. Risius B, Zelch MG, Graor RA, et al: Catheter-directed low dose streptokinase infusion: A preliminary experience. *Radiology* 1984; 150:349–355.
27. Brewer ML, Kinnison ML, Perler BA, White RI, Jr: Blue toe syndrome: Treatment with anticoagulants and delayed percutaneous transluminal angioplasty. *Radiology* 1988; 166:31–36.
28. Paulson EK, Miller FJ: Embolization of cardiac mural thrombus: Complication of intraarterial fibrinolysis. *Radiology* 1988; 168:95–96.
29. Marder VJ, Sherry S: Thrombolytic therapy: Current status (part 1). *N Engl J Med* 1988; 318:1512–1520.
30. Grabenwöger F, Dock W, Appel W, Pinterits F: Fibrinolysetherapie thromboembolischer gefäßverschlüsse: Primäre erfolgsrate und langzeitergebnisse. *Rofo* 1988; 148:615–618.
31. Browse DJ, Torrie EPH, Galland RB: Early results and 1-year follow-up after intraarterial thrombolysis. *Br J Surg* 1993; 80:194–197.
32. Lammer J, Pilger E, Justich E, et al: Fibrinolysis in chronic arteriosclerotic occlusions: Intrathrombotic injections of streptokinase. *Radiology* 1985; 157:45–50.
33. Wilms GE, Verhaeghe RH, Pouillon MM, et al: Local thrombolysis in femoropopliteal occlusion: Early and late results. *Cardiovasc Intervent Radiol* 1987; 10:272–275.
34. Spengel FA, Küffer G, Stiegler H: Efficacy and tolerance of recombinant tissue-type plasminogen activator in patients with thrombotic or embolic occlusions of leg-arteries. *Clin Investig* 1993; 71:323–326.
35. Do-dai-Do, Mahler F, Triller J, Nachbur B: Combination of short- and long-term catheter thrombolysis for peripheral arterial occlusion. *Eur J Radiol* 1987; 7:235–238.
36. LeBlang SD, Becker GJ, Benenati JF, et al: Low-dose urokinase regimen for the treatment of lower extremity arterial and graft occlusions: Experience in 132 cases. *J Vasc Interv Radiol* 1992; 3:475–483.
37. Gardiner GA, Jr, Harrington DP, Koltun W, et al: Salvage of occluded arterial bypass grafts by means of thrombolysis. *J Vasc Surg* 1989; 9:426–431.
38. Smith CM, Yellin AE, Weaver FA, et al: Thrombolytic therapy for arterial occlusion: A mixed blessing. *Am Surg* 1994; 60:371–375.
39. Bookstein JJ, Moser KM, Hougie C: Coagulative interventions during angiography. *Cardiovasc Intervent Radiol* 1982; 5:46–56.
40. Belkin M, Belkin B, Bucknam CA, et al: Intra-arterial fibrinolytic therapy: Efficacy of streptokinase vs urokinase. *Arch Surg* 1986; 121:769–773.
41. Matsumoto AH, Selby JB, Tegtmeyer CJ, et al: Recent development of rigors during infusion of urokinase: Is it related to an endotoxin? *J Vasc Interv Radiol* 1994; 5:433–438.
42. Pernes JM, Vitoux JF, Brenoit P, et al: Acute peripheral arterial and graft occlusion: Treatment with selective infusion of urokinase and lysyl plasminogen. *Radiology* 1986; 158:481–485.

43. Risius B, Graor RA, Geisinger MA, et al: Thrombolytic therapy with recombinant human tissue-type plasminogen activator: A comparison of two doses. *Radiology* 1987; 164:465–468.
44. Traughber PD, Cook PS, Micklos TJ, Miller FJ: Intraarterial fibrinolytic therapy for popliteal and tibial artery obstruction: Comparison of streptokinase and urokinase. *Am J Roentgenol* 1987; 149:453–456.
45. Gardiner GA, Jr, Koltun W, Kandarpa K, et al: Thrombolysis of occluded femoropopliteal grafts. *Am J Roentgenol* 1986; 147:621–626.
46. Ouriel K, Shortell CK, Azodo MVU, et al: Acute peripheral arterial occlusion: Predictors of success in catheter-directed thrombolytic therapy. *Radiology* 1994; 193:561–566.
47. McNamara TO: The use of lytic therapy with endovascular "repair" of the failed infrainguinal graft. *Semin Vasc Surg* 1990; 3:59–65.
48. McNamara T: Technique and results of "higher-dose" infusion. *Cardiovasc Intervent Radiol* 1988; 11:S48–S57.
49. Fiessinger J-N, Vitoux J-F, Pernes J-M, et al: Complications of intraarterial urokinase-lys-plasminogen infusion therapy in arterial ischemia of lower limbs. *Am J Roentgenol* 1986; 146:157–159.
50. Valji K, Roberts AC, Davis GB, Bookstein JJ: Pulse-spray thrombolysis of arterial and bypass graft occlusions. *Am J Roentgenol* 1991; 156:617–621.
51. Valji K, Bookstein JJ, Roberts AC, Sanchez RB: Occluded peripheral arteries and bypass grafts: Lytic stagnation as an end point for pulse-spray pharmaco-mechanical thrombolysis. *Radiology* 1993; 188:389–394.
52. Kandarpa K, Chopra PS, Aruny JE, et al: Intraarterial thrombolysis of lower extremity occlusions: Prospective, randomized comparison of forced periodic infusion and conventional slow continuous infusion. *Radiology* 1993; 188:861–867.
53. Yusuf SW, Whitaker SC, Gregson RHS, et al: Experience with pulse-spray technique in peripheral thrombolysis. *Eur J Vasc Surg* 1994; 8:270–275.
54. Meyerovitz MF, Goldhaber SZ, Reagan K, et al: Recombinant tissue-type plasminogen activator versus urokinase in peripheral arterial and graft occlusions: A randomized trial. *Radiology* 1990; 175:75–78.
55. Krause F-J, Endsin O: Lokale Katheterlyse der Femoralarterie: rt-PA versus Urokinase. *Rofo* 1993; 158:46–48.
56. Rutherford RB, Becker GJ: Standards for evaluating and reporting the results of surgical and percutaneous therapy for peripheral vascular disease. *J Vasc Interv Radiol* 1991; 2:169–174.
57. LeBolt SA, Tisnado J, Cho S-R: Treatment of peripheral arterial obstruction with streptokinase: Results in arterial vs graft occlusions. *Am J Roentgenol* 1988; 151:589–592.
58. Katzen BT, VanBreda A: Low dose streptokinase in the treatment of arterial occlusions. *Am J Roentgenol* 1981; 136:1171–1178.
59. Delcour C, Bellens B, Vandenbosch G, et al: Long-term follow-up of intraarterial infusion of streptokinase in acute lower limb ischemia. *Vasc Surg* 1987; 21:339–343.
60. Clouse ME, Stokes KR, Perry LJ, Wheeler HG: Percutaneous intraarterial thrombolysis: Analysis of factors affecting outcome. *J Vasc Interv Radiol* 1994; 5:93–100.

61. Cragg AH, Smith TP, Corson JD, et al: Two urokinase dose regimens in native arterial and graft occlusions: Initial results of a prospective, randomized clinical trial. *Radiology* 1991; 178:681–686.
62. Zwaan M, Rinast E, Kummer-Kloess D, et al: Thrombotische und thromboembolische Beinarterien- und Bypassverschlüsse: Kurzzeit- versus Langzeitlyse. *Rofo* 1993; 158:536–541.
63. McNamara TO, Bomberger RA: Factors affecting initial and 6 month patency rates after intraarterial thrombolysis with high dose urokinase. *Am J Surg* 1986; 152:709–712.
64. Pratesi C, Michelagnoli S, Pulli R, et al: Late graft occlusion: Thrombolytic treatment. *Vasc Surg* 1991; 25:708–718.
65. Young AT, Hunter DW, Castañeda-Zuñiga WR, et al: Thrombosed synthetic hemodialysis access fistulas: Failure of fibrinolytic therapy. *Radiology* 1985; 154:639–642.
66. Beathard GA: Mechanical versus pharmacomechanical thrombolysis for the treatment of thrombosed dialysis access grafts. *Kidney Int* 1994; 45:1401–1406.
67. Fankuchen EI, Neff RA, Collins RA, et al: Urokinase infusion for axillary-subclavian vein thrombosis. *Cardiovasc Intervent Radiol* 1984; 7:90–93.
68. Fraschini G, Jadeja J, Lawson M, et al: Local infusion of urokinase for the lysis of thrombosis associated with permanent central venous catheters in cancer patients. *J Clin Oncol* 1987; 5:672–678.
69. Galland RB, Earnshaw JJ, Baird RN, et al: Acute limb deterioration during intraarterial thrombolysis. *Br J Surg* 1993; 80:1118–1120.
70. Lauer CG, Burge R, Tang DB, et al: Effect of ultrasound on tissue-type plasminogen activator induced thrombolysis. *Circulation* 1992; 86:1257–1264.
71. Wagner H-J, Starck EE, Reuter P: Long-term results of percutaneous aspiration embolectomy. *Cardiovasc Intervent Radiol* 1994; 17:241–246.
72. Vorwerk D, Günther RW, Clerk C, et al: Percutaneous embolectomy: In vitro investigations of the self-expanding tulip sheath. *Radiology* 1992; 182:415–418.
73. Drasler WJ, Jenson ML, Wilson GJ, et al: Rheolytic catheter for percutaneous removal of thrombus. *Radiology* 1992; 182:263–267.
74. Tadavarthy SM, Murray PD, Inampudi S, et al: Mechanical thrombectomy with the Amplatz device: Human experience. *J Vasc Interv Radiol* 1994; 5:715–724.

12

Embolotherapy

KEY CONCEPTS

1. Embolization can be used for control of bleeding, closing of arteriovenous malformations or fistulae, tumor palliation, organ ablation, and treatment of varicocele.
2. Choice of agent depends on the size of the vessel to be occluded, desirability of infarction, permanency of occlusion, and ease of catheter placement.
3. Knowledge of vascular anatomy, variations, and collateral vessels is essential for the prevention of complications.
4. The postembolization syndrome of fever, pain, and leukocytosis may last for several days, and soft tissue gas is often present.
5. Antibiotics are absolutely necessary for splenic embolization.

INDICATIONS

The most widely accepted indication for percutaneous transcatheter embolization is treatment of hemorrhage from trauma or unresectable neoplasm. In cases of pelvic injury involving extensive fractures, surgery is largely ineffective for controlling bleeding, and embolization can be a lifesaving procedure.[1-3] Other situations for which embolotherapy offers distinct advantages over surgery include uncontrollable gastric bleeding, arterial hemorrhage due to pancreatitis, and unremitting hemobilia.[4-8]

In bowel with limited collateral circulation, such as the colon and small bowel, embolization can control massive bleeding as a temporizing measure. Operative mortality is greatly decreased if a patient can undergo transfusion and be stabilized prior to surgery.[9] Embolotherapy eliminates the need for exploration in some cases, but it must be anticipated that bowel ischemia may result.[10,11] Although bleeding from gastric and esophageal varices has been aggressively treated by percutaneous transhepatic occlusive interventions, results have been almost uniformly disappointing.[12-14] Esophageal sclerotherapy is presently the preferred method of controlling acute variceal hemorrhage. Transjugular intrahepatic portosystemic shunt (TIPS) placement has become a widely accepted practice for prevention of recurrent variceal bleeding. Transcatheter embolization is often combined with TIPS through the access to the varices provided by the shunt. However, if the post-TIPS portosystemic gradient is low enough, embolization is usually unnecessary.

Catheter embolization has been effective in controlling massive hemoptysis due to tuberculosis, sarcoidosis, or other inflammatory disease.[15] It is also a primary treatment for pulmonary arteriovenous malformations (AVMs), which are dangerous even when asymptomatic.[16] Traumatic AV fistulae can be occluded, and AVMs can be palliated by embolotherapy alone or in conjunction with surgery.[17-20]

Embolization for neoplasm can alleviate the symptoms of those with metastatic islet cell or other secreting endocrine tumors, prolong life in patients with unresectable primary or metastatic hepatic malignancies, and relieve intractable pain.[21-27] It can also be employed preoperatively to diminish blood loss in very vascular renal, osseous, or other tumors undergoing resection.[28] Embolization has been effective in treating painful aneurysmal bone cysts and giant cell tumors not amenable to resection.[29]

Other indications for which embolotherapy has been used successfully include hypersplenism, recurrent hyperparathyroidism from mediastinal adenomas, malignant hypertension or nephrotic syndrome in end-stage renal disease, priapism, and varicocele.[30-34] When surgery has been difficult or impossible, percutaneous techniques have been employed to occlude aneurysms and pseudoaneurysms.[35-37]

Over the years, interventional radiologists have learned the hazards and limitations of embolotherapy. At the same time, however, experience gained has stimulated the continued development of new embolic agents, delivery systems, and applications.

BEFORE PROCEEDING

Therapeutic Goals and Choice of Materials

Before therapeutic embolization is attempted for an individual patient, the objectives should be clearly defined. The interventional radiologist must determine the level and permanency of vascular occlusion needed and the materials most appropriate to the situation at hand (Table 12-1).

For traumatic hemorrhage the aim of embolization is not to cause tissue infarction but rather to diminish perfusion to the point that endogenous hemostatic mechanisms stop the bleeding. On the one hand, too distal an occlusion, such as that produced by powders, microspheres, or polymerizing fluids, can produce necrosis and major complications. On the other hand, large particles, when used alone, may occlude a vessel feeding the site of

Table 12-1   Materials for Transcatheter Vascular Occlusion

Category	Arteriolar/Precapillary Occlusion	Duration of Occlusion	Inflammatory Response
Particulates			
Autologous clot	–	Hours	None
Surgical gelatin (Gelfoam)	+ (powder)	Days to weeks	Moderate
Oxidized cellulose (Oxycel)	–	Days to weeks	Moderate
Microfibrillar collagen (Avitene)	+	Days to weeks	?
Polyvinyl alcohol (Ivalon)	+ (powder)	Permanent	Minimal
Silicone spheres	+	Permanent	None
Mechanical			
Steel coils with fiber	–	Permanent	Dependent on fiber
Steel "spiders"	–	Permanent	None?
Detachable balloons	–	Permanent	Minimal
Polymerizing Fluids			
Isobutyl-2-cyanoacrylate (Bucrylate)*	+/–†	Permanent	Long-term effects Controversial
Silicone rubber*	+	Permanent	Minimal
Polyurethane*	+	Permanent	Severe
Other			
Absolute ethanol	+	Permanent	Minimal

*Investigational.
†Level of occlusion depends on amount injected and mode of delivery.
From Wojtowycz M, Miller FJ: *Semin Intervent Radiol* 1984; 1:2; with permission.

extravasation centrally, only to permit the hemorrhage to continue through collateral vessels (a problem common to surgical ligation). As a matter of principle, the agent used should be deposited as selectively and as close to the site of bleeding as possible. The embolizing particles should be appropriate to the size of vessel injured. A nonpermanent material such as gelatin sponge (Gelfoam) is preferable. Ideally, the vessel should be occluded long enough to provide healing, but it should eventually recanalize and provide optimal tissue perfusion for the long term. For example, a man treated for pelvic trauma by bilateral hypogastric artery embolization may suffer erectile dysfunction as a result.[2] Such risks can be minimized (but not eliminated) by knowledge of materials available and by careful attention to technique.

For unresectable malignant neoplasms, complete tissue ablation is usually the goal, although rarely attained in practice. Depending on the organ involved, embolization with small, permanent particles can be used to prevent tumor viability from being maintained by collateral vessels. In hepatic tumors it is unwise to place coils or other large permanent particles in the proper hepatic artery. Repeat embolotherapy may be rendered much more difficult, if not impossible, as a result. Absolute ethanol is extremely toxic, but its careful application in cases of renal cell carcinoma can occasionally produce complete tumor necrosis and clinical remission.[38]

High-flow AV fistulae are best occluded with large, permanent devices, such as detachable balloons, metallic "spiders," or coils.[8,17,39] In contrast, AVMs in an extremity typically have multiple feeding arteries. Occlusion of large vessels leads to recurrence, often through myriad collateral vessels. Lasting palliation requires obliteration of the "nidus" at the core of most AVMs, and small permanent particles, tissue adhesives, and sclerosing agents produce the best results.[19,20] Judicious application of alcohol may also be effective,[40] and it may be considered the treatment of choice in symptomatic cavernous hemangiomas of the extremities. A more detailed discussion of specific pathologic and anatomic considerations for various indications can be found later in this chapter.

Postembolization Syndrome
When tumor or other tissue necrosis takes place, both physician and patient should be aware of its expected consequences. The postembolization syndrome (PES) consists of pain, fever, leukocytosis, nausea, and vomiting.[22,23,41] Symptoms arise shortly after embolotherapy, and usually resolve within 3 days, but may persist up to 1 week. Leukocytosis may be marked. Only close clinical observation and use of blood cultures can distinguish PES from a complicating infection. Generally, pain can be controlled with intravenous or oral analgesics. Patient-controlled analgesia intravenous pumps should be ordered for those whose embolizations are likely to produce severe pain, such as hepatic or renal tumors.

A potentially confusing finding after embolization is the presence of gas in the infarcted soft tissues; sometimes even pneumoperitoneum can be seen. The origin of this gas has been debated. Although some microbubbles are injected during every procedure, particularly when porous materials (gelatin sponge or polyvinyl alcohol) are used, most of the gas evidently arises from the necrotic tissue itself.[38,42,43] Precisely because of devascularization of the affected tissues, gas resorption may take several weeks.

Staged Procedures

Complications and patient discomfort may be reduced by performing therapeutic embolization in stages. In many cases, diagnostic angiography should be performed separately in order to reduce the duration of a given procedure and the amount of contrast medium administered at one time. For multiple lesions, particularly pulmonary AVMs or hepatic tumors, or for large pelvic or extremity AVMs, staged embolizations are preferable.[16,22,23,40]

Potential Complications

Complications of embolization include infection and undesired ischemia and/or infarction, in addition to the host of problems that can arise from angiography alone, such as hemorrhage at the puncture site, acute renal failure, and anaphylactic shock.[44,45] The incidence of complications is dependent on many factors. Experience of the operators, general condition of the patient, lesion treated, choice of materials, and anatomic variants all contribute to outcome. As in any procedure, the patient should be fully informed of potential adverse effects before consent is obtained.

An absolutely essential prerequisite for all occlusive interventions is high-resolution, high-quality diagnostic angiography. The vessels feeding the lesion to be treated must be identified. Large AV communications must be recognized. Anatomy and possible variants must be well understood, and potential problems identified, before embolization is undertaken. If a kidney is to undergo embolization with ethanol, careful attention should be paid to the location of adrenal and gonadal branches of the renal artery.[32] In bronchial artery embolization for hemoptysis, anterior spinal branches must be identified to prevent the disastrous complication of paraplegia.[15] Complications specific to particular lesions, organs, and embolic materials are addressed as these items are discussed.

Use of Antibiotics

Antibiotics have not been given routinely prior to embolotherapy for most indications, but they are indispensable for certain situations. Partial splenic ablation, in particular, demands administration of broad-spectrum antibiotics and strict attention to aseptic technique to prevent splenic abscess formation.[30,45] Renal abscess can arise if an embolized kidney is associated with stones or an untreated urinary tract infection.[41] Recent reports indicate that unrecognized bacteremia occurs in many angiographic interventions, and sepsis is a leading cause of death directly attributable to therapeutic embolization.[45,46] For this reason, patients treated for hepatic neoplasms should routinely receive preprocedural parenteral antibiotics.[45]

MATERIALS AND METHODS

Delivery Systems

In virtually any embolic intervention it is advisable to use a vascular sheath. Particles and tissue adhesives may jam or occlude a catheter, and a sheath allows its easy replacement. Administering catheters should not contain sideholes. Greater control is afforded by injection through an endhole catheter, and the possibility of unrecognized particles lodging within a sidehole, with subsequent unintended embolization, can be avoided. When its selective placement is possible, an occlusion balloon catheter adds a margin of safety.[32,47] Not only is reflux prevented but also the degree of devascularization can also be considerably enhanced.

Coaxial catheter systems have been developed for superselective angiography and vessel occlusion. One that offers distinct advantages over previous designs is the Tracker (Target Therapeutics, Los Angeles).[19,48] It is a semirigid, 3 Fr polyethylene catheter tapered to a softer 2.7 Fr tip, easily passed through standard selective catheters, and it has great flexibility while retaining a good degree of torque control. A radiopaque marker at the end of the Tracker makes it readily visible; without a marker, small catheters can be very difficult to see on even the highest-resolution fluoroscopic monitors. The Tracker is capable of delivering small particles of gelatin sponge or polyvinyl alcohol, tissue adhesives, and fluids. Other manufacturers are now producing catheters with similar characteristics.

Flow-directed catheters, such as the Kerber calibrated-leak balloon catheter, are also useful for superselective placement.[49] However, only fluids can be injected through this device. Removable-core, injectable guidewires are capable of infusing powders as well as fluids. No doubt there will be further technical developments for improved selective and superselective embolotherapy.

In certain cases, direct percutaneous fine needle puncture of a lesion is the best or only nonoperative approach possible. Ethanol, bucrylate, and thrombin have been safely injected directly into aneurysms, vascular malformations, and tumors.[20,35,40,50]

The mode of delivery chosen depends on the nature of the lesion being treated, its location, and vascular anatomy. Operator experience and preferences are additional factors. Whatever method is used, placement of the access device must be stable, and the device must accept the occluding agent. If there is any question about catheter–embolizing agent compatibility, the combination should be checked in vitro.

Particulate Agents

Particles are the most commonly employed agents in embolotherapy, as well as the most versatile. The earliest materials used were endogenous: autologous clot, lyophilized dura mater, and fascia lata. Autologous clot is immediately available at the time of embolization, but its effect may be quite transient, even if it is reinforced by the application of exogenous thrombin. Dura mater and fascia produce more lasting occlusion, but neither is as readily available as many other materials.

Gelatin Sponge (Gelfoam)

A gelatin sponge provided in sheets or powder (Gelfoam) is the most frequently used temporary occlusive material. Sheets can be cut to any desired size, with 2-mm cubes or 2-mm × 2-mm × 6-mm "torpedos" easily injectable through standard diagnostic catheters. Particles are soaked in contrast medium diluted with saline and then drawn up in small syringes. Although the particles may jam within a catheter, forceful injection or passage of a guidewire can often clear the lumen. If the catheter tip is not advanced well into the desired vessel or if flow is stagnant, an occlusion balloon should be used to prevent reflux. Gelfoam is quite thrombogenic, and occlusion can be expected to last at least 1 to 2 weeks. Although Gelfoam powder is available, it presents a much greater risk of causing unintended ischemia. Skin necrosis, neural injury, and gallbladder infarction have been reported with the use of powder.[51,52]

Gelfoam is inherently radiolucent, a problem common to many agents. Mixture with water-soluble contrast material permits monitoring of Gelfoam injection. Tantalum and Lipiodol (iodized oil contrast agent) have also been used to provide radiopacity, which at best is only transient. Once a vessel is occluded, great care must be taken to avoid forceful catheter flushing or selective injection of contrast material into the vessel because particle reflux can result. If repeat embolotherapy is not a consideration, placement of a central coil can produce permanent occlusion and may prevent delayed retrograde embolization of Gelfoam.[53]

Polyvinyl Alcohol (Ivalon)

Ivalon, like Gelfoam, is supplied as sheets or as small particles. Unlike Gelfoam, it produces a permanent occlusion. Plugs can be cut from sheets, which are constituted of compressed material. Such particles expand on exposure to blood or other fluids. One mode of administration involves the advance preparation of a plug of Ivalon compressed, dried, and mounted on the tip of a guidewire.[54] At the time of embolization, the stability of catheter position can be checked by passage of a dummy wire before the Ivalon wire is introduced. After the plug expands, it can be stripped from the wire by the introducing catheter.

The small particles are available in a variety of diameters from 0.25 mm to 1 mm. Care should be taken to mix particles well within 5-ml syringes; otherwise, they have a tendency to aggregate and jam within the catheter. To keep the particles in suspension, two syringes may be joined by a segment of clear connecting tubing, with to-and-fro injection between syringes. Administration into the embolization catheter can follow immediately through a three-way stopcock connection. Ivalon, too, is radiolucent and must be mixed with contrast medium. Because of problems with homogeneity of size, small Ivalon particles should not be used if a substantial degree of AV shunting is suspected.

Other Particles
Many of the problems attendant with the handling and delivery of gelatin sponge and polyvinyl alcohol are common to other particulate agents. Oxidized cellulose (Oxycel) and microfibrillar collagen (Avitene) are similar in effect to Gelfoam, and occlusions produced last days to weeks. A newer agent under investigation, glutaraldehyde cross-linked collagen (GAX), produces a longer-lasting occlusion and less of an inflammatory tissue response than most other particulates.[55] It is suspended in contrast medium, can be injected through 2 Fr catheters or open-ended guidewires, and produces small vessel occlusion. Silicone microspheres occlude small vessels permanently and have been used in the treatment of AVMs. Microspheres, Avitene, and GAX, by their distal site of action, are more likely to produce infarction and necrosis, and neural damage is a possible complication.[44]

Radioactive Emboli
One variation in the transcatheter treatment of tumors is the use of radioactive agents. Yttrium 90 has been incorporated into glass microspheres, and Lipiodol (a fluid) has been labeled with iodine 131 to administer local radiation to hepatic tumors.[56,57] These therapies are investigational, and their effectiveness remains unproven. However, Lang and Sullivan have shown that unresectable renal cell carcinomas can be embolized with iodine-125 seeds, with palliation as good as that provided by any other currently available treatment.[58]

Metallic Coils and Spiders
Since their introduction in the mid-1970s, Gianturco coils have been a mainstay of embolotherapy for occlusion of large vessels. Originally, wool

strands were attached at the tip to enhance thrombosis, but Dacron was later substituted because of the marked granulomatous reactions produced by wool.[44] Dispersal of the fibers along the length of the wire coils has made jamming within the catheter less of a problem. In high-flow situations or when a patient's coagulation is impaired, coils do not necessarily thrombose,[59] and combination with gelatin sponge or thrombin injection may be needed.

Coils are now produced in various sizes, and many can be introduced through standard tapered catheters by standard guidewires. In fact, microcoils and brushes designed for introduction through the Tracker catheter are now available. Close attention must be paid to the manufacturer's instructions for embolization. As noted earlier, if there is any question as to the compatibility of a catheter-coil-guidewire introducer combination, the system should be tested before its use in a patient. Because coils are introduced by guidewires or pushers, catheter position stability is more critical than it is for many other embolic agents. The introducing wire should be passed through the catheter into the vessel being occluded as a test before the coil is inserted.

Coils should be carefully matched in size to the vessel being treated. A coil that is too large is deposited in an elongated configuration and may project into a feeding vessel. It can potentially erode through vessel wall, resulting in pseudoaneurysm. If a coil is too small, it may fail to lodge, causing unintended embolization by reflux into other vessels. In experienced hands, embolotherapy with coils is quite safe. Chuang and Wallace noted only eight major complications in more than 1200 patients treated.[60] Even when their coils strayed, they were able to retrieve several by means of intravascular snares.

In cases of large AV fistula, coils alone may be too small to treat the lesion. A metallic "spider" has been designed to serve as a baffle to trap coils or other large particles.[39] Spiders are available in 10-mm and 15-mm diameters, and barbed feet serve to anchor them in vessel wall. Introduction with a special threaded guidewire permits precise positioning before release of the spider.

Detachable Balloons

Detachable balloons are most useful in the management of large AV communications, such as traumatic AV fistulae or pulmonary AVMs, and of varicocele.[8,16,61] Their principal advantage is that the operator can check the position and adequacy of occlusion before balloon detachment, and partial balloon inflation can flow-direct the balloon to the site of AV communication. Various balloon systems using coaxial catheter introduction have been described. Silicone balloons should be inflated with an isotonic contrast agent because silicone is semipermeable. Premature deflation may lead to unintended embolization.[44]

Polymers and Tissue Adhesives

Advantages of polymers include the ability to be injected through small catheters or open-ended guidewires, production of occlusion in vessels of various sizes, and predictable control of bleeding in patients whose coagulation is impaired. Disadvantages are the rather cumbersome preparations necessary for administration of these agents and the investigational nature of the polymers developed thus far.

Bucrylate

Bucrylate (isobutyl-2-cyanoacrylate) has been most the widely investigated tissue adhesive in the United States. Its capability of penetrating into small vessels has made it quite useful for obliterating AVMs.[19] However, because of reported carcinogenic effects in animals, bucrylate has been withdrawn from the market.[62] Related compounds developed in Europe, such as n-butyl cyanoacrylate (Histacryl), are presently undergoing clinical studies in the United States. A feature common to the compounds of this class is rapid polymerization and adhesion on exposure to ionic fluids. For this reason, delivery systems must be flushed with nonionic dextrose solutions.

Bucrylate must be opacified with agents such as tantalum powder, and the speed of polymerization can be controlled by careful mixture with various amounts of iophendylate (Pantopaque). Polymerization time after injection into a vessel is approximately half that of a given mixture as measured in vitro, and this factor must be taken into account before embolization.[19] Tissue adhesives must be administered through coaxial catheters (or open-ended wires), and the catheter should be withdrawn immediately after the compound is injected. A complication unique to these agents is the possibility of gluing a catheter in place! Experience in the administration of tissue adhesives is best obtained in the laboratory before one proceeds to clinical application.

Nonadhesive Polymers

Low-viscosity silicone rubber and polyurethane are two other polymerizing fluids that have been studied. As with bucrylate, care must be taken to control the polymerization time so that only the vessels desired undergo embolization. Penetration of capillaries by silicone rubber can result in ischemic skin changes or neural injury.[63] These compounds have not caused the tissue inflammatory responses noted with bucrylate. Lack of tissue adhesion is seen in retraction of the polymers from the vessel wall with time.[63] The nonadhesive nature of silicone rubber may also have contributed to the report of a case of pulmonary embolization during treatment of an AVM in an extremity.[64]

Sclerosing and Locally Toxic Fluids

These agents have the property of producing vascular occlusion or tissue infarction by virtue of their direct effects at high concentration. In dilution the effects are substantially decreased. As fluids, they are not as dependent on large catheters or special delivery apparatus as are particulate emboli.

Ethanol

Absolute ethanol produces tissue necrosis directly, with vascular occlusion consequent to stasis.[65] This makes ethanol a very attractive agent for the treatment of unresectable renal tumors.[32] It has also been applied with success in cases of AVM, obliterating the nidus of the lesion.[20,40] Its very toxicity limits its use, for serious complications have arisen from penetration of pure ethanol into collateral vessel beds or reflux into the aorta or other vessels.[66–68] Ethanol lacks radiopacity, and a small amount of nonionic contrast agent may be mixed without negating the toxic tissue effects. However, use of an occlusion balloon affords greater control of ethanol administration and is highly recommended. Ethanol should never be injected into mesenteric arteries and must be used with particular care in the extremities.

Other Sclerosants

Sodium tetradecyl sulfate (Sotradecol) and hypertonic glucose have long been injected into varicose veins of the lower extremities, and they have also been applied directly to gastroesophageal varices.[12] In Europe a fatty acid of cod liver oil (Varicocid) has been used successfully to occlude internal spermatic veins associated with varicocele.[34] Ionic contrast material in a concentration of 76% has been effective in ablating parathyroids and kidney.[31,69] Again, use of an occlusion balloon is advisable, not only to prevent reflux of the sclerosant but also to prevent dilution by inflowing blood.

Other Methods of Vascular Occlusion

Iodinated contrast medium heated to 100 °C occludes vessels by its thermal effects.[70] A particular advantage is that one can fluoroscopically monitor the tissues treated. Electrocoagulation probes also cause thrombosis by heating.[71] Thrombin injection may enhance the effect of other injected agents, or it can precipitate coagulation on its own.[18,35] Thrombin works best in the presence of stasis; when flow is rapid, it is quickly diluted and inactivated.

SPECIFIC ANATOMIC CONSIDERATIONS

Bronchial and Pulmonary Interventions

Massive Hemoptysis

Untreated massive hemoptysis has high mortality, and embolization of bronchial arteries is an effective treatment that can obviate major surgical intervention. Tuberculosis and other inflammatory diseases are the most common causes of massive hemoptysis. Bronchial arteries are variable in number and distribution (see Chapter 7 entitled Thoracic Aortography and Bronchial Angiography), but there are usually no more than two to each lung, and most arise from the descending thoracic aorta at the level of T5-6. A normal bronchial artery is no larger than 3 mm in diameter. Enlargement can be taken as presumptive evidence of hemorrhagic source, if the origin of bleeding has not been identified bronchoscopically. Active extravasation on angiography is rarely recognizable. Peripheral inflammatory lesions can also receive blood supply from intercostal arteries and other chest wall vessels. Innominate, subclavian, and internal thoracic artery injections may be needed for complete evaluation. Pleural thickening should alert one to the presence of such collateral vessels, and embolization of lesions associated with pleural thickening is less likely to result in the long-term control of hemoptysis.[72] Massive bleeding from the pulmonary arterial circulation is distinctly unusual, but a tuberculous pseudoaneurysm is one possible source.[73]

Embolization has stopped pulmonary hemorrhage in 75% to 90% of patients, but there is a 20% rate of rebleeding within 6 months.[15] Patients with aspergillomas are most likely to suffer recurrent hemoptysis, and intracavitary treatment by direct instillation of amphotericin through a catheter placed percutaneously should be considered.[74] Patients with cystic fibrosis may suffer chronic intermittent hemoptysis of a moderate degree that can be controlled for 1 year or longer by embolization.[75]

The most feared complication of bronchial artery embolization is spinal cord injury. For this reason, careful angiography prior to embolization should identify a possible anterior spinal branch. A right intercostobronchial trunk is most likely to give rise to such a vessel.[15] Each patient should have a neurologic examination before embolization, with possible monitoring of somatosensory evoked potentials during the procedure. Uflacker and colleagues have treated nine patients with spinal branches from the bleeding vessel.[76] They increased the size of gelatin sponge pledgets injected to 3 mm × 10 mm, producing a more proximal occlusion. Although no neurologic damage occurred, such a procedure should be seen as quite risky.

Bronchial arteries have rich anastomotic connections to pulmonary arteries ranging in size from 72 to 325 µm. Use of small particles or fluids such as alcohol can result in bronchial infarction and death.[67]

Pulmonary Arteriovenous Malformations

Pulmonary AVMs not only can produce problems with blood oxygen desaturation and high-output cardiac failure but also are likely to cause cerebral emboli and brain abscess. For the latter reasons, even asymptomatic lesions should be treated by embolotherapy. The great majority of these patients have Rendu-Osler-Weber syndrome (hereditary hemorrhagic telangiectasia). White and associates have had a high degree of success in occluding 276 lesions in 76 patients with detachable balloons.[16] By closing all feeding vessels larger than 3 mm, they have seen no recurrence of symptoms in up to 5 years of follow-up.

Most lesions are found in the lower lobes and are fed by a single artery. If the vessel is larger than 9 mm, a nest of large coils must be constructed before balloon deposition. The balloon should be placed as peripherally as possible, and the effectiveness of occlusion must be checked by digital subtraction angiography or fluoroscopy before release of the balloon.

Renal Embolization

Embolization has been used in kidneys to palliate tumors, as well as to decrease operative blood loss at nephrectomy for carcinoma. In cases of end-stage renal disease, ablation can help control hypertension or protein loss from nephrotic syndrome. For these indications, complete infarction is desirable. For bleeding or AV fistulae, more directed embolization with larger particles is generally needed.

Wallace and colleagues suggested that there was prolongation of life in those patients with renal cell carcinoma who underwent embolization before nephrectomy, compared to those having nephrectomy alone.[41] However, this study was not controlled, and there has been no subsequent confirmation of any significant effect in such patients. In most institutions, routine preoperative embolization of renal tumors has fallen out of favor. Because of the danger of inadvertent intraoperative embolization of the opposite kidney,[77] any coils placed preoperatively should be several centimeters from the renal artery origin. The surgeon should be aware of the number and position of coils, and the specimen must be examined immediately to verify their removal.

Ethanol is quite useful for producing renal infarction, but it has been implicated in the complications of colonic and testicular infarction.[66,78] Alcohol can also cause massive release of catecholamine if it enters the adrenal circulation.[79] If ethanol is employed, an occlusion balloon must be placed to prevent reflux. It should remain inflated for several minutes after ethanol injection, and a check with contrast medium should be performed before the balloon is deflated. Ethanol may cause considerable pain when injected into the renal vascular bed, but pain may be prevented to some extent by prior injection of lidocaine through the catheter. Ethanol has been associated with less severe postembolization symptoms than other agents.[38]

Although use of an occlusion balloon can prevent reflux, penetration of collateral channels may be responsible for some cases of colonic infarction. The renal artery very commonly has multiple retroperitoneal anastomoses. The most common of these are transcapsular and adrenal, but aortic, iliac, gonadal, and inferior mesenteric artery connections have been observed.[80] Therefore, caution is still justified with the use of ethanol and other toxic agents.

Hepatic Embolotherapy

For embolization, a most important consideration is the dual hepatic blood supply. Tumors receive their blood almost entirely from hepatic artery, whereas normal liver parenchyma derives most of its blood from the portal vein. As long as the portal vein is open and flow is hepatopedal, embolization can be performed without great danger, but arterial embolization in the face of portal occlusion or hypotension can be fatal.[53,81] Nevertheless, portal vein thrombosis is not an absolute contraindication, as long as collateral circulation is present. Pentecost and associates performed chemoembolization in nine such patients without producing hepatic infarction or insufficiency.[82] Those with jaundice or massive replacement of liver by tumor should not be treated because of the risk of hepatic failure. Staged embolization is advisable for many patients with widespread neoplasm. Combining embolic agents with chemotherapeutic drugs has theoretical advantages in exposing tumor cells to high doses of the drugs for a prolonged period of time, while potentiating the local toxicity through ischemia.

Embolotherapy has been shown to prolong life in patients with unresectable hepatocellular carcinoma, and it is more effective than chemotherapy alone.[23,81] Lipiodol injected intraarterially tends to accumulate in primary hepatic tumors and can be used to deliver chemotherapy or local radiation.[57] For small hepatocellular carcinomas not amenable to resection, a promising treatment is percutaneous ethanol injection therapy (PEIT) through a fine needle placed with ultrasound or computed tomography guidance. Five-year survival of 38%, comparable to that of resective surgery, has been achieved in one large series.[50] Unfortunately, because hepatocellular carcinoma tends to be a multifocal disease, tumor recurrence is common after operation or PEIT.[83] Those with one to three lesions, none larger than 3 cm in diameter, are most appropriate for PEIT, which is a procedure usually staged over days to weeks. Related methods of achieving focal tumor destruction by tissue freezing or heating with laser probes or other means are being investigated.[84–86]

Secreting islet cell tumors and carcinoid tumors unresponsive to medical management can be controlled by embolization in most cases.[21,22,25,26] Premedication, such as with the somatostatin analogue octreotide for carcinoid tumors, is very important for preventing morbidity from massive hormone release.[87] Although these tumors tend to be indolent in their course, embolization may very well prolong life. Other metastatic tumors, such as colorectal metastases, may show regression in the majority of patients, but treatment has little effect on survival.[27]

If the catheter cannot be advanced selectively into the proper hepatic artery or its branches, use of an occlusion balloon can reverse flow in the gastroduodenal artery (GDA) and prevent its embolization. An alternate strategy is to place a coil into the proximal GDA to protect its distal circulation. Direct manual compression over the GDA can also stop antegrade flow, allowing embolization to proceed from the common hepatic artery.[88] The cystic artery is often occluded in the course of hepatic embolization. Even so, clinical cholecystitis is rarely severe, unless a powder is used.[52]

Splenic Embolization

Embolization of the splenic artery has been used to treat hypersplenism and its attendant hematologic abnormalities, while preserving some splenic tissue and function.[89,90] Painful splenic enlargement can also be resolved by embolization, although complete response may take several weeks.[91] Splenic artery aneurysms can be occluded by careful selective placement of coils or large particles, as long as collateral flow is maintained to the spleen itself.[36,37] A similar strategy can be applied when arterial bleeding complicates splenic trauma.[92]

Splenic rupture has been reported as a complication by early investigators,[93] but the overriding danger in splenic embolization is the susceptibility of the organ to abscess if parenchyma is infarcted.[45,53] Spigos and colleagues developed a highly aseptic procedure, including full-body povidone-iodine baths for the patient prior to embolotherapy, broad-spectrum antibiotic coverage, and injection of Gelfoam particles soaked in an antibiotic solution.[30] As long as strict attention to sterility is observed and no more than two thirds of the spleen is infarcted, risk of infection is low. Potent analgesia or epidural anesthesia may be needed to control pain for several days after treatment. Powder should not be injected into the splenic artery, for it can evoke the complication of pancreatitis.

A more central splenic artery embolization can be performed as an adjunct to surgical splenectomy, several hours prior to operation. It is most useful in patients with massive splenomegaly from myeloproliferative disorders.[94] In those without massive organ enlargement, careful coil placement can assist the new technique of laparoscopic splenectomy.[95]

Mesenteric Procedures

Most gastric hemorrhage is self-limited, and only rarely does such bleeding not respond to conservative measures. In the past, selective vasopressin infusion of the left gastric artery has proved useful for controlling otherwise refractory bleeding from gastritis or other small vessel lesions.[5] Catheter embolization was applied only to those patients who continued to lose blood despite infusion. However, more than 70% of such patients could be managed by immediate embolization with fewer complications and fewer episodes of rebleeding.[4,5] Therefore, embolization with gelatin sponge can be considered a primary interventional treatment for continuing gastric hemorrhage. Even if the bleeding source is not found, embolization of the left gastric artery is recommended (as long as the gastric circulation is not otherwise compromised), for it decreases the risk of recurrence.[96] The left gastric artery is the vessel supplying the great majority of major upper gastrointestinal bleeds.

If an upper gastrointestinal bleeding source is fed by other vessels, such as the gastroduodenal artery, control by embolization is much less likely. Occlusion of the gastroduodenal artery causes immediate collateral perfusion from the superior mesenteric artery by way of the pancreaticoduodenal arcades. Thus, fewer than half of patients with duodenal ulcer bleeding respond to embolotherapy, although the use of tissue adhesives may improve results.[14] As noted earlier, transhepatic occlusion of bleeding gastroesophageal varices is at best a temporizing procedure and has been abandoned in most institutions.

Arterial hemorrhage from erosion by a pancreatic pseudocyst is less common than peptic disease. The splenic or gastroduodenal arteries are most often affected. In this situation embolization with large particles or coils has proved quite effective.[7]

Embolization of small bowel or colonic vessels has been performed with success, although the need for such treatment is exceptional. One must reckon with a 13% to 22% risk of ischemic complications.[9–11,96] No more than one major mesenteric vessel should undergo embolization, and the effect of each administered particle must be examined serially by injection of contrast material. Embolization should not be continued if extravasation has ceased. Although some feel that vessels distal to the marginal arcades must not be embolized, Guy and associates found that injection of polyvinyl alcohol particles directly into the arteria recta through a Tracker catheter controlled bleeding without resulting in undue ischemia.[97] Small bowel vessels do not respond readily to selective arterial vasopressin infusion, but infusion should be attempted in those with colonic bleeding.[14]

Before embolization of even the left gastric artery, note should be made of any compromise to collateral circulation, such as severe atherosclerosis or previous surgery. The danger of bowel infarction is elevated in those with limited collaterals.[2,4] For the same reason, vasopressin infusion should not be reinstituted after embolization therapy, even if bleeding has not stopped.

Pelvic and Retroperitoneal Hemorrhage

Pelvic trauma requires angiographic evaluation for hemorrhage in fewer than 10% of cases, but pelvic bleeding can be deadly.[3] Mortality for patients with pelvic fractures who present in shock has been reported as 42%, compared to 3% in similar patients who are hemodynamically stable.[1] Indications for angiography and embolization include transfusion requirement of more than 4 units over 24 hours, more than 6 units over 48 hours, open pelvic fractures, or expanding hematoma found at laparotomy.[1] In severe blunt trauma such as fall from a height, major bleeding can arise from lumbar arteries, especially in the presence of vertebral fractures.[98]

Evaluation includes abdominal aortography followed by selective injections within the internal iliac arteries, as well as lumbar and other arteries that appear to be possible bleeding sources. As in any suspected case of hemorrhage, filming should be carried out to at least 30 seconds to allow extravasation to be recognized. Arterial stasis and vertebral body "stain" are indirect signs of bleeding.[98] Bleeding can often be controlled by gelatin sponge embolization, but central placement of coils decreases the chance of recurrence. If a bleeding site is found and occluded, clinical stabilization can be expected in 85% to 95% of patients, but a large number may die of associated injuries.[1,3]

Pelvic embolization is also useful when there is bleeding from bladder, rectal, or uterine neoplasms. In addition, palliation of pain caused by tumor invasion of sacral nerves can be achieved. Because of rich collateral communications, bilateral internal iliac embolization is often necessary in many patients with traumatic or neoplastic bleeding. Powders or deeply penetrating fluids are best avoided because of the risk of neural injury.[51]

Arteriovenous Malformations in Extremities
Treatment of AVMs in an extremity is best reserved for symptomatic lesions, for many AVMs may assume a more aggressive behavior after intervention. Amputation is a last resort, but a real risk when a lesion is large. Vascular occlusion should be directed to sites associated with pain, bleeding, or ulceration. The small-vessel core or nidus must be obliterated for lasting results. Small particles of polyvinyl alcohol or other permanent agents should be directed as selectively as possible, whether through 3 Fr catheters or direct needle puncture.[19,20] Good results have also been obtained with bucrylate and the judicious staged application of ethanol.[19,40] Blood pressure cuffs or direct compression is used to slow flow and maximize the desired sclerosis. If skin becomes discolored, treatment must be stopped or tissue sloughing may occur.[20] Cavernous hemangiomas can be most thoroughly evaluated by venography. They may be treated by direct needle puncture of the venous spaces and sclerosis with alcohol.

In any AVM one must be aware of major AV communications, in order to avoid passing small particles to the pulmonary circulation. Major risks of small vessel occlusion in the extremities include tissue ischemia and nerve palsies.[20]

Varicoceles

Varicocele may be treated for local symptoms or because of its possible effect on fertility. It has been termed the most common correctable cause of male infertility. Traditional treatment has been surgical ligation of the internal spermatic vein, but recurrence has been fairly high after surgery. The left side is much more commonly abnormal.

Selective internal spermatic venography (by way of the left renal vein) allows detailed delineation of vessel incompetence and anatomy. Venography can show duplications or anomalous communications, which are present in most patients with varicocele.[34] The vein can then be occluded at a location that will not allow reflux through duplications or retroperitoneal communicators. Sclerosing agents, coils, and balloons have been safely applied with long-term clinical and venographic success in up to 97% of cases.[34,44,61] The greatest challenge with treatment of varicocele is successful selective placement of the administering catheter. A minimally invasive urologic alternative has been developed in which a sclerosing agent is delivered antegrade through a vein isolated by scrotal cutdown.[99]

REFERENCES

1. Mucha P, Jr, Welch TJ: Hemorrhage in major pelvic fractures. *Surg Clin North Am* 1988; 68:757–773.
2. Jander HP, Russinovitch NAE: Transcatheter Gelfoam embolization in abdominal, retroperitoneal and pelvic hemorrhage. *Radiology* 1980; 136:337–344.
3. Matalon TSA, Athanasoulis CA, Margolies MN, et al: Hemorrhage with pelvic fractures: Efficacy of transcatheter embolization. *Am J Roentgenol* 1979; 133:859–864.
4. Rösch J, Keller FS, Kozak B, et al: Gelfoam powder embolization of the left gastric artery in treatment of massive small-vessel gastric bleeding. *Radiology* 1984; 151:365–370.
5. Eckstein MR, Kelemouridis V, Athanasoulis CA, et al: Gastric bleeding: Therapy with intraarterial vasopressin and transcatheter embolization. *Radiology* 1984; 152:643–646.
6. Kuroda C, Kawamoto S, Hori S, et al: Pancreatic pseudocyst hemorrhage controlled by transcather embolization. *Cardiovasc Intervent Radiol* 1983; 6:167–169.
7. Huizinga WKJ, Kalideen JM, Bryer JV, et al: Control of major haemorrhage associated with pancreatic pseudocysts by transcatheter arterial embolization. *Br J Surg* 1984; 71:133–136.
8. Mitchell SE, Shuman LS, Kaufman SL, et al: Biliary catheter drainage complicated by hemobilia: Treatment by balloon embolotherapy. *Radiology* 1985; 157:645–652.
9. Uflacker R: Transcatheter embolization for treatment of acute lower gastrointestinal bleeding. *Acta Radiol* 1987; 28:425–430.
10. Palmaz JC, Walter JF, Cho KJ: Therapeutic embolization of the small-bowel arteries. *Radiology* 1984; 152:377–382.

11. Rosenkrantz H, Bookstein JJ, Rosen RJ, et al: Postembolic colonic infarction. *Radiology* 1982; 142:47–51.

12. Benner KG, Keefe EB, Keller FS, Rösch J: Clinical outcome after percutaneous transhepatic obliteration of esophageal varices. *Gastroenterology* 1983; 85:146–153.

13. Yune HY, O'Connor KW, Klatte EC, et al: Ethanol thrombotherapy of esophageal varices: Further experience. *Am J Roentgenol* 1985; 144:1049–1053.

14. Feldman L, Greenfield AJ, Waltman AC, et al: Transcatheter vessel occlusion: Angiographic results versus clinical success. *Radiology* 1983; 147:1–5.

15. Stoll JF, Bettman MA: Bronchial artery embolization to control hemoptysis: A review. *Cardiovasc Intervent Radiol* 1988; 11:263–269.

16. White RI, Jr, Lynch-Nyhan A, Terry P, et al: Pulmonary arteriovenous malformations: Techniques and long-term outcome of embolotherapy. *Radiology* 1988; 169:663–669.

17. Clark RA, Gallant TE, Alexander ES: Angiographic management of traumatic arteriovenous fistulas: Clinical results. *Radiology* 1983; 147:9–13.

18. Laffey KJ, Bixon R, Martin EC: Thrombin as an adjunct to embolisation in high flow arteriovenous fistulae. *J Intervent Radiol* 1988; 3:27–30.

19. Widlus DM, Murray RR, White RI, Jr, et al: Congenital arteriovenous malformations: Tailored embolotherapy. *Radiology* 1988; 169:511–516.

20. Gomes AS: Embolization therapy of congenital arteriovenous malformations: Use of alternate approaches. *Radiology* 1994; 190:191–198.

21. Mitty HA, Warner RRP, Newman LH, et al: Control of carcinoid syndrome with hepatic artery embolization. *Radiology* 1985; 155:623–626.

22. Ajani JA, Carrasco CH, Charnsangavey C, et al: Islet cell tumors metastatic to liver: Effective palliation by sequential hepatic artery embolization. *Ann Intern Med* 1988; 108:340–344.

23. Lin D-Y, Liaw Y-F, Lee T-Y, Lai C-M: Hepatic arterial embolization in patients with unresectable hepatocellular carcinoma: A randomized controlled trial. *Gastroenterology* 1988; 94:453–456.

24. O'Keeffe FN, Carrasco CH, Charnsangavej C, et al: Arterial embolization of adrenal tumors: Results in nine cases. *Am J Roentgenol* 1988; 151:819–822.

25. Hajarizadeh H, Ivancev K, Mueller CR, et al: Effective palliative treatment of metastatic carcinoid tumors with intra-arterial chemotherapy/chemoembolization combined with octreotide acetate. *Am J Surg* 1992; 163:479–483.

26. Moertel CG, Johnson CM, McKusick MA, et al: The management of patients with advanced carcinoid tumors and islet cell carcinomas. *Ann Intern Med* 1994; 120:302–309.

27. Pentecost MJ: Transcatheter treatment of hepatic metastases. *Am J Roentgenol* 1993; 160:1171–1175.

28. Rossi C, Ricci S, Boriani S, et al: Percutaneous transcatheter arterial embolization of bone and soft tissue tumors. *Skeletal Radiol* 1990; 19:555–560.

29. Chuang VP, Soo CS, Wallace S, Benjamin RS: Arterial occlusion: Management of giant cell tumor and aneurysmal bone cyst. *Am J Roentgenol* 1981; 136:1127–1130.

30. Spigos DG, Jonasson O, Mozes M, Capek V: Partial splenic embolization in the treatment of hypersplenism. *Am J Roentgenol* 1979; 132:777–782.

31. Miller DL, Doppman JL, Chang R, et al: Angiographic ablation of parathyroid adenomas: Lessons from a 10-year experience. *Radiology* 1987; 165:601–607.
32. Keller FS, Coyle M, Rösch J, Dotter CT: Percutaneous renal ablation in patients with end-stage renal disease: Alternative to surgical nephrectomy. *Radiology* 1986; 159:447–451.
33. Crummy AB, Ishizuka J, Madsen PO: Posttraumatic priapism: Successful treatment with autologous clot embolization. *Am J Roentgenol* 1979; 133:329–330.
34. Seyferth W, Jecht E, Zeitler E: Percutaneous sclerotherapy of varicocele. *Radiology* 1981; 139:335–340.
35. Cope C, Zeit R: Coagulation of aneurysms by direct percutaneous thrombin injection. *Am J Roentgenol* 1986; 147:383–387.
36. Uflacker R: Transcatheter embolisation of arterial aneurysms. *Br J Radiol* 1986; 59:317–324.
37. Baker KS, Tisnado J, Cho S-R, Beachley MC: Splanchnic artery aneurysms and pseudoaneurysms: Transcatheter embolization. *Radiology* 1987; 163:135–139.
38. Ekelund L, Ek A, Forsberg L, et al: Occlusion of renal arterial tumor supply with absolute ethanol: Experience with 20 cases. *Acta Radiol (Diag)* 1984; 25:195–201.
39. Lund G, Cragg AH, Rysavy JA, et al: Detachable stainless-steel spider: A new device for vessel occlusion. *Radiology* 1983; 148:567–568.
40. Yakes WF, Haas DK, Parker SH, et al: Symptomatic vascular malformations: Ethanol embolotherapy. *Radiology* 1989; 170:1059–1066.
41. Wallace S, Chuang VP, Swanson D, et al: Embolization of renal carcinoma. *Radiology* 1981; 138:563–570.
42. Carroll BA, Walter JF: Gas in embolized tumors: An alternative hypothesis for its origin. *Radiology* 1983; 147:441–444.
43. Rankin RN: Gas formation after renal tumor embolization without abscess: A benign occurrence. *Radiology* 1979; 130:317–320.
44. Wojtowycz M, Miller FJ: Complications of transcatheter embolization. *Semin Intervent Radiol* 1984; 1:179–188.
45. Hemingway AP, Allison DJ: Complications of embolization: Analysis of 410 procedures. *Radiology* 1988; 166:669–672.
46. Meyer P, Reizine D, Aymard A, et al: Septic complications in interventional angiography: Evaluation of risk and preventive measures—preliminary studies. *J Intervent Radiol* 1988; 3:73–75.
47. Greenfield A, Athanasoulis CA, Waltman AC, LeMoure ER: Transcatheter embolization: Prevention of embolic reflux using balloon catheters. *Am J Roentgenol* 1978; 131:651–655.
48. Matsumoto AH, Suhocki PV, Barth KH: Technical note: Superselective Gelfoam embolotherapy using a highly visible small caliber catheter. *Cardiovasc Intervent Radiol* 1988; 11:303–306.
49. Kerber C: Balloon catheter with a calibrated leak. *Radiology* 1976; 120:547–550.
50. Shiina S, Tagawa K, Niwa Y, et al: Percutaneous ethanol injection therapy for hepatocellular carcinoma: Results in 146 patients. *Am J Roentgenol* 1993; 160:1023–1028.

51. Hare WSC, Holland CJ: Paresis following internal iliac artery embolization. *Radiology* 1983; 146:47–51.

52. Kuroda C, Iwasaki M, Tanaka T, et al: Gallbladder infarction following hepatic transcatheter arterial embolization. *Radiology* 1983; 149:85–89.

53. Trojanowski JQ, Harrist JT, Athanasoulis CA, Greenfield AJ: Hepatic and splenic infarctions: Complications of therapeutic transcatheter embolization. *Am J Surg* 1980; 139:272–277.

54. Tadavarthy SM, Castañeda-Zuñiga W, Zollikofer C, et al: Angiodysplasia of the right colon treated by embolization with Ivalon (polyvinyl alcohol). *Cardiovasc Intervent Radiol* 1981; 4:39–42.

55. Strother CM, Laravuso R, Rappe A, et al: Glutaraldehyde cross-linked collagen (GAX): A new material for therapeutic embolization. *AJNR* 1987; 8:509–515.

56. Herba MJ, Illescas FF, Thirlwell MP, et al: Hepatic malignancies: Improved treatment with intraarterial Y-90. *Radiology* 1988; 169:311–314.

57. Bretagne J-F, Raoul J-L, Bourguet P, et al: Hepatic artery injection of I-131-labeled lipiodol: Part II—Preliminary results of therapeutic use in patients with hepatocellular carcinoma and liver metastases. *Radiology* 1988; 168:547–550.

58. Lang EK, Sullivan J: Management of primary and metastatic renal cell carcinoma by transcatheter embolization with iodine 125. *Cancer* 1988; 62:274–282.

59. Rao VR, Mandalam RK, Joseph S, et al: Embolization of large saccular aneursyms with Gianturco coils. *Radiology* 1990; 175:407–410.

60. Chuang VP, Wallace S, Gianturco C, Soo CS: Complications of coil embolization: Prevention and management. *Am J Roentgenol* 1981; 137:809–813.

61. Kaufman SL, Kadir S, Barth KH, et alr: Mechanisms of recurrent varicocele after balloon occlusion or surgical ligation of the internal spermatic vein. *Radiology* 1983; 147:435–440.

62. Suby-Long T, Bos GD, Rösch J: Biopsy proven eradication of an aneurysmal bone cyst treated by superselective embolization: A case report. *Cardiovasc Intervent Radiol* 1988; 11:292–295.

63. Miller FJ, Jr, Rankin RS, Gliedman JB, Nakashima E: Experimental internal iliac artery embolization: Evaluation of low viscosity silicone rubber. Isobutyl 2-cyanoacrylate, and carbon microspheres. *Radiology* 1978; 129:51–58.

64. Capan LM, Lardizabal S, Sinha K, et al: Acute pulmonary embolism during therapeutic arterial embolization with silicone fluids. *Anesthesiology* 1983; 58:569–571.

65. Buchta K, Sands J, Rosenkrantz H, Roche WD: Early mechanism of action of arterially infused alcohol U. S. P. in renal devitalization. *Radiology* 1982; 145:45–48.

66. Siniluoto TMJ, Hellström PA, Päivänsalo MJ, Leinonen ASS: Testicular infarction following ethanol embolization of a renal neoplasm. *Cardiovasc Intervent Radiol* 1988; 11:162–164.

67. Ivanick MJ, Thorwarth W, Donohue J, et al: Infarction of the left main-stem bronchus: A complication of bronchial artery embolization. *Am J Roentgenol* 1983; 141:535–537.

68. Mulligan BD, Espinosa GA: Bowel infarction: Complication of ethanol ablation of a renal tumor. *Cardiovasc Intervent Radiol* 1983; 6:55–57.

69. Siragusa RJ, Merandi S, Hanner JS, et al: Renal ablation with iodinated contrast medium: Initial clinical experience. *Semin Intervent Radiol* 1988; 5:146–148.
70. Cragg AH, Rosel P, Rysavy JA, et al: Renal ablation using hot contrast medium: An experimental study. *Radiology* 1983; 148:683–686.
71. Brunelle F, Kunstlinger F, Quillard J: Endovascular electrocoagulation with a bipolar electrode and alternating current: A follow-up study in dogs. *Radiology* 1983; 148:413–415.
72. Tamura S, Kodama T, Otsuka N, et al: Embolotherapy for persistent hemoptysis: The significance of pleural thickening. *Cardiovasc Intervent Radiol* 1993; 16:85–88.
73. Remy-Jardin M, Wattine L, Remy J: Transcatheter occlusion of pulmonary arterial circulation and collateral supply: Failures, incidents, and complications. *Radiology* 1991; 180:699–705.
74. Shapiro MJ, Albelda SM, Mayock RL, McLean GK: Severe hemoptysis associated with pulmonary aspergilloma: Percutaneous intracavitary treatment. *Chest* 1988; 94:1225–1231.
75. Tonkin ILD, Hanissian AS, Boulden TF, et al: Bronchial arteriography and embolotherapy for hemoptysis in patients with cystic fibrosis. *Cardiovasc Intervent Radiol* 1991; 14:241–246.
76. Uflacker R, Kaemmerer A, Neves C, Picon PD: Management of massive hemoptysis by bronchial artery embolization. *Radiology* 1983; 146:627–634.
77. Wirthlin LS, Gross WS, James TP, Sadiq S: Renal artery occlusion from migration of stainless steel coils. *JAMA* 1980; 243:2064–2065.
78. Cox GG, Lee KR, Price HI, et al: Colonic infarction following ethanol embolization of renal-cell carcinoma. *Radiology* 1982; 145:343.
79. Fink IJ, Girton M, Doppman JL: Absolute ethanol injection of the adrenal artery: Hypertensive reaction. *Radiology* 1985; 154:357–358.
80. Wilkins RA, Sandin B, Price A, Twomey B: Extrarenal arterial connections of the normal renal artery. *Cardiovasc Intervent Radiol* 1986; 9:119–122.
81. Yamada R, Sato M, Kawabata M, et al: Hepatic artery embolization in 120 patients with unresectable hepatoma. *Radiology* 1983; 148:397–401.
82. Pentecost MJ, Daniels JR, Teitelbaum GP, Stanley P: Hepatic chemoembolization: Safety with portal vein thrombosis. *J Vasc Interv Radiol* 1993; 4:347–351.
83. Kotoh K, Sakai H, Sakamoto S, et al: The effect of percutaneous ethanol injection therapy on small solitary hepatocellular carcinoma is comparable to that of hepatectomy. *Am J Gastroenterol* 1994; 89:194–198.
84. Amin Z, Bown SG, Lees WR: Liver tumor ablation by interstitial laser photocoagulation: Review of experimental and clinical studies. *Semin Intervent Radiol* 1993; 10:88–100.
85. Kane RA: Ultrasound-guided hepatic cryosurgery for tumor ablation. *Semin Intervent Radiol* 1993; 10:132–142.
86. Kopecky KK, Yang R, Sanghvi NT, Rescorla FJ: Liver tumor ablation with high-intensity focused ultrasound. *Semin Intervent Radiol* 1993; 10:125–131.
87. Coldwell DM, Stokes KR, Yakes WF: Embolotherapy: Agents, clinical applications, and techniques. *RadioGraphics* 1994; 14:623–643.

88. Kubota H, Nimura Y, Hayakawa N, Shionoya S: Hepatic transcatheter arterial embolization with gastroduodenal artery blocking by finger compression. *Radiology* 1989; 170:562–563.

89. Kumpe DA, Rumack CM, Pretorius DH, et al: Partial splenic embolization in children with hypersplenism. *Radiology* 1985; 155:357–362.

90. Sangro B, Bilbao I, Herrero I, et al: Partial splenic embolization for the treatment of hypersplenism in cirrhosis. *Hepatology* 1993; 18:309–314.

91. Grassi CJ, Boxt LM, Bettman MA: Partial splenic embolization for painful splenomegaly. *Cardiovasc Intervent Radiol* 1987; 10:291–294.

92. Sclafani SJA, Weisberg A, Scalea TM, et al: Blunt splenic injuries: Nonsurgical treatment with CT, arteriography, and transcatheter arterial embolization of the splenic artery. *Radiology* 1991; 181:189–196.

93. Wholey MH, Chamorro HA, Rao G, Chapman W: Splenic infarction and spontaneous rupture of the spleen after therapeutic embolization. *Cardiovasc Radiol* 1978; 1:249–253.

94. Fujitani RM, Johs SM, Cobb SR, et al: Preoperative splenic artery occlusion as an adjunct for high risk splenectomy. *Am Surg* 1988; 54:602–608.

95. Poulin E, Thibault C, Mamazza J, et al: Laparoscopic splenectomy: Clinical experience and the role of preoperative splenic artery embolization. *Surg Laparosc Endosc* 1993; 3:445–450.

96. Lang EV, Wittich G: Therapeutic and prophylactic transcatheter therapy in patients with massive arterial upper gastrointestinal haemorrhage. *Minimal Invasive Ther* 1993; 2:173–180.

97. Guy GE, Shetty PC, Sharma RP, et al: Acute lower gastrointestinal hemorrhage: Treatment by superselective embolization with polyvinyl alcohol particles. *Am J Roentgenol* 1992; 159:521–526.

98. Sclafani SJA, Florence LO, Phillips TF, et al: Lumbar arterial injury: Radiologic diagnosis and management. *Radiology* 1987; 165:709–714.

99. Tauber R, Johnsen N: Antegrade scrotal sclerotherapy for the treatment of varicocele: Technique and late results. *J Urol* 1994; 151:386–390.

13

Lower Extremity Venography

KEY CONCEPTS

1. Contrast venography is no longer the primary imaging study for the diagnosis of deep venous thrombosis, but it remains indispensable in evaluating patients with chronic venous disease or whose duplex ultrasound findings are equivocal.
2. Presence of an intraluminal filling defect is necessary for confirmation of acute deep venous thrombosis. Failure to opacify deep veins and sharp cutoffs are less specific signs.
3. Proper technique is essential to prevent artifacts and false-positive studies.
4. Low-osmolality contrast media and heparinized saline flush minimize the risk of postvenographic phlebitis.
5. Descending venography can be used to assess valvular competence in patients with symptoms of venous stasis.

INDICATIONS

Over the past few years venography has been displaced as the gold standard for detecting lower extremity deep venous thrombosis (DVT).[1] In our department the number of lower extremity venograms has dropped by more than 90% since the late 1980s. Nevertheless, venography continues to play a valuable role in evaluating patients with chronic or recurrent DVT or in whom sonographic examination is difficult or equivocal. In such situations venography is commonly called upon to enable the diagnosis of acute DVT, for clinical examination can be notoriously deceptive. Conditions capable of mimicking DVT are lymphedema, congestive heart failure, Baker's cyst, pelvic tumor, and muscular injury. Other occasional indications for venography include evaluation of deep venous insufficiency, a condition that is often a long-term consequence of thrombophlebitis; varicose veins (the deep veins must be shown to be patent before the saphenous or other major superficial veins are ligated or stripped), and determination of the suitability of the greater saphenous vein as a potential arterial graft. However, venous duplex ultrasound has largely replaced contrast venography for these indications as well.

ANATOMY

The deep veins of the leg and pelvis parallel the course of the arterial supply (Figs. 13-1 and 13-2). The anterior tibial, posterior tibial, and peroneal veins are paired. Popliteal and superficial femoral veins may be duplicated, partially or completely, but in most cases they are single vessels. Muscular veins from the gastrocnemius and soleus are also part of the deep venous system.

A variable number of valves are present in deep veins inferior to the inguinal ligament. These valves permit flow of blood to the heart while preventing distal transmission of the great hydrostatic pressure that an uninterrupted column of fluid can produce.

The greater and lesser saphenous veins are part of the superficial venous network. Blood normally flows from the superficial veins into the deep venous system by way of short perforating veins that contain valves for the prevention of backflow.

TECHNIQUE FOR ASCENDING PHLEBOGRAPHY

Many techniques and variations have been devised for lower extremity venography, most of them designed to provide good fill of the deep veins in order to detect clots.[2-9] For DVT studies, venipuncture of the foot is preferable, and many radiologists recommend that the needle

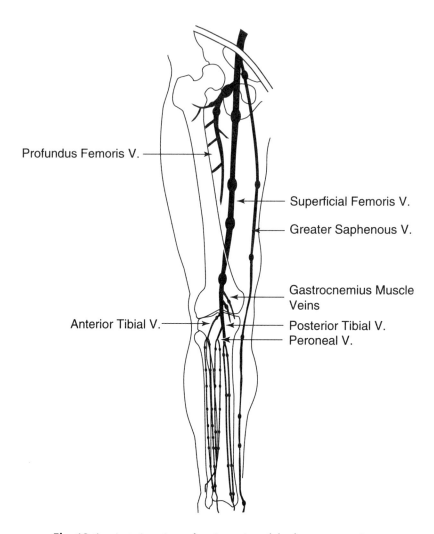

Fig. 13-1 Anterior view of major veins of the lower extremity.

tip be directed distally (toward the toes). "Downhill" puncture may produce better opacification of the deep venous system and allows study of pedal veins.

Semiupright Venography
Semiupright technique is widely used in those patients who are able to stand. With this method of examination, contrast material is less likely to layer and incompletely fill the vein, and chances for misinterpretation are reduced. Because contrast material does not clear out as rapidly as when

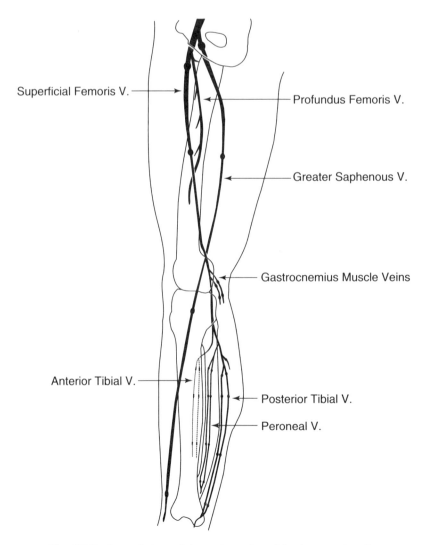

Fig. 13-2 Lateral view of the major veins of the lower extremity.

the patient is supine, continuous infusion is unnecessary with the semi-upright technique, and the examiner has more time to perform various maneuvers to best demonstrate any abnormalities present.

The patient is placed on a fluoroscopic table tilted 45° from the horizontal and bears weight on the foot not being examined. The injected extremity should be completely relaxed; any muscle contraction can impede filling of the deep veins. Because the normal direction of blood flow in the leg is from the superficial into the deep veins, tourniquets are not absolutely necessary in semiupright venography; in fact, they can obstruct filling of some veins, particularly the anterior tibial, soleal, and gastrocnemius veins. Nevertheless, tourniquets are routinely applied in many institutions, often one placed above the ankle and another above the knee.

Injection of contrast material may be performed by hand, slow power injection, or drip infusion. Manual injection provides the most immediate control. Observation of flow of the contrast material by fluoroscopy allows optimal timing of film exposure and permits the best projections to be selected. At least two projections of the calf and knee are obtained, including a lateral view. Plantar veins should be examined if there are any symptoms specific to the foot, but most venographers do not routinely study the foot. A single anteroposterior view of the thigh and pelvic vessels is ordinarily sufficient. When used, tourniquets should be released for better filling of the femoral veins. Immediately before filming the iliac veins and distal inferior vena cava, the table is lowered to a horizontal position and the patient's leg is elevated. Large film format, such as 14 × 17 inches with two or three exposures on one film, makes interpretation of the study easier. After filming is complete, heparinized saline (5000 to 10,000 units in 100 to 250 ml of normal saline) is infused through the needle, and the leg maintained in elevation to reduce the risk of postvenography thrombophlebitis. Contrast medium of 43% concentration provides adequate opacification for diagnosis, inducing less discomfort than a 60% concentration and probably decreasing the possibility of thrombosis after venography. Nonionic contrast agents share these advantages over 60% ionic media. The total volume injected per leg is usually on the order of 100 ml.

Methods ancillary to semiupright venography for DVT include calf compression and the Valsalva maneuver for more complete filling of the thigh and pelvic vessels, especially the internal iliac vein and profunda femoris. The theoretical possibility of inducing pulmonary embolization by these procedures exists, but Thomas has never encountered such an episode despite performing compression and Valsalva in more than 600 studies.[3] If extensive varicose veins are present, the leg can be wrapped in an elastic bandage, permitting better deep venous filling without injection of an excessive total volume of contrast material. An elastic bandage can also aid in demonstration of the soleal sinusoids after they have been initially emptied through compression. If the bandage is removed during injection, the sinusoids fill retrograde from the posterior tibial veins.[10] Digital subtraction venography may be helpful in some cases, but multiple projections cannot be obtained during a single injection. High-resolution unsubtracted digital imaging, however, can be used to great advantage in a "spot-film" mode.

Supine Venography

Venography with the patient supine is preferable for the examination of debilitated or severely ill patients. Most of the technical details are much the same as for semiupright studies, but tourniquets should be used, and continuous infusion of contrast is recommended.[8] Recently, Smith and colleagues have described the use of common femoral vein compression to decrease the amount of contrast material needed for supine leg venography.[7] They have also applied the technique at the conclusion of lower extremity runoff arteriography in order to evaluate the saphenous vein for possible use as a potential in situ graft.

If DVT is found in one extremity, the other leg need not be studied unless there are compelling reasons. However, routine bilateral simultaneous venography has its advocates.[9]

IF NO FOOT VEIN CAN BE FOUND

Prolonged elevation of the leg, compressive bandages, or blood pressure cuffs over the foot have been used to displace edema fluid and to uncover foot veins. If these steps do not work, the standard approach has been surgical cutdown venotomy over the dorsum of the foot. Another alternative from the early decades of venography is intraosseous injection, but the need for general anesthesia or heavy sedation, as well as the risk of fat embolization, make this an unattractive option. More recently, high-intensity fiber-optic transillumination and high-resolution ultrasound have been used to detect and guide catheterization of pedal veins when standard methods have failed.[11,12]

Puncture of a distal superficial vein or varicosity, with the needle tip directed distally and a tight tourniquet applied proximally, can reliably produce diagnostic deep venous studies up through the iliac veins.[4,5] Meticulous care must be taken to flush away any residual contrast medium afterward, for varicose veins are very susceptible to thrombosis.

PHLEBOGRAPHIC FINDINGS IN DEEP VENOUS THROMBOSIS

The venographic sine qua non of clot demonstration is evidence of a filling defect in the contrast material column. Less specific is the finding of an abrupt termination of fill at a constant site. Failure of deep venous filling despite attention to proper technique, particularly in association with a network of collateral channels, is also indicative of thrombosis.

The appearance of thrombus depends on its age (Fig. 13-3). Small clots may lyse within a matter of days. Fresh "free-floating" thrombus indicates formation within the previous week. After the first week, the

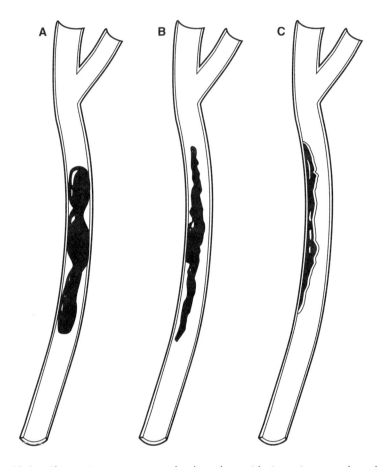

Fig. 13-3 Change in appearance of a thrombus with time: **A,** acute thrombus forms cast of vein; **B,** retraction of subacute clot; **C,** chronic residual mural irregularity.

clot begins to organize, with retraction and mural adherence.[13] This change represents cellular invasion from the vessel wall and capillary proliferation.[14] If adherence is circumferential, the vein becomes occluded. Over the course of weeks to months the vessel may recanalize; the resulting channel often shows irregular walls, loss of valves, and longitudinal "membranes."

The accuracy of venography is difficult to determine, for lack of a more reliable control in vivo. Lund and associates studied 199 lower limbs by postmortem venography followed by meticulous dissection of veins.[15] Thrombi were found in 65 limbs, with the sensitivity and specificity of venography in this context 97% and 95%, respectively.

SOME CLINICALLY RELEVANT INFORMATION

Deep venous thrombosis is a major clinical problem, with an incidence of 56 per 100,000 for a first diagnosis, according to the Worcester DVT study.[16] The incidence of recurrent disease is of the same order of magnitude. In the same study, 40% of patients were obese, 32% had cancer, and recent surgery was a contributing factor for 19%. Additional risk factors for DVT included congestive heart failure, myocardial infarction, stroke, trauma, and chronic obstructive pulmonary disease; 80% of all patients had at least three of the risk factors present, and the case-fatality rate was 5%.[16] The risk of DVT climbs with age.

Deep venous thrombosis has a high incidence in some surgical patients, such as those undergoing total hip replacement. One prospective study of immobilized trauma patients not treated by any prophylactic measures found thrombus in 24 of 38 patients (63%), with clot extending above the knee in 12 patients.[17] Even patients on medical wards (10% to 14%) may develop DVT during hospitalization.[18] Those with congestive heart failure or pneumonia are at substantially higher risk.

Radionuclide fibrinogen studies indicate that the majority of lower extremity thrombi arise in the calf. The work of Nicolaides and colleagues suggests that clot often forms in the muscular veins of the soleus.[10] In fact, in 18% of their positive venograms, thrombus was confined to the soleus. Although foot veins have been implicated as instrumental in the genesis of DVT, Glanz and Gordon failed to detect any plantar vein thrombosis in isolation in 200 venograms, and routine foot filming does not appear indicated.[19] Untreated DVT is likely to propagate proximally, and although half of pulmonary emboli are said to form in the calf, those arising from more proximal thrombi are much more important clinically. Even so, about 13% to 15% of fatal pulmonary emboli may come from calf veins.[20] Smaller clots pose much greater risk to those with limited cardiopulmonary reserve.

Most patients with clot limited to the calf have low-probability ventilation-perfusion scans, but 35% to 40% of those with thrombus extending above the calf have evidence of segmental or larger pulmonary emboli, even in the absence of symptoms.[21,22] The proximal extent of thrombosis commonly determines both the need for therapy and its duration.

Another clinical point of importance is that occluded femoral and iliac veins are less likely to recanalize and are more likely to result in severe debilitation than occluded calf veins.[13,14] In serious iliofemoral thrombosis, surgery may be considered for clot removal. However, extensive adherence of thrombus can make such a procedure quite difficult, and reocclusion is apt to occur from the intimal trauma involved in thrombectomy.[13] Thrombolysis is a therapeutic alternative for iliofemoral occlusion.[23]

Most patients with documented pulmonary emboli show clot in the lower extremity on venography, but a venogram negative for clot cannot reasonably exclude the possibility of embolus from the diagnosis.[24]

VENOUS INCOMPETENCE AND DESCENDING VENOGRAPHY

The postphlebitic syndrome can be an extremely debilitating condition characterized by edema, pain, varicosities, skin changes, and ulceration resulting from venous stasis and high transmitted venous pressures. These symptoms are the result of valvular thickening, shortening, and incompetence after DVT. Similar symptoms can also be seen as a primary condition in which major valves have stretched and dilated.[25] In fact, primary valvular incompetence appears to be more common than postphlebitic venous stasis.[26] Surgical treatment involves resuspending proximal valves or anastomosing an incompetent vein to another with proximal competent valves in an end-to-side manner (e.g., incompetent superficial femoral vein to intact saphenous). Duplex sonography is now widely used for evaluation, and it appears more reliable than venography for the demonstration of distal valvular incompetence.[27] At times, descending venography may be ordered for further characterization of disease.

Descending venography may be performed through a catheter placed from the arm or from the opposite femoral vein,[28,29] but it can also be done through a needle or cannula placed directly into the common femoral vein of the involved side. A small amount of contrast medium (about 15 ml) is injected, and the reflux is observed fluoroscopically and graded. The exam proceeds with the patient either upright on a tilt table or supine and performing the Valsalva maneuver. Grading is from 0 to 5, grade 0 representing no reflux and grade 5 representing reflux to the level of the ankle. Even asymptomatic legs can show reflux to the knee, depending on the technique employed, so surgery is reserved for those with more extensive valvular incompetence.[30]

VARICOSE VEINS

Varicose veins may be secondary to chronic deep venous disease, or they may be primary in origin. Primary varicose veins are associated with saphenous vein incompetence and are treated by proximal saphenous vein ligation or stripping.[31] Saphenous vein incompetence is easily assessed by duplex sonography, and descending saphenous venography is rarely requested today. The latter procedure is identical to descending phlebography as described earlier, but grading of insufficiency is unnecessary. The very presence of any valvular incompetence determines the need for surgery.

In individuals with recurrent varicose veins, identification of incompetent perforating veins is generally accomplished with sonography. Incompetent perforators may also be identified by conventional ascending venography, but direct puncture of a varicose group (varicography) can provide a clearer and more complete demonstration.[32] A radiopaque ruler should be placed next to the leg to relate the site of disease to bony landmarks. Spot films are obtained during filling, and it is essential that they be exposed early in the examination before overlapping vessels confuse interpretation. Several venipunctures of isolated varicose groups may be necessary for a complete study, with care taken to flush out contrast material from the previous injection by infusion of heparinized saline before further study. Heparin infusion and use of low-osmolality contrast medium are of utmost importance for the prevention of superficial thrombophlebitis after varicography.

EVALUATING THE SAPHENOUS VEIN AS DONOR VESSEL FOR GRAFT

When the saphenous vein is examined preoperatively, it is useful to do what is explicitly avoided for phlebography in suspected DVT; namely, the distal saphenous is punctured directly, the needle is pointed cephalad, no tourniquets are used with the patient supine, and the patient is instructed to engage the quadriceps and calf muscles in sustained isometric contraction against resistance.[6] The result is better opacification of the greater saphenous vein at the expense of deep and muscular venous filling. The addition of a Valsalva maneuver is also helpful. Venous ultrasound has now made this technique all but obsolete.

TECHNICAL PROBLEMS AND PITFALLS

Errors in diagnosis are commonly the result of incomplete filling of vessels. Defects in the contrast material column are often from the inflow of unopacified blood from a tributary vessel. With fluoroscopy and multiple projections, it can be seen that flow defects, unlike thrombi, are inconstant. Fluoroscopy is essential to establish that contrast medium has reached the vessels being filmed and that opacification is adequate. Otherwise, the timing of filming can be a hit-or-miss proposition. As mentioned, improper needle placement in a superficial vein, weightbearing or muscle contraction by the patient, or use of tourniquets can produce artifacts of poor filling that must be recognized.

COMPLICATIONS AND THEIR PREVENTION

As in any study using iodinated radiographic contrast medium, hypersensitivity reactions occasionally occur during venography. Most are mild, but the examiner must be prepared to treat life-threatening situations. Because of the high volumes injected for most studies, especially if bilateral phle-bography is necessary, careful attention must be paid to renal function and hydration. Note must be made of diabetes mellitus, multiple myeloma, hyperuricemia, and advanced age, all of which increase the risk of acute renal failure.

Extravasation of contrast medium may occur, and most small extrava-sations (less than 10 ml) do not pose a problem. However, tissue necrosis and ulceration have been reported, and risk is higher in those with arterial insufficiency.[33] Plastic cannulas are less subject to extravasation. Saline should be infused through a well-secured needle or cannula prior to injec-tion of contrast material, and the injection site must be regularly checked during its infusion. If extravasation does occur, the leg should be elevated and a cold compress applied.[34] Low-osmolality contrast media are unlike-ly to produce tissue necrosis, even when large volumes are extravasated.[34]

The complication most specific to leg venography is postprocedural thrombophlebitis. Its incidence is related to the concentration and osmo-lality of the contrast agent and to the duration of its contact with the venous endothelium. Positive radionuclide-labeled fibrinogen studies have been reported after venography in up to 60% of individuals with initially normal venograms, but addition of 10,000 units of heparin to 100 ml of normal saline infusion immediately following phlebography reduces this to 3%.[35] A reduced-osmolality contrast agent is also less likely to produce this com-plication.[36] No matter what technique or contrast medium is used, it is advisable to keep examination time as short as possible and to elevate a patient's leg immediately after venography.

ALTERNATIVE METHODS FOR DIAGNOSING DEEP VEIN THROMBOSIS

Impedance plethysmography is a noninvasive technique that measures changes in electrical impedance in the leg that result from changes in blood and/or fluid volume. It is very sensitive in the detection of proximal (femoral and above) venous occlusion, but subocclusive thrombi or thrombi in the presence of large collaterals or duplicated channels can be missed.[37]

A complementary technique is iodine-125 fibrinogen scanning for active thrombus formation. Fibrinogen scanning requires 2 days to com-plete and is not a good diagnostic tool for determining proximal clot, but it is well suited for evaluating the popliteal and calf veins. Hull and asso-ciates have found the combination of fibrinogen scanning and impedance plethysmography to be cost-effective, particularly when obtained on an outpatient basis, and virtually as accurate as venography.[38]

Doppler examination (without ultrasound imaging) is useful when there is an abnormality, but it lacks sensitivity.[39] Duplex sonography of lower extremity veins, combining real-time ultrasonic imaging and Doppler (or color-flow Doppler imaging), improves sensitivity to 95% with a specificity of 98%, and it has largely displaced venography as a screening measure for DVT.[1] Imaging of calf veins can also be performed with high accuracy but is much more dependent on equipment, operator training, and meticulous technique.[40] Even so, not all investigators are convinced that duplex ultrasound merits designation as the new gold standard. Davidson and associates found its sensitivity and positive predictive value to be 38% and 26%, respectively, in a group of patients at high risk for DVT.[41] Patients with chronic venous disease pose particular problems.

Preliminary studies with magnetic resonance imaging (MRI) highlight its potential for detecting DVT.[42] Although MRI may be shown to be accurate, the cost of examination is likely to limit its application.

REFERENCES

1. Cronan JJ: Venous thromboembolic disease: The role of ultrasound. *Radiology* 1993; 186:619–630.
2. Rabinov K, Paulin S: Roentgen diagnosis of venous thrombosis in the leg. *Arch Surg* 1972; 104:134–144.
3. Thomas ML: Phlebography. *Arch Surg* 1972; 104:145–151.
4. Tisnado J, Tsai FY, Beachley MC: An alternate technique for lower extremity venography. *Radiology* 1979; 133:787–788.
5. Gordon DH, Glanz S, Stillman R, Sawyer PN: Descending varicose venography. *Radiology* 1982; 145:832–834.
6. Sapala JA, Szilagyi DE: A simple aid in greater saphenous phlebography. *Surg Gynecol Obstet* 1975; 140:265–267.
7. Smith TP, Cardella JF, Darcy MD, et al: Lower-extremity venography: Value of femoral-vein compression. *Am J Roentgenol* 1986; 147:1025–1026.
8. Kramer FL, Teitelbaum G, Merli GJ: Panvenography and pulmonary angiography in the diagnosis of deep venous thrombosis and pulmonary thromboembolism. *Radiol Clin North Am* 1986; 24:397–418.
9. Rampton JB, Armstrong JD Jr: Bilateral venography of the lower extremities. *Radiology* 1977; 123:802–804.
10. Nicolaides AN, Kakkar VV, Field ES, Renney JTG: The origin of deep vein thrombosis: A venographic study. *Br J Radiol* 1971; 44:653–663.
11. Bhargava R, Millward SF: Contrast venography in patients with very edematous feet: Use of transdermal illumination to aid in vein puncture. *Radiology* 1991; 179:583.
12. Johns CM, Sumkin JH: US-guided venipuncture for venography in the edematous leg. *Radiology* 1991; 180:573.
13. Thomas ML, McAllister V: The radiological progression of deep venous thrombus. *Radiology* 1971; 99:37–40.
14. Lipchik EO, DeWeese JA, Rogoff SM: Serial long-term phlebography after documented lower leg thrombosis. *Radiology* 1976; 120:563–566.

15. Lund F, Diener L, Ericsson JLE: Postmortem intraosseous phlebography as an aid in studies of venous thromboembolism. *Angiology* 1969; 20:155–176.

16. Anderson FA, Wheeler HB, Goldberg RJ, et al: A population-based perspective of the hospital incidence and case-fatality rates of deep vein thrombosis and pulmonary embolism: The Worcester DVT study. *Arch Intern Med* 1991; 151:933–938.

17. Kudsk KA, Fabian TC, Baum S, et al: Silent deep vein thrombosis in immobilized multiple trauma patients. *Am J Surg* 1989; 158:515–519.

18. Kierkegaard A, Norgren L, Olsson C-G, et al: Incidence of deep venous thrombosis in bedridden non-surgical patients. *Acta Med Scand* 1987; 222:409–414.

19. Glanz S, Gordon DH: Utility of foot venography as part of the routine lower-extremity venogram: A prospective study. *Cardiovasc Intervent Radiol* 1986; 9:15–16.

20. Giachino A: Relationship between deep-vein thrombosis in the calf and fatal pulmonary embolism. *Can J Surg* 1988; 31:129–130.

21. Dorfman GS, Cronan JJ, Tupper TB, et al: Occult pulmonary embolism: A common occurrence in deep venous thrombosis. *Am J Roentgenol* 1987; 148:263–266.

22. Moser KM, Fedullo PF, Littlejohn JK, Crawford R: Frequent asymptomatic pulmonary embolism in patients with deep venous thrombosis. *JAMA* 1994; 271:223–225.

23. Turpie AGG, Levine MN, Hirsh J, et al: Tissue plasminogen activator (rt-PA) vs heparin in deep vein thrombosis: Results of a randomized trial. *Chest* 1990; 97:S172–S175.

24. Hull RD, Hirsh J, Carter CJ, et al: Pulmonary angiography, ventilation lung scanning, and venography for clinically suspected pulmonary embolism with abnormal perfusion lung scan. *Ann Intern Med* 1983; 98:891–899.

25. Kistner RL: Primary venous valve incompetence of the leg. *Am J Surg* 1980; 140:218–224.

26. Train JS, Schanzer H, Peirce EC, et al: Radiologic evaluation of the chronic venous stasis syndrome. *JAMA* 1987; 258:941–944.

27. Valentin LI, Valentin WH, Mercado S, Rosado CJ: Venous reflux localization: Comparative study of venography and duplex scanning. *Phlebology* 1993; 8:124–127.

28. Herman RJ, Neiman HL, Yao JST, et al: Descending venography: A method of evaluating lower extremity venous valvular function. *Radiology* 1980; 137:63–69.

29. Taheri SA, Sheehan F, Elias S: Descending venography. *Angiology* 1983; 34:299–305.

30. Thomas ML, Keeling FP, Ackroyd JS: De scending phlebography: A comparison of three methods and an assessment of the normal range of deep vein reflux. *J Cardiovasc Surg (Torino)* 1986; 22:27–30.

31. Thomas ML, Bowles JN: Descending phlebography in the assessment of long saphenous vein incompetence. *Am J Roentgenol* 1985; 145:1255–1257.

32. Thomas ML, Bowles JN: Incompetent perforating veins: Comparison of varicography and ascending phlebography. *Radiology* 1985; 154:619–623.

33. Spigos DG, Thane TT, Capek V: Skin necrosis following extravasation during peripheral phlebography. *Radiology* 1977; 123:605–606.
34. Elam EA, Dorr RT, Lagel KE, Pond GD: Cutaneous ulceration due to contrast extravasation: Experimental assessment of injury and potential antidotes. *Invest Radiol* 1991; 26:13–16.
35. Minar E, Ehringer H, Sommer G, et al: Prevention of postvenographic thrombosis by heparin flush: Fibrinogen uptake measurements. *Am J Roentgenol* 1984; 143:629–632.
36. Murphy WA, Destouet JM, Gilula LA, et al: Hexabrix as a contrast agent for ascending leg phlebography. *Am J Roentgenol* 1985; 144:1279–1281.
37. Ramchandani P, Soulen RL, Fedullo LM, Gaines VD: Deep vein thrombosis: Significant limitations of non-invasive tests. *Radiology* 1985; 156:47–49.
38. Hull R, Hirsch J, Sackett DL, Stoddart G: Cost effectiveness of clinical diagnosis, venography, and noninvasive testing in patients with symptomatic deep-vein thrombosis. *N Engl J Med* 1981; 304:1561–1567.
39. Langsfeld M, Hershey FB, Thorpe L, et al: Duplex B-mode imaging for the diagnosis of deep venous thrombosis. *Arch Surg* 1987; 122:587–591.
40. Yucel EK, Fisher JS, Egglin TK, et al: Isolated calf venous thrombosis: Diagnosis with compression US. *Radiology* 1991; 179:443–446.
41. Davidson BL, Elliott CG, Lensing AWA: Low accuracy of color Doppler ultrasound in the detection of proximal leg vein thrombosis in asymptomatic high-risk patients. *Ann Intern Med* 1992; 117:735–738.
42. Evans AJ, Sostman HD, Knelson MH, et al: Detection of deep venous thrombosis: Prospective comparison of MR imaging with contrast venography. *Am J Roentgenol* 1993; 161:131–139.

14

Pulmonary Angiography

KEY CONCEPTS

1. Ventilation-perfusion scans can direct pulmonary arteriography to the region of greatest suspicion for pulmonary embolism.
2. Initial noninvasive evaluation for lower extremity DVT reduces the need for pulmonary arteriography by 50%.
3. Beware of patients with severe pulmonary hypertension or left bundle branch block.
4. Selective and subselective arteriography are clearly superior to main pulmonary artery or atrial injections.
5. For unequivocal diagnosis of acute pulmonary embolus, intraluminal clot or an abrupt vascular cutoff must be defined.
6. A negative high-quality pulmonary arteriogram excludes clinically significant pulmonary embolus.
7. Pulmonary arteriography is needed for planning operative treatment of chronic pulmonary embolism.

INDICATIONS

Pulmonary arteriography remains the standard for making the diagnosis of acute pulmonary embolism, which is by far the most common indication for the procedure. Magnetic resonance imaging and spiral computed tomography may modify its application in the future, but these methods are still undergoing development and evaluation. Occasionally, pulmonary angiography is used to plan or follow treatment for a variety of other conditions, including chronic pulmonary embolism, developmental abnormalities, arterial hypoplasia or stenosis, pulmonary sequestration, aneurysms, arteriovenous malformations, vasculitides, and vascular occlusion by tumor or inflammatory disease. Rarely, catheterization may be used in massive pulmonary embolism for suction embolectomy or other emergency transcatheter intervention.

WHAT TO KNOW ABOUT THE PATIENT BEFORE STARTING

For an invasive study often performed in very ill patients, pulmonary angiography is quite safe. However, appropriate performance of the study with minimum risk to the patient requires knowledge of the patient's clinical presentation—including onset of symptoms, presence of known underlying pulmonary or cardiac disease (especially left bundle branch block), renal insufficiency, diabetes mellitus, multiple myeloma or other risk factors for acute renal failure from exposure to radiographic contrast media, and, naturally, any history of hypersensitivity to iodinated contrast material. If left bundle branch conduction block is present, there is real danger of inducing total heart block during catheterization, and a temporary cardiac pacemaker should be placed before the catheter is introduced into the pulmonary artery.

Chest radiographs and radionuclide examinations must be reviewed, with particular attention to location of any focal disease or perfusion abnormalities. A radionuclide ventilation-perfusion scan should be obtained when possible in any patient suspected of pulmonary embolus, because the findings may either obviate angiography or direct the study to the area most likely to provide the diagnosis. Heparin should be discontinued at least 1 hour before angiography is performed, but its administration may be resumed immediately afterward.

TECHNIQUE

Catheterization can be performed from a brachial or jugular approach, but the route most commonly used is the common femoral vein. In the latter location, the femoral artery should be palpated and local anesthetic infiltrated just medial to the pulse. Either a double-wall puncture with a

Seldinger needle or a single-wall puncture with a hollow, thin-wall, 18-gauge needle can be used to gain entry. With the single-wall technique, inadvertent passage through the artery is less likely. In both techniques, the needle is placed under gentle suction as it is advanced (hollow needle) or withdrawn (Seldinger). Free return of venous blood indicates that the tip is within the vessel. The guidewire should not be advanced above the common iliac vein before catheter insertion, in case of a major clot in the inferior vena cava. Patency of the iliac vein and inferior vena cava is checked by hand injections of contrast material under fluoroscopic guidance as the catheter is advanced into the right atrium.

The catheter placed should be of large bore (7 Fr or greater), with multiple sideholes and a pigtail tip. Large catheter caliber allows the rapid injection necessary to obtain adequate vascular opacification, and it makes catheter recoil less violent. Straight endhole catheters have been known to cause myocardial injury and pericardial extravasation through recoil and jet effect.

Grollman-type catheters are fairly stiff, have good torque control, and have a sidearm that may be directed through the tricuspid valve. Once the right ventricle is entered, such a catheter is rotated 180° to direct the tip toward the pulmonic valve. The catheter is then advanced into the pulmonary circulation. An alternative method employs a soft pigtail catheter (such as a 7 Fr Kifa) and a tip-deflecting guidewire. The guidewire tip is placed to the level of the pigtail but not beyond the catheter tip. In the atrium the deflecting wire can be used to direct the catheter through the tricuspid valve by fixing the curve of the wire and feeding the catheter forward off the wire (Fig. 14-1). Once into the right ventricle, the catheter and wire are rotated 180°, and deflection is repeated toward the pulmonic valve. Similar manipulations can then place the catheter into the right or left pulmonary artery as desired. Occasionally the catheter may coil in an enlarged atrium as attempts are made to advance it; in such an event the catheter can be straightened by introducing the stiff end of a guidewire up to the pigtail. The catheter may then be slipped off the wire and advanced without buckling.

During all manipulations in the right side of the heart, an observer must constantly monitor the patient's electrocardiogram and call out any induced ectopic beats. If a run of ventricular tachycardia is encountered, it can usually be reversed by immediately withdrawing the catheter and instructing the patient to cough. Rarely, pharmacologic infusion (lidocaine or other antiarrhythmic agent) or electroversion may be necessary. The examiner must always be prepared to treat a possible cardiac or pulmonary arrest.

The catheter tip is best placed initially within the lower lobe pulmonary arterial trunk, unless the major abnormality seen on prior radionuclide studies involves the upper lobe. Pulmonary arterial pressure readings are obtained, and a hand injection of contrast material is used to gauge blood flow. For full-lung opacification in a relatively healthy individual, between

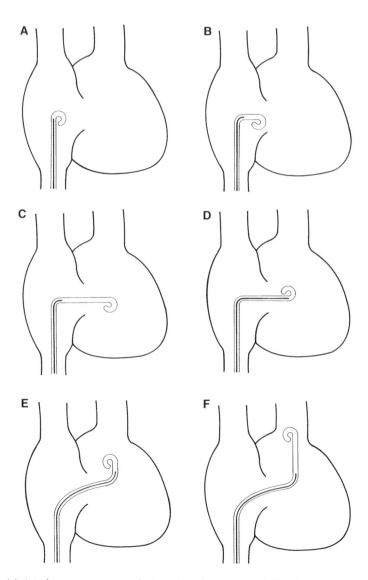

Fig. 14-1 Pulmonary artery catheterization by use of a deflecting wire. **A,** Pigtail catheter and wire in right atrium; **B,** activation of deflecting wire; **C,** catheter advanced through tricuspid valve as wire is held stationary with active deflection; **D,** wire advanced and catheter rotated 180°; **E,** activation of deflecting wire; **F,** catheter fed off deflecting wire through pulmonic valve.

30 and 45 ml of 76% contrast medium is injected at a rate of 20 to 35 ml/second, depending on cardiac output. In patients with severe underlying cardiac or pulmonary disease, the amount and rate of injection should be decreased accordingly. The equipment used must allow a rapid exposure sequence of 14 × 14-inch films. A typical study may include three films per second for 3 seconds, followed by one film per second for the next 6 seconds. Such a sequence normally provides opacification of the pulmonary veins, left side of the heart, and aorta (revealing any unsuspected vascular abnormality, such as aortic dissection). On subsequent injections in a given lung, the last three films may be omitted.

At least two views of each lung should be obtained. Simultaneous biplane filming can decrease the length of the study and the amount of contrast material injected. The ipsilateral posterior oblique view tends to produce the least amount of vascular overlap. If any injection demonstrates embolus, the examination can usually be stopped. In difficult cases, the pigtail catheter may be replaced with a straight or occlusion balloon catheter over an exchange guidewire, and subselective studies performed with magnification filming. Balloon occlusion studies may be more sensitive than conventional angiograms.[1] At some institutions, such injections with magnification are performed routinely in the region of greatest perfusion scan abnormality, if selective injections fail to reveal embolus.[2] Single-projection angiograms with main pulmonary artery or right atrial injection are inadequate to exclude pulmonary embolus.[3]

There are various alternatives to these techniques. The use of cineangiography has some advantages, including the recognition of to-and-fro motion of emboli and the ability to resolve problems with overlap by using respiratory motion,[4] but these are balanced by the smaller field size, lower spatial resolution, and higher radiation dose. Rapid-frame rate, high-resolution digital angiography provides the same advantages without the major drawbacks. It can be used either with or without subtraction, and supplements conventional film studies when they are equivocal. Digital angiography is very well suited for high-risk patients for whom the concentration and amount of contrast material per injection can be decreased, particularly if radionuclide study suggests larger central emboli. One technique to be avoided is "bedside" pulmonary angiography through indwelling central venous catheters. In one comparison of conventional pulmonary angiography and injection of wedge catheters in 21 patients, the latter had a sensitivity of 19%, specificity of 60%, and accuracy of 29% for detection of pulmonary embolus.[5]

ACUTE PULMONARY EMBOLISM

The estimated incidence of pulmonary embolism in the United States is about 600,000, and perhaps 90% survive the initial insult.[6] Anderson and colleagues found that a first episode of recognized pulmonary embolism occurred at an annual rate of 23 per 100,000.[7] Risk is particularly high in certain groups—over 5% in patients with acute spinal cord injury.[8] Pulmonary embolism is found in nearly 20% and massive embolism in 5% of autopsies.[9] In the 1950s only 12% of major emboli were diagnosed antemortem, and although diagnosis has improved, more recent large autopsy series indicate that no more than 30% are currently being recognized.[9,10] The elderly and those with concomitant pneumonia or congestive heart failure are much less likely to be given the correct diagnosis. An Italian survey found pulmonary embolism suspected in only 5% of elderly patients dying with massive emboli.[9] About a third of those with pulmonary embolus have recurrent emboli, and mortality in untreated patients has been reported from 18% to 38%.[2] With proper treatment, mortality can be reduced to less than 3%, and recurrence of clinically evident emboli can be dropped to 8%.[11] Clinical signs and symptoms, laboratory results, and chest radiographs have been notoriously unreliable in securing the diagnosis.

A confident diagnosis of pulmonary embolus is required because therapy has its own risks. Standard treatment comprises intravenous administration of heparin, followed in 1 week by oral warfarin (Coumadin), the latter being continued for 3 to 6 months. Heparin may be the leading cause of drug reaction in hospitalized patients, and anticoagulation in the treatment of pulmonary embolus results in major hemorrhage in 4% to 10% of patients.[12,13]

The development of radionuclide lung scanning has provided clinicians with a useful, low-morbidity tool to screen for embolic disease. In a prospective comparison of radionuclide scanning, pulmonary angiography, and venography in 139 patients, Hull and associates found 30 of the 35 patients with at least one segmental or larger ventilation-perfusion mismatch to have embolus on angiographic study.[14] Refined criteria for scan interpretation have produced a sensitivity of 97%, a specificity of 94%, and accuracy of 96% for readings of high or low probability in another series of patients.[6] The Prospective Investigation of Pulmonary Embolism Diagnosis (PIOPED) study of more than 750 patients found that when clinical assessment and high-probability scan were congruent, 96% of those patients had emboli.[15] In the face of a normal or near-normal perfusion scan, the likelihood of pulmonary embolus was very low, 4%. Others have confirmed the high predictive value and accuracy of a normal perfusion scan.[16] Unfortunately, the great majority of patients investigated have inconclusive radionuclide studies.

Lower extremity venography in patients suspected of suffering pulmonary embolus is helpful in the institution of treatment only if fresh thrombus is found above the knee. A large percentage of those with acute thrombus extending proximally have embolus, even if no pulmonary symptoms are evident.[17] Conversely, absence of thrombus on leg venography does not exclude pulmonary embolus. Up to 18% of those with documented pulmonary embolus have no evidence of leg clot, and noninvasive examinations (less sensitive for deep venous thrombosis than venography) may be normal in more than half.[18] Potential other sources for embolization of thrombus include the pelvic, renal, and subclavian veins. Confounding the issue still further is the observation that 15% of patients found to have thrombotic-embolic disease have a pulmonary arteriogram that is negative for disease, but a positive leg venogram.[14]

Because of the difficulties posed by low- or intermediate-probability readings for most ventilation-perfusion scans, various strategies have been proposed for further noninvasive imaging. A combination of the degree of clinical suspicion, radionuclide study findings, and noninvasive evaluation (serial duplex sonography or impedance plethysmography) for lower extremity deep venous thrombosis (DVT) can cut the need for pulmonary angiography by at least half without sacrificing accuracy, while at the same time containing costs.[19,20] By refraining from placing patients with nondiagnostic radionuclide examinations on anticoagulant medication, as long as serial noninvasive studies remained negative for DVT, Hull and associates encountered evidence of thromboembolic disease in fewer than 2% of such patients on long-term follow-up.[21] Still, not everyone agrees on dispensing with pulmonary arteriography entirely.[20,22] The most prudent course may be to subject those individuals without evidence of DVT and with equivocal ventilation-perfusion scans to pulmonary arteriography.

Pulmonary angiography remains the standard by which all other studies are judged. To make the diagnosis of pulmonary embolus angiographically, intraluminal filling defects or abrupt vascular cutoffs must be identified. Indirect signs, such as diminished capillary stain or delayed opacification, are very nonspecific. Common conditions in those found by angiography not to have pulmonary embolus include congestive heart failure, angina, myocardial infarct, pneumonia, atelectasis, pleurisy, bronchospasm, and bronchiectasis.[2,23] Angiographically, atelectasis is shown by crowded vessels and an intense capillary stain; pneumonia produces markedly slowed blood flow with intrinsically normal vessels and no marked blush.[23] Pulmonary hypertension can produce occasional arterial occlusion from intimal and medial hypertrophy, but such occlusions arise in vessels less than 0.5 mm in diameter. Bronchiectasis is characterized by slow flow or nonopacification because of bronchial artery communications. Emphysematous blebs displace vessels, and there is decreased arborization. Patients with carcinoma may have flow slowed to the entire involved lung, independent of arterial encasement or obliteration.[23]

Injections into the main pulmonary artery may demonstrate emboli as small as 2 mm in diameter, but superselective and magnification techniques can enable detection of clots as small as 0.5 to 1 mm.[2,24] Interobserver agreement is very good for segmental or larger emboli, but interpretation of angiograms is more difficult for subsegmental filling defects.[25]

In a study of 180 patients followed at least 6 months after negative high-quality pulmonary arteriograms, none had signs or symptoms of recurrent embolization.[2] In the PIOPED study, only 4 of 675 patients with arteriograms interpreted as negative were later shown to have emboli.[26] These results support the contention that pulmonary angiography is highly sensitive for detection of clinically relevant pulmonary embolus, and a patient should not be placed on anticoagulants in the face of an angiogram negative for embolus (assuming there is no other indication for anticoagulation).

In obtaining a pulmonary arteriogram, one must be aware of when the patient's symptoms arose. Fred and associates have reported that emboli can lyse completely in 1 to 3 weeks.[27] Another study with 15 patients undergoing serial angiography showed little change in findings in the first week and only rare disappearance of clots before 2 weeks.[28] In any event, it is rarely necessary to perform angiography for diagnosis in the early morning hours unless there is a contraindication to anticoagulation with heparin.

Pulmonary infarction does not occur with large central occluding emboli, but rather with distal occlusions, and is probably related to increased segmental bronchial artery blood flow.[29] True pulmonary infarction is less common than embolus with pulmonary hemorrhage. The latter tends to resolve quickly, whereas the former almost never occurs in the absence of heart disease. It is felt that elevated pulmonary venous pressure is required to produce a true infarction.

In massive pulmonary embolism, catheter methods may be the most expeditious means of saving a patient's life. Catheter embolectomy using a special suction device has been successfully used in individuals in shock or cardiopulmonary arrest.[30] Alternative ways of quickly improving pulmonary perfusion include breaking up central thrombi with the catheter, guidewire, or angioplasty balloon catheter.[31] Experimental work is being done on devices designed for rapid and virtually complete dispersion of large pulmonary clots.[32]

If a patient is not in shock, thrombolysis may be attempted, but several hours are needed to obtain improved perfusion.[33,34] Central pulmonary arterial infusion of thrombolytic agents has not shown any benefit over peripheral venous infusion. If effective thrombolytic protocols are established, the treatment of pulmonary embolism may mirror that presently used for acute myocardial infarction.

CHRONIC PULMONARY EMBOLISM

Chronic pulmonary embolism presents a different clinical and angiographic picture (Fig. 14-2). Symptoms of progressive exertional dyspnea, right-sided heart failure, and cyanosis arise insidiously. Anticoagulants are not an effective treatment, and surgical embolectomy is recommended.[35] The condition may be very difficult to distinguish clinically from primary pulmonary hypertension, but ventilation-perfusion radionuclide scans are virtually always diagnostic.[36,37] Preoperative pulmonary and bronchial angiograms may be obtained to demonstrate anatomy and the likelihood of postoperative improvement. Chronic pulmonary embolism is manifested by arterial webs, stenoses, irregular occlusions, wall-scalloping, and "pouching" defects (a concave edge of thrombus facing the opacified lumen).[23,38]

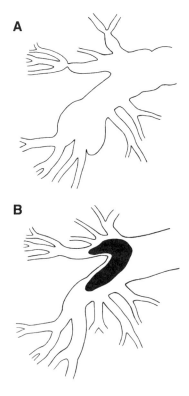

Fig. 14-2 Chronic and acute pulmonary embolism. **A,** Chronic embolism can produce webs, scalloped mural irregularities, and outpouchings. **B,** Unequivocal demonstration of acute embolism requires a filling defect produced by contrast medium flowing around and outlining a thrombus.

PULMONARY ANGIOGRAPHY IN NONEMBOLIC DISEASE

Arteriography can be used to confirm the presence of pulmonary arteriovenous malformations, which can be effectively treated by transcatheter embolization. Untreated lesions can produce cyanosis, hemoptysis, and systemic emboli (often septic). Mycotic or other pulmonary arterial aneurysms may require angiographic evaluation.[39]

Rarely, Takayasu's arteritis can present with occlusion of major pulmonary arterial branches.[40,41] Primary or metastatic intraluminal tumors can simulate pulmonary embolism.[41] Congenital webs, enlarged nodes, or fibrosing mediastinitis can produce pulmonary venous obstruction and secondary pulmonary arterial hypertension. In such cases segmental injections and measurement of pulmonary wedge pressures may be vital for making the correct diagnosis.[42]

COMPLICATIONS

Reactions to contrast material are similar in incidence and severity to those elicited by excretory urography or other contrast infusion studies. In the PIOPED study there were 5 deaths in 1111 patients undergoing pulmonary arteriography; another 1% had severe complications and 5% had minor complications.[26] The incidence of renal failure afterwards was 1%, including 3 patients who needed dialysis. In a review of 1350 procedures at Duke University hospitals, 11 episodes of hypersensitivity to contrast material were noted, including 4 severe reactions.[43] In the same review there were 11 significant arrhythmias and 5 cardiac arrests; all patients were successfully resuscitated.

At Duke, three deaths have been directly attributable to pulmonary angiography (mortality of 0.2%), all in patients with pulmonary arterial systolic pressures greater than 70 mm Hg and with right ventricular end-diastolic pressures of at least 20 mm Hg. These individuals suffered irreversible right-heart failure after angiography. Risk of mortality in such patients is 2% to 3% and does not appear related to the site and amount of injection.[43,44] One similar death has been reported after a single subselective injection of 10 ml of contrast medium by hand.[45] By contrast, Auger and colleagues encountered no fatal complications in their series of 250 patients with chronic pulmonary embolism; the mean pulmonary systolic pressure in their series was 77 mm Hg.[38] In any event, prudence dictates that high-risk patients be studied by subselective injections in which small amounts of contrast material are used. Nonionic or dilute contrast agents may be safer. Special care should be exercised in patients who have been given amiodarone for cardiac arrhythmias.[46]

The risk of performing pulmonary angiography in any given patient must be weighed against the risk of inappropriate treatment. As noted earlier, long-term anticoagulation can cause life-threatening hemorrhage, and the decision to assume anticoagulant therapy should not be made lightly.

REFERENCES

1. Ferris EJ, Smith PL, Lim WN, et al: Radionuclide-guided balloon occlusion pulmonary cineangiography: An adjunct to pulmonary arteriography. *Am Heart J* 1984; 108:539–542.
2. Novelline RA, Baltarowich OH, Athanasoulis CA, et al: The clinical course of patients with suspected pulmonary embolism and a negative pulmonary arteriogram. *Radiology* 1978; 126:561–567.
3. Price L: False negative angiogram in pulmonary embolism. *Chest* 1985; 88:139–141.
4. Meyerovitz MF, Levin DC, Harrington DP, et al: Evaluation of optimized biplane pulmonary cineangiography. *Invest Radiol* 1985; 20:945–949.
5. LePage JR, Gracia RM: The value of bedside wedge pulmonary angiography in the detection of pulmonary emboli: A predictive and prospective evaluation. *Radiology* 1982; 144:67–73.
6. Spies WG, Burstein SP, Dillehay GL, et al: Ventilation-perfusion scintigraphy in suspected pulmonary embolism: Correlation with pulmonary angiography and refinement of criteria for interpretation. *Radiology* 1986; 159:383–390.
7. Anderson FA, Wheeler HB, Goldberg RJ, et al: A population-based perspective of the hospital incidence and case-fatality rates of deep vein thrombosis and pulmonary embolism: The Worcester DVT study. *Arch Intern Med* 1991; 151:933–938.
8. Rogers FB, Shackford SR, Wilson J, et al: Prophylactic vena cava filter insertion in severely injured trauma patients: Indications and preliminary results. *J Trauma* 1993; 35:637–642.
9. Bussani R, Cosatti C: L'embolia polmonare: Analisi epidemiologica su 27,410 sogetti sottoposti ad autopsia nel corso di 10 anni. *Med-Ital* 1990; 10:40–43.
10. Goldhaber SZ, Hennekens CH, Evans DA, et al: Factors associated with correct antemortem diagnosis of major pulmonary embolism. *Am J Med* 1982; 73:822–826.
11. Carson JL, Kelley MA, Duff A, et al: The clinical course of pulmonary embolism. *N Engl J Med* 1992; 326:1240–1245.
12. Glenny RW: Pulmonary embolism: Complications of therapy. *South Med J* 1987; 80:1266–1276.
13. Gurwitz JH, Goldberg RJ, Holden A, et al: Age-related risks of long-term oral anticoagulant therapy. *Arch Intern Med* 1988; 148:1733–1736.
14. Hull RD, Hirsh J, Carter CJ, et al: Pulmonary angiography, ventilation lung scanning, and venography for clinically suspected pulmonary embolism with abnormal perfusion lung scan. *Ann Intern Med* 1983; 98:891–899.
15. PIOPED Investigators: Value of the ventilation/perfusion scan in acute pulmonary embolism: Results of the prospective investigation of pulmonary embolism diagnosis (PIOPED). *JAMA* 1990; 263:2753–2759.

16. Hull RD, Raskob GE, Coates G, Panju AA: Clinical validity of a normal perfusion lung scan in patients with suspected pulmonary embolism. *Chest* 1990; 97:23–26.
17. Moser KM, Fedullo PF, Littlejohn JK, Crawford R: Frequent asymptomatic pulmonary embolism in patients with deep venous thrombosis. *JAMA* 1994; 271:223–225.
18. Scigala EM, McDonnell AM, Hadcock WE, et al: Prevalence of deep venous thrombosis in patients with proven pulmonary embolism. *Bruit* 1984; 8:222–224.
19. Stein PD, Hull RD, Saltzman HA, Pineo G: Strategy for diagnosis of patients with suspected acute pulmonary embolism. *Chest* 1993; 103:1553–1559.
20. Oudkerk M, van Beek EJR, van Putten WLJ, Büller HR: Cost-effectiveness analysis of various strategies in the diagnostic management of pulmonary embolism. *Arch Intern Med* 1993; 153:947–954.
21. Hull RD, Raskob GE, Ginsberg JS, et al: A noninvasive strategy for the treatment of patients with suspected pulmonary embolism. *Arch Intern Med* 1994; 154:289–297.
22. Quinn RJ, Nour R, Butler SP, et al: Pulmonary embolism in patients with intermediate probability lung scans: Diagnosis with doppler venous US and D-Dimer measurement. *Radiology* 1994; 190:509–511.
23. Bookstein JJ, Silver TM: The angiographic differential diagnosis of acute pulmonary embolism. *Radiology* 1974; 110:25–33.
24. Bookstein JJ, Feigin DS, Seo KW, Alazraki NP: Diagnosis of pulmonary embolism: Experimental evaluation of the accuracy of scintigraphically guided pulmonary arteriography. *Radiology* 1980; 136:15–23.
25. Quinn MF, Lundell CO, Klotz TA, et al: Reliability of selective pulmonary arteriography in the diagnosis of pulmonary embolism. *Am J Roentgenol* 1987; 149:469–471.
26. Stein PD, Athanasoulis C, Alavi A, et al: Complications and validity of pulmonary angiography in acute pulmonary embolism. *Circulation* 1992; 85:462–468.
27. Fred HL, Axelrad MA, Lewis JM, Alexander JK: Rapid resolution of pulmonary thromboemboli in man. *JAMA* 1966; 196:1137–1139.
28. Dalen JE, Banas JS Jr, Brooks HL, et al: Resolution rate of acute pulmonary embolism in man. *N Engl J Med* 1969; 280:1194–1199.
29. Dalen JE, Haffajee CI, Alpert JS, et al: Pulmonary embolism, pulmonary hemorrhage, and pulmonary infarction. *N Engl J Med* 1977; 296:1431–1435.
30. Timsit J-F, Reynaud P, Meyer G, Sors H: Pulmonary embolectomy by catheter device in massive pulmonary embolism. *Chest* 1991; 100:655–658.
31. Brady AJB, Crake T, Oakley CM: Percutaneous catheter fragmentation and distal dispersion of proximal pulmonary embolus. *Lancet* 1991; 338:1186–1189.
32. Schmitz-Rode T, Günther RW: New device for percutaneous fragmentation of pulmonary emboli. *Radiology* 1991; 180:135–137.
33. Rosenthal D, Evans RD, Borrero E, et al: Massive pulmonary embolism: Triple-armed therapy. *J Vasc Surg* 1989; 9:261–270.
34. Goldhaber SZ: Thrombolysis in venous thromboembolism: An international perspective. *Chest* 1990; 97:S176–S181.

35. Mills SR, Jackson DC, Sullivan DC, et al: Angiographic evaluation of chronic pulmonary embolism. *Radiology* 1980; 136:301–308.
36. Moser KM, Page GT, Ashburn WL, Fedullo PF: Perfusion lung scans provide a guide to which patients with apparent primary pulmonary hypertension merit angiography. *West J Med* 1988; 148:167–170.
37. Chapman PJ, Bateman ED, Benatar SR: Primary pulmonary hypertension and thromboembolic pulmonary hypertension: Similarities and differences. *Respir Med* 1990; 84:485–488.
38. Auger WR, Fedullo PF, Moser KM, et al: Chronic major-vessel thromboembolic pulmonary artery obstruction: Appearance at angiography. *Radiology* 1992; 182:393–398.
39. SanDretto MA, Scanlon GT: Multiple mycotic pulmonary artery aneurysms secondary to intravenous drug abuse. *Am J Roentgenol* 1984; 142:89–90.
40. Hayashi K, Nagasaki M, Matsunaga N, et al: Initial pulmonary artery involvement in Takayasu arteritis. *Radiology* 1986; 159:401–403.
41. Cassling RJ, Lois JF, Gomes AS: Unusual pulmonary angiographic findings in suspected pulmonary embolism. *Am J Roentgenol* 1985; 145:995–999.
42. Bowen JS, Bookstein JJ, Johnson AD, et al: Wedge and subselective pulmonary angiography in pulmonary hypertension secondary to venous obstruction. *Radiology* 1985; 155:599–603.
43. Mills SR, Jackson DC, Older RA, et al: The incidence, etiologies, and avoidance of complications of pulmonary angiography in a large series. *Radiology* 1980; 136:295–299.
44. Perlmutt LM, Braun SD, Newman GE, et al: Pulmonary arteriography in the high-risk patient. *Radiology* 1987; 162:187–189.
45. Marsh JD, Glynn M, Torman HA: Pulmonary angiography: Application in a new spectrum of patients. *Am J Med* 1983; 75:763–770.
46. Wood DL, Osborn MJ, Rooke J, Holmes DR: Amiodarone pulmonary toxicity: Report of two cases associated with rapidly progressive fatal adult respiratory distress syndrome after pulmonary angiography. *Mayo Clin Proc* 1985; 60:601–603.

15

Vena Caval Filters

KEY CONCEPTS

1. Inferior vena cava (IVC) filters are used to prevent pulmonary emboli (PE) in those who have recurrent PE on anticoagulants or in whom anticoagulation is contraindicated.
2. Caval size, patency, and the presence of any venous anomalies must be documented prior to filter insertion.
3. Infrarenal placement, as close as possible to the lowest renal vein, is optimal.
4. Use of a guidewire and meticulous attention to technique prevent the most serious complication: accidental filter discharge or embolization into the heart.
5. Recurrent PE and IVC occlusion are rare after proper placement of a caval filter.

INDICATIONS

Standard therapy for pulmonary embolism (PE) or lower extremity deep venous thrombosis (DVT) is intravenous heparin followed by longer-term oral warfarin (Coumadin). Such a regimen may reduce the estimated 30% mortality of untreated PE to 2.5%.[1] Patients in dire straits from massive embolization or with large iliofemoral thromboses may be treated more aggressively by systemic thrombolytic drugs. However, there are many patients for whom anticoagulant and thrombolytic therapy are contraindicated or have failed to prevent recurrent PE.

Anticoagulation is contraindicated in the presence of active or recent hemorrhage, especially intracranial bleeding. Peptic ulcer disease and alcoholism predispose patients on warfarin to major bleeding problems. Up to 28% of patients presenting with venous thromboembolic disease may have peptic ulcers or erosion.[2] Although some might dispute the risks posed to those with primary or metastatic intracranial tumors, most physicians would avoid anticoagulation drugs in such patients.[3] Recent or planned surgery may be complicated by the need for anticoagulation, and some patients, such as those undergoing hip arthroplasty in the face of a previous history of DVT, are particularly vulnerable to postoperative thromboembolic disease. Others whose problems are difficult to manage by anticoagulation alone include those with malignant tumors and paraplegia.[4]

Furthermore, 8% to 28% of those on drug therapy for PE may have recurrent emboli.[1,5,6] Often they can be attributed to poor control and inadequate anticoagulation, but there are cases in which the best medical management is ineffective.

It is primarily for these indications that surgical and nonsurgical interventions have been devised to interrupt the path between peripheral thrombi and the pulmonary circulation. With the introduction of easily placed and effective caval filters, some have extended the indications for filter placement to include prophylaxis for those with low cardiopulmonary reserve, spinal cord injury, or extensive femoropelvic fractures combined with head trauma.[7–9] Others, noting a 30-day mortality as high as 26%, question the wisdom of routine insertion of caval filters in patients with advanced malignancy or severe heart disease.[10] Despite the ease of filter placement, clinical judgment and proper documentation of the reason for intervention should be applied in every instance.

BACKGROUND

The first surgical approaches to thromboembolic prophylaxis included bilateral femoral vein ligation below the junction with saphenous vein, but recurrent emboli were still observed. Some surgeons have not yet abandoned the procedure, although 11% of their patients have suffered subsequent PE.[11] Inferior vena cava (IVC) ligation similarly resulted in clinical failure in 4% to 50%, while causing venous stasis problems in a large number of patients.[12] These procedures did not address the problem of collateral drainage. Collateral veins (pelvic and lumbar) enlarge markedly with time and can thus provide an alternate pathway for large embolizing clots. For this same reason, balloon occlusion of the vena cava might be expected to have limited efficacy, although Hunter and associates have reported a large series of patients without any late deaths attributable to recurrent PE.[13] In any event, the percutaneously placed Hunter-Sessions balloon has not achieved widespread clinical acceptance.

Surgical techniques for caval fenestration by sutures or specially designed clips were developed in order to maintain IVC flow through a set of smaller parallel channels. Recurrent PE was reduced to the order of 4%, and caval patency was maintained in 76% to 80% of patients.[12] However, long-term problems with venous stasis were not overcome by caval fenestration. Moreover, ligation or clip placement requires major surgery with its attendant morbidity in patients who are often seriously ill. Reported mortality of IVC plication patients has been 12%.[14]

CAVAL FILTERS

The problems of recurrent emboli, caval patency–venous stasis, and operative risk have been addressed by the design of a number of caval filtering devices (Fig. 15-1). Several features desired of any venous filter include ease and stability of placement, efficacy of clot trapping, long-term patency, and lack of associated complications (caval perforation, migration, infection, or thrombosis of the access vein). An ideal filter would also be removable percutaneously, thus permitting use for temporary indications such as protection of the pulmonary circulation during thrombolysis of a large central venous thrombus.[15]

Mobin-Uddin Filter

The first filter to receive widespread application was the Mobin-Uddin "umbrella," which was introduced in 1967.[14] It was the first to allow introduction through a peripheral venous cutdown, which posed much less risk to the patient than an abdominal operation. The initial filter was 23 mm in diameter, which was quickly increased to 28 mm when migration was found to be a major problem. Although the instances of migration were decreased to less than 1%, IVC thrombosis occurred in 33% to 85% of patients.[16]

The Stainless Steel (Original) Greenfield Filter

The Greenfield filter represented a major improvement over the Mobin-Uddin. The original Greenfield filter, which is still available (primarily for

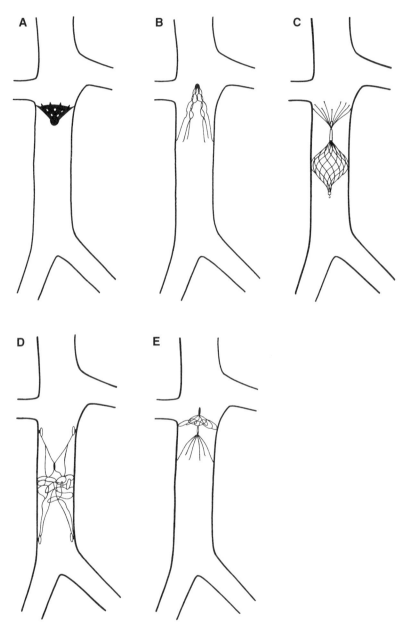

Fig. 15-1 Various inferior vena caval filters in place inferior to the renal veins: **A,** Mobin-Uddin; **B,** Greenfield; **C,** Günther; **D,** bird's nest; **E,** Simon nitinol.

intraoperative placement during pulmonary thrombectomy or other surgical procedure), is composed of six stainless-steel wires joined at the hub and radiating in a cone of 35° with the hook-tipped wires 6 mm apart at the base. The hub points in the direction of blood flow, and trapped emboli are directed toward the center of the vessel. This design has the effect of maintaining flow through the IVC and subjecting the trapped clot to endogenous thrombolysis. The more open design of the filter has resulted in a 1-year caval patency rate of 96%, while decreasing the incidence of recurrent PE to 4%.[17] In a recently published study using venacavography, filter patency at a mean of more than 2.5 years of follow-up was 90%; 3% of the patients died of recurrent pulmonary embolism.[18]

The efficacy of the Greenfield filter is dependent on proper alignment with the vena cava. A tilt of 10° to 20° with respect to IVC axis may make the filter completely ineffective for all but the largest emboli.[19] Significant tilting has been observed in 12% to 16% of patients,[16,20] and has been directly implicated in cases of recurrent PE.[21]

Methods for percutaneous insertion of both Mobin-Uddin and stainless-steel Greenfield filters were devised, obviating the need for surgical cutdown and greatly speeding placement, but the methods needed large venotomies to accommodate the 24 Fr insertion capsules.[14,22] The large capsule sizes limited the sites of potential venous access, and the trauma of insertion commonly led to thrombosis of the access vein. At our institution the last percutaneous insertion of a stainless-steel Greenfield filter resulted in the laceration of a small common iliac vein and emergency surgery. Fortunately, the new generation of filters now available has made percutaneous introduction faster and much less traumatic.

The Titanium Greenfield Filter
Modification of the original Greenfield design resulted in a slightly longer titanium device, also slightly broader at the base, which is inserted by a 12 Fr carrier passed through a 14 Fr sheath.[23,24] Addition of a trigger release has simplified discharge. The initial titanium Greenfield filters had an unacceptable 30% rate of migration, tilting, and IVC penetration, but a revision of the hook design has largely overcome these problems.[24] Reported incidence of recurrent PE has been 0 to 3%, and caval patency is 89% to 91% at 1 year.[9,24,25]

Bird's Nest Filter
The bird's nest filter is descriptively named. After discharge, it forms a tangle of wires resembling a nest. The filter is composed of four fine stainless-steel wires that can be inserted through a 12 Fr sheath.[26] It is fixed in place by pairs of cranial and caudal hooks and can be released in larger-diameter IVCs than the Greenfield or other filters can. Control

during filter discharge is maintained by a guidewire-pusher with a button release at its end. The button is protected by a peel-away cover that prevents unintended discharge. Reported incidences of IVC thrombosis and recurrent pulmonary embolism are comparable to those occurring after Greenfield filter placement.[26,27] An advantage of this filter is the ability to deploy it safely in an IVC as large as 40 mm in diameter.[28] It is also the only available filter designed to be removed or repositioned after partial discharge. Nevertheless, after optimal deployment, the bird's nest filter covers about 70 mm, twice the length of other available devices. Since the redesign of the anchoring struts before the FDA approval of the filter, there have been very isolated reports of filter migration, and those have been associated with trapping of massive emboli.[29] At the University of Wisconsin–Madison, we have inserted more than 250 of these filters with satisfactory results.

Simon Nitinol Filter

The Simon filter is composed of nitinol, a nickel-titanium alloy that has a heat-dependent memory.[30] The configuration is somewhat similar to that of the Greenfield filter, but with the addition of an overlapping open-wire cap to the hub. The cap permits the filter to align itself with the IVC immediately upon discharge. As long as the filter is cooled in iced water it is quite pliable and can be straightened in its 8 Fr carrier. Exposure to body temperature at the time of placement causes the filter to resume the shape it "memorized" at manufacture.

Early evaluation has shown a 7% rate of IVC thrombosis, and one fourth of the patients examined by caval imaging at follow-up had signs of thrombi trapped by the filter.[30] The Simon nitinol filter has the advantage of having the smallest carrier of any commercially available device, and it can be inserted through a brachial vein, if necessary. There have been instances of filter migration to the heart and pulmonary arteries, perhaps a consequence of the filter's lack of penetrating anchoring hooks.[25,31]

Vena Tech LGM Filter

This filter is a stamped, six-pronged cone made of stainless steel.[32] It is prepackaged in a loading syringe and inserted through a 12 Fr sheath. One-year caval patency has been 92%, and recurrent PE has been noted in 2%.[32] A longer-term study by Crochet and colleagues has shown 92% patency at 2 years and 70% patency at 6 years follow-up.[33]

Amplatz Filter

This filter is composed of 18 wires formed into a "spider"; it is capable of insertion through a 14 Fr sheath.[34] The Amplatz filter is positioned from above by a threaded guidewire or from the femoral approach by a snare fastened to a hook. The Amplatz filter has the advantage of possible retrieval through the common femoral vein, as long as retrieval is attempted within 2 weeks of placement. Filters left in position for a longer period become permanently fixed within the IVC. McCowan and associates reported a 7% incidence of recurrent PE and 23% caval occlusion rate with this filter by clinical follow-up criteria.[35] The Amplatz filter is not commercially available.

Günther Basket Filter
The Günther filter consists of 12 heparin-coated stainless-steel wires formed into a basket and placed through a 10 Fr catheter.[36] This filter was also designed to permit its removal within 10 days of insertion by means of a snare from the femoral route. Because of very high rates of caval perforation (some struts penetrating aorta and bowel), as well as filter breakage and disruption, this device (never available in the United States) has been withdrawn from the market.[37]

TECHNIQUE OF PERCUTANEOUS FILTER PLACEMENT

Before placing an IVC filter, some would advocate documenting the lower extremities as source of emboli in all cases.[6] However, absence of leg clots on venography does not necessarily exclude a lower extremity source, and some PEs undoubtedly arise in pelvic veins. Therefore, the decision to perform lower extremity venography before filter placement should be made on an individual basis. Similarly, some radiologists recommend pulmonary arteriography in every patient.[22] In all events, the risks of DVT and PE, their documentation by imaging studies, and the contraindications to conventional medical therapy must all be taken into consideration.

The various filters designed for percutaneous placement are usually inserted through the right femoral vein or right internal jugular vein, but, should the need arise (because of insertion site thrombosis or anatomic anomaly), the left femoral and jugular veins may be used. The Simon nitinol filter may be placed through a brachial venous access. McCowan and associates have had success placing filters through the right external jugular vein in 13 patients using an Amplatz superstiff guidewire to straighten the course of the vein during insertion.[38]

Whatever approach or filter is used, an IVC cavogram is obtained initially to document caval patency and size. If a very large IVC or megacava (over 30 mm in size) is encountered, a bird's nest filter should be used as long as the IVC diameter is not greater than 40 mm. An alternative would be to leave a filter in both common iliac veins. If a duplication of the IVC is uncovered, a filter may be deployed in each of the vessels.

The location of the renal veins must also be documented. Ideal filter position is immediately inferior to the renal veins. If the IVC should occlude at the site of filter placement, renal vein obstruction would not necessarily follow. An anatomic variant that must be kept in mind is the circumaortic renal vein, a venous ring found in up to 11% of renal venograms.[39] The retroaortic segment often drains into the IVC at the level of L3. If a filter were placed between the two segments of the ring, a large, unfiltered collateral pathway to the pulmonary circulation would be immediately available to emboli. When necessary, such as with renal vein thrombi or caval occlusion to the level of the kidneys, filters can be safely placed in the suprarenal IVC.[16,40]

The use of a Bell-Thompson ruler, or radiopaque letters or numbers taped to the patient's back, permits the level of renal veins to be determined at a glance. The precise technique of filter discharge varies from simple trigger mechanisms for the titanium Greenfield and LGM filters to somewhat more elaborate placement methods for the Simon nitinol and bird's nest devices. Different carriers are needed for each type of filter, depending on a femoral versus jugular or upper extremity approach.

Femoral Approach

Placement from a femoral vein is preferred by many radiologists, who find it a more familiar and comfortable approach than the jugular vein. Also, patient comfort, as well as field sterility, may be maintained more easily. Air embolus is much less likely to occur with transfemoral insertion. Disadvantages of the approach include the possibility of iliofemoral thrombus obstructing the vein, possible IVC thrombus extension, and the occasional difficulty in advancing the filter introducer sheath beyond the crossing right common iliac artery if a left femoral access is used. A rapid and limited ultrasound evaluation of the femoral vein is often useful before access is attempted.

When the femoral vein is entered, the guidewire and catheter should not be inserted very far. Injection of contrast medium permits the presence of obstructing or nonobstructing thrombus to be identified. If no iliac clot is encountered, a pigtail catheter is placed to the level of the confluence of iliac veins, and an IVC study is performed. Once the diagnostic films have been obtained, the introducer sheath and filter carrier are advanced over a wire to the level of desired deployment.

If one is unfamiliar with the introduction and release of the particular filter to be placed, the manufacturer's instructions should be carefully read and the procedure rehearsed (without actually discharging the device). The filter carrier should be flushed as directed by the manufacturer before it is inserted through the sheath. Once the filter is discharged, attempts at heroic manipulations to alter its position or configuration are not advised, for filter embolization or caval wall laceration could result. An exception is the gentle probing with a J-tipped guidewire or catheter. This is sometimes needed to unhook crossed filter legs with the titanium Greenfield filter.

Abdominal radiographs and/or repeat cavography should always be obtained after filter placement. The position and configuration are documented, allowing comparison with subsequent films if any late problem or question of filter displacement arises.

Jugular Placement
Use of the right jugular vein for access avoids the possibility of trying to catheterize an occluded femoral vein. Symptomatic jugular vein occlusion is less likely to occur after percutaneous filter placement than postinsertion femoral vein thrombosis. However, extra care must be taken to prevent air embolism by placing the patient in a Trendelenburg position or by elevating the legs, and by having the patient perform a Valsalva maneuver during insertion of the sheath and carrier assembly.

The eustachian valve (valve of the IVC) at the junction of the right atrium and the IVC can occasionally cause some difficulties. After the diagnostic cavogram is obtained, a stiff exchange wire should be used, and its tip securely positioned in an iliac vein to ensure filter discharge in the IVC. Mistaken filter placement into hepatic, renal, or even gonadal veins has occurred.[34] If a stiff guidewire and careful fluoroscopic observation are not employed, the wire and filter can buckle into the right ventricle. Fluoroscopy is mandatory; the great majority of misplacements into the heart have resulted from lack of radiologic guidance.[41]

As noted, the filter carriers needed for a transjugular or upper extremity insertion differ from those of a femoral filter introducer. In other respects, the steps in filter placement are similar to those previously described for the femoral approach.

FOLLOW-UP, COMPLICATIONS, AND OTHER CONSIDERATIONS

After filter placement, the patient should be kept at bedrest and observed for 2 to 4 hours to minimize the chance of puncture site bleeding. Although puncture site thrombosis can complicate insertion, with the smaller introducers now available it has become less of a problem. Patients who develop new or worsening extremity edema or signs of venous stasis may be examined with duplex sonography or catheter contrast venography to assess possible deep venous thrombosis or caval occlusion. Magnetic resonance imaging is useful in the examination of patients with titanium or nitinol filters, but other stainless-steel devices cause considerable artifact.[28]

Over the long term, many symptoms of stasis are consequent to the patient's underlying venous disease and postphlebitic valvular incompetence, rather than to IVC obstruction.[27,33,42] Anticoagulation may be resumed within several hours, but use of thrombolytics should be avoided after filter placement.[43]

If a Greenfield or LGM filter is severely tilted (or if thrombus is found to arise from the filter or more proximal IVC), another filter may be placed above it, in the suprarenal cava. Cases of inappropriate filter discharge can sometimes be managed conservatively, but filters within the heart should be removed. There have been reports of percutaneous retrieval,[25,44] but most patients with intracardiac filters need open-heart surgery.[29] Once a filter has been released, catheterization through it is possible,[45] but it should be performed only as a last resort.

Placement of a Greenfield filter in the superior vena cava (SVC) has been reported in conjunction with documented pulmonary emboli from an upper extremity source.[46] We have placed an LGM filter in the SVC of a similar patient, but the circumstances demanding such a procedure are quite rare.

Distal migration of Greenfield filters (up to 2 cm) has been commonly observed with time, as has perforation of the IVC wall by filter struts.[47] Migration and decrease in filter span should raise the suspicion of IVC thrombosis.[48] Distal migration and caval perforation have been very common with Günther filters.[36,37] Although caval wall perforation is usually innocuous, it may lead to adhesions, bowel obstruction, or peritonitis, particularly in quadriplegic patients engaging in vigorous maneuvers during pulmonary physical therapy.[47] No matter which particular device is chosen, the risk of filter disruption or disintegration over time should make one circumspect about leaving any filter in a young patient without malignant disease.[37,49]

In vitro characteristics of various filters have been compared by Katsamouris and colleagues by using clots of 2-mm to 7-mm diameter.[19] In their study the Mobin-Uddin and Greenfield filters were ineffective when tilted and caused the most turbulent downstream flow. The other filters all captured clots larger than 2-mm diameter, whether or not filter configuration was optimal. The Mobin-Uddin and Amplatz filters produced the largest pressure gradients after trapping a few clots, whereas the bird's nest filter accommodated the most thrombi before causing a pressure rise. Despite the implications of these data, the Greenfield filter has been quite effective clinically, and it reliably captures thrombi 6 to 8 mm in diameter in vivo, even when tilted.[50] To this point, the newer filters available in the United States (titanium Greenfield, bird's nest, Vena Tech LGM, Simon nitinol) appear to be safe and demonstrate comparable efficacy.

REFERENCES

1. Carson JL, Kelley MA, Duff A, et al: The clinical course of pulmonary embolism. *N Engl J Med* 1992; 326:1240–1245.

2. Monreal M, Boix J, Humbert P, et al: Gastroduodenal ulcer incidence in patients with venous thromboembolism. *Gastrointest Endosc* 1989; 35:386–388.
3. Olin JW, Young JR, Graor RA, et al: Treatment of deep venous thrombosis and pulmonary emboli in patients with primary and metastatic brain tumors: Anticoagulants or inferior vena cava filter? *Arch Intern Med* 1987; 147:2177–2179.
4. Golueke PJ, Garrett WV, Thompson JE, et al: Interruption of the vena cava by means of the Greenfield filter: Expanding the indications. *Surgery* 1988; 103:111–117.
5. Monreal M, Ruiz J, Salvador R, et al: Recurrent pulmonary embolism: A prospective study. *Chest* 1989; 95:976–979.
6. Glenny RW: Pulmonary embolism: Complications of therapy. *South Med J* 1987; 80:1266–1276.
7. Rohrer MJ, Scheidler MG, Wheeler HB, Cutler BS: Extended indications for placement of an inferior vena cava filter. *J Vasc Surg* 1989; 10:44–50.
8. Pomper SR, Lutchman G: The role of intracaval filters in patients with COPD and DVT. *Angiology* 1991; 42:85–89.
9. Rogers FB, Shackford SR, Wilson J, et al: Prophylactic vena cava filter insertion in severely injured trauma patients: Indications and preliminary results. *J Trauma* 1993; 35:637–642.
10. Arnold TE, Karabinis VD, Mehta V, et al: Potential of overuse of the inferior vena cava filter. *Surg Gynecol Obstet* 1993; 177:463–467.
11. Louagie Y, Vanruyssevelt P, Elhammouti F, et al: Ligation of the superficial femoral vein in prevention of pulmonary embolism: An old fashion procedure. *J Cardiovasc Surg (Torino)* 1990; 31:416–423.
12. Coleman CC: Overview of interruption of the inferior vena cava. *Semin Intervent Radiol* 1986; 3:175–187.
13. Hunter JA, DeLaria GA, Goldin MD, et al: Inferior vena cava interruption with the Hunter-Sessions balloon: Eighteen years' experience in 191 cases. *J Vasc Surg* 1989; 10:450–456.
14. Coleman CC, Castañeda-Zuñiga WR, Amplatz K: Mobin-Uddin vena caval filters. *Semin Intervent Radiol* 1986; 3:193–195.
15. Chavan A, Gulba D, Schaefer C, et al: The Filcard temporary, removable vena cava filter: Use in local thrombolytic therapy. *Z Kardiol* 1993; 82:191–193.
16. Kanter B, Moser KM: The Greenfield vena cava filter. *Chest* 1988; 93:170–175.
17. Greenfield LJ, Michna BA: Twelve-year clinical experience with the Greenfield vena caval filter. *Surgery* 1988; 104:706–712.
18. Lang W, Schweiger H, Hofmann-Preiss K: Results of long-term venacavography study after placement of a Greenfield vena caval filter. *J Cardiovasc Surg (Torino)* 1992; 33:573–578.
19. Katsamouris AA, Waltman AC, Deichatsios MA, Athanasoulis CA: Inferior vena cava filters: In vitro comparison of clot trapping and flow dynamics. *Radiology* 1988; 166:361–366.
20. Greenfield LJ, Peyton R, Crute S, Barnes R: Greenfield vena cava filter experience: Late results in 156 patients. *Arch Surg* 1981; 116:1451–1456.

21. Schanzer H, Knight R: Recurrent pulmonary embolism from thrombi in Greenfield filter: Case report. *Vasc Surg* 1988; 22:110–113.

22. Denny DF, Cronan JJ, Dorfman GS, Esplin C: Percutaneous Kimray-Greenfield filter placement by femoral vein puncture. *Am J Roentgenol* 1985; 145:827–829.

23. Greenfield LJ, Cho KJ, Pais O, Van Aman M: Preliminary clinical experience with the titanium Greenfield vena caval filter. *Arch Surg* 1989; 124:657–659.

24. Greenfield LJ, Cho KJ, Proctor M, et al: Results of a multicenter study of the modified hook titanium Greenfield filter. *J Vasc Surg* 1991; 14:253–257.

25. Ferris EJ, McCowan TC, Carver DK, McFarland DR: Percutaneous inferior vena caval filters: Follow-up of seven designs in 320 patients. *Radiology* 1993; 188:851–856.

26. Roehm JOF Jr, Johnsrude IS, Barth MH, Gianturco C: The bird's nest inferior vena cava filter: Progress report. *Radiology* 1988; 168:745–749.

27. Lord RSA, Benn I: Early and late results after bird's nest filter placement in the inferior vena cava: Clinical and duplex ultrasound follow up. *Aust N Z J Surg* 1994; 64:106–114.

28. Dorfman GS: Percutaneous inferior vena caval filters. *Radiology* 1990; 174:987–992.

29. Rogoff PA, Hilgenberg AD, Miller SL, Stephan SM: Cephalic migration of the bird's nest inferior vena caval filter: Report of two cases. *Radiology* 1992; 184:819–822.

30. Simon M, Athanasoulis CA, Kim D, et al: Simon nitinol inferior vena cava filter: Initial clinical experience. *Radiology* 1989; 172:99–103.

31. LaPlante JS, Contractor FM, Kiproff PM, Khoury MB: Migration of the Simon nitinol vena cava filter to the chest. *Am J Roentgenol* 1993; 160:385–386.

32. Ricco JB, Crochet D, Sebilotte P, et al: Percutaneous transvenous caval interruption with the "LGM" filter: Early results of a multicenter trial. *Ann Vasc Surg* 1988; 3:242–247.

33. Crochet DP, Stora O, Ferry D, et al: Vena Tech-LGM filter: Long-term results of a prospective study. *Radiology* 1993; 188:857–860.

34. Darcy MD, Hunter DW, Lund GB, Cardella JF: Amplatz retrievable vena caval filter. *Semin Intervent Radiol* 1986; 3:214–219.

35. McCowan TC, Ferris EJ, Carver DK, Baker ML: Amplatz vena caval filter: Clinical experience in 30 patients. *Am J Roentgenol* 1990; 155:177–181.

36. Fobbe F, Dietzel M, Korth R, et al: Günther vena caval filter: Results of long-term follow-up. *Am J Roentgenol* 1988; 151:1031–1034.

37. Romaniuk P, Thieme T, Miersch G, et al: Zur Implantation von Vena-cava-Filtern bei akuten Lungenembolien. *Z Kardiol* 1993; 82:35–40.

38. McCowan TC, Ferris EJ, Carver DK, Harshfield DL: Use of external jugular vein as a route for percutaneous inferior vena cava filter placement. *Radiology* 1990; 176:527–530.

39. Beckmann CF, Abrams HL: Circumaortic venous ring: Incidence and significance. *Am J Roentgenol* 1979; 132:561–565.

40. Greenfield LJ, Cho KJ, Proctor MC, et al: Late results of suprarenal Greenfield vena cava filter placement. *Arch Surg* 1992; 127:969–973.

41. Villard J, Detry L, Clermont A, Pinet F: Huit filtres de Greenfield dans les cavités cardiaques droites: Traitement chirurgical. *Ann Radiol (Paris)* 1987; 30:102–104.
42. Dorfman GS, Cronan JJ, Paolella LP, et al: Iatrogenic changes at the venotomy site after percutaneous placement of the Greenfield filter. *Radiology* 1989; 173:159–162.
43. Novelline RA: Practical points on transvenous insertion of inferior vena cava filters. *Cardiovasc Intervent Radiol* 1980; 3:319–324.
44. Tsai FY, Myers TV, Ashraf A, Shah DC: Aberrant placement of a Kimray-Greenfield filter in the right atrium: Percutaneous retrieval. *Radiology* 1988; 167:423–424.
45. Hansen ME, Geller SC, Yucel EK, et al: Transfemoral venous catheterization through inferior vena caval filters: Results in seven cases. *Am J Roentgenol* 1991; 157:967–970.
46. Pais SO, De Orchis DF, Mirvis SE: Superior vena caval placement of a Kimray-Greenfield filter. *Radiology* 1987; 165:385–386.
47. Balshi JD, Cantelmo NL, Menzoian JO: Complications of caval interruption by Greenfield filter in quadraplegics. *J Vasc Surg* 1989; 9:558–562.
48. Messmer JM, Greenfield LJ: Greenfield caval filters: Long-term radiographic follow-up study. *Radiology* 1985; 156:613–618.
49. Lang W, Schweiger H, Fietkau R, Hofmann-Preiss K: Spontaneous disruption of two Greenfield vena caval filters. *Radiology* 1990; 174:445–446.
50. Thompson BH, Cragg AH, Smith TP, et al: Thrombus-trapping efficiency of the Greenfield filter in vivo. *Radiology* 1989; 172:979–981.

16
Lymphography

KEY CONCEPTS

1. Computed tomographic imaging has largely displaced lymphography in the staging of tumors, but the latter study is still occasionally used for Hodgkin lymphoma and testicular tumors.
2. For best accuracy, both lymphatic flow and nodal patterns must be analyzed together.
3. Tumors can produce obstruction, marginal filling defects, enlargement, and diffuse "foamy" patterns.
4. Central defects are often the result of scar or fatty replacement.
5. Diffuse enlargement with homogeneous uptake of contrast material may represent benign "reactive" hyperplasia.
6. For the diagnosis of lymphedema, lymphoscintigraphy is a more suitable study.

Lymphography has been in clinical use for more than 40 years, and for much of that time it was the only way, short of surgery, to evaluate non-palpable lymph nodes. In more recent years it has been superseded to a large extent by computed tomography (CT) and ultrasonography. Magnetic resonance imaging, lymphoscintigraphy, and interstitial lymphangiography are now under investigation, and the development of monoclonal antibody–radionuclide conjugates holds promise for detection of small metastases.[1]

Lymphography has been virtually abandoned at many institutions because it is an invasive procedure demanding considerable time and technical skill.[2] Even so, it maintains a role in oncologic centers and teaching hospitals, for lymphography remains the sole imaging study that has demonstrated consistent utility for detecting neoplastic involvement of nonenlarged nodes.

Bipedal lymphography is best suited for conditions that may affect femoral, inguinal, external or common iliac, and paraaortic nodes. The thoracic duct and some mediastinal nodes can also be imaged. However, internal iliac, high paraaortic, retrocrural, and mesenteric nodes are usually poorly opacified, if at all. Lymphography does not enable detection of pathologic processes in renal or hepatic hilar nodes, and it does not provide information about possible extranodal disease. Then again, lymphographic contrast material may persist for 1 or 2 years, allowing tumor response to treatment (or relapse) to be followed easily and inexpensively by periodic abdominal and pelvic radiographs.[3]

INDICATIONS

Hodgkin Lymphoma

In patients with Hodgkin lymphoma presenting for staging, up to 10% have lymph nodes of normal size containing tumor.[4] Because CT criteria of abnormality are based on size alone, disease in these patients would be staged inaccurately if CT scan were not followed by lymphography or surgery. Lymphography can be quite sensitive. Castellino and colleagues reported no false-negative examinations in 111 patients undergoing surgical node dissection after a lymphogram interpreted as showing no malignant disease.[5] Overall accuracy for lymphography in Hodgkin lymphoma has been reported between 82% and 95%, compared to CT accuracy of 75% to 84%.[6] Nevertheless, North and associates recently reviewed 61 patients undergoing both CT scan and lymphography and found that staging was correct in 96% of patients by either study considered alone.[7] It now appears that CT scan is adequate for staging the majority of Hodgkin lymphoma patients. Lymphography may be used selectively for patients with negative CT examinations when the referring oncologist feels further imaging is needed.

Non-Hodgkin Lymphoma

Staging laparotomy is seldom necessary for non-Hodgkin lymphoma today. Because of the tendency of this disease to involve retrocrural, high paraaortic, and mesenteric nodes, as well as liver, spleen, and other organs, CT scan is the initial diagnostic procedure of choice. Lymphography may be reserved for those with normal or equivocal CT findings, in whom the results would affect therapy.[8] The increased use of combination chemotherapy and radiotherapy for these tumors makes this situation much less likely to arise.[7]

Pelvic Malignancies

In testicular tumors, lymphography has a lower sensitivity, ranging from 54% to 89%, and a specificity on the order of 88%.[9] Although CT scan does not improve sensitivity to nodal mestastases, it is superior at the level of the thoracolumbar junction.[10] More bulky metastases are generally seen in patients with embryonal carcinoma. Positive studies can be confirmed by needle biopsy. Lymphograms can direct surgical dissection or radiation portals, and their continued use in evaluating testicular tumors is still favored by some.[9,11,12] Nevertheless, lymphography is falling into disuse in some institutions because many physicians treat stage I patients as though they have stage II disease, and combining CT and lymphographic staging is not felt to be cost-effective.[13] Lymphography has the disadvantages of not opacifying "sentinel" nodes and, at times, inducing reactive hyperplasia and fibrosis that may make lymphadenectomy more difficult.

For prostatic carcinoma, both CT scan and lymphography are quite specific, but sensitivity is lacking, generally less than 60%.[9,14] Patients with positive nodes can be spared lymphadenectomy, and Flanigan and colleagues assert that outpatient lymphography with directed needle biopsy can save costs compared to CT screening.[14]

The benefits of screening are more controversial in cervical carcinoma. With 18% to 25% sensitivity, lymphography may be worse at clinical staging than physical examination alone.[15,16] Nevertheless, some have reported acceptable overall accuracy (91%) and continue to use lymphography on a routine basis.[17] The value of the study in various other pelvic tumors, such as vulvar carcinoma and bladder carcinoma, remains in debate.[18,19]

Thoracic Duct Injury

Posttraumatic or postsurgical chylothorax can have serious consequences. Sachs and associates found lymphography very useful in determining which patients needed operative repair, as well as for showing the exact site of thoracic duct disruption prior to surgery.[20]

Extremity Lymphedema

Extremity lymphedema may be primary or secondary (consequent to infection, inflammation, malignancy, radiotherapy, surgery, or other trauma) and has often been a diagnosis of exclusion, once deep venous thrombosis or other likely causes have been ruled out. Occasionally, positive confirmation of an underlying lymphatic abnormality is desired. To this end, lymphoscintigraphy (especially dynamic quantitative lymphoscintigraphy) has demonstrated its value.[21] Interstitial lymphangiography with an investigational dimeric water-soluble contrast agent has been quite accurate for making the diagnosis in more advanced cases of lymphedema, and it may play a role in the future.[22] Neither lymphoscintigraphy nor interstitial lymphangiography requires incisions or direct injection of lymphatic vessels. Administration of the relevant imaging agent is by intradermal or subcutaneous injection. In any case, conventional oil-based lymphographic contrast media should not be used to examine patients with suspected lymphedema, for tissue reaction to the contrast medium can exacerbate the lymphedema.[1]

TECHNIQUE

Because some degree of venous embolization of the oily contrast medium is encountered in all patients, lymphography should be avoided in those with severe pulmonary disease or intracardiac shunts. Older individuals with marked tremors may be impossible to study.

Prior to lymphography, patients should be questioned about any hypersensitivity reactions on previous exposure to iodinated contrast materials or vital dyes. They should be advised that lymphography is a 2-day test, requiring up to 4 or 5 hours on the first day for isolation of lymphatic vessels, cannulation, and injection, as well as a return the following day for filming of the static nodal phase. They should also be warned of the temporary discoloration produced by the vital dye (Evans blue, methylene blue, isosulfan blue, among others used) injected into the feet. Because of the length of time required for contrast injection, patients should void before being placed on the procedure table, and they may bring reading material to occupy the time.

Vital dye is injected intradermally into the webs between the toes. A 25-gauge needle is used to administer about 0.5 ml at each site. The webs between the first three toes or the most medial and lateral webs may be chosen. Having the patient then walk about for several minutes may improve opacification of lymphatics in the foot. After 10 to 15 minutes, both feet are sterilely prepared and draped.

The course of lymphatic channels is made evident by uptake of dye, and a vessel over the dorsum of the foot can be selected. After generous administration of 1% lidocaine, a shallow transverse incision is made, with care taken not to cut completely through dermis over the lymphatic. A hemostat can be passed gently under the incompletely incised portion from the margin of the incision. The scalpel can then cut down upon the hemostat, avoiding inadvertent injury to the lymphatic vessel. The vessel is isolated by meticulous dissection with blunt forceps. Spreading a hemostat repeatedly under the vessel may help clean fat from its surface.

A sterile hairclip may be used to isolate and stabilize the vessel for cannulation. Ligatures can also be placed, but they are not absolutely necessary. The lymphatic may be distended by "milking" the dorsum of the foot by compressing skin distally to proximally with a blunt instrument. A 30-gauge needle with connecting tubing filled with iodized oil contrast agent (Lipiodol or Ethiodol) is advanced, bevel up, into the channel. Gentle injection confirms intraluminal placement by absence of leakage. If a few small air bubbles are in the line, they may help recognition of successful cannulation.[23]

With satisfactory needle placement, the clip is closed and the connecting tubing secured by sterile tape. The contrast agent is then injected by means of a 10-ml syringe placed under a 10-lb weight. The patient is monitored every 15 minutes during injection, and an early film over the lower leg is obtained to confirm lymphatic filling and exclude the possibility of lymphatic-venous communication. Injection is complete when 6 to 10 ml of contrast medium per foot have been introduced. A slightly larger amount may be given if cannulation is successful in one side but not the other. There is normally some cross-filling of periaortic lymphatics, an effect that may provide adequate information about abdominal nodes from a unilateral injection.

After injection and needle removal, incisions are closed by interrupted sutures and dressed. Anteroposterior (AP) and oblique films of the pelvis and abdomen are obtained, in addition to a lateral view of the abdomen and an AP chest. These allow assessment of lymphatic channels, including displacement or collateral formation. The same films are repeated the following day for evaluation of lymph node characteristics. The studies may be repeated at intervals of several months for up to a year or more to detect new or recurrent disease in opacified nodes.

Adverse reactions are rare. Other than hypersensitivity reactions to the iodized oil or vital dye, major risks include local infection at the incision site or massive oil embolism if venous communications are present. Normally, patients may experience mild fever and cough the night after the procedure.

INTERPRETATION

Normal lymph nodes are oval or kidney-shaped and may vary in length from 2 mm to 30 mm.[24] Lymph nodes are composed of follicles (predominantly located in the cortex) and sinuses that drain the afferent channels entering at the periphery. Lymph from the afferent channels enters marginal sinuses and flows through a reticular network of medullary sinuses into the hilum of the node. The hilum gives rise to the efferent channels. Oily lymphographic contrast material is normally homogeneously distributed throughout a node, which has a fine reticular appearance.

Pathologic nodes may be enlarged or normal in size, with focal or diffuse filling defects. In general, nodes with all diameters greater than 2 cm are abnormal, although size criteria do vary somewhat between chains.11 Particular care must be made in interpreting inguinal nodes, which are prone to repeated or chronic inflammation.

Nonneoplastic disease can produce patterns that confound interpretation. Nodes may normally develop central scarring or fat deposition, and experienced lymphographers can usually recognize such cases of fibrolipomatosis. Many false-positive examinations are caused by sinus histiocytosis (packing of sinuses by proliferating histiocytes) and follicular hyperplasia. These conditions are grouped under the term *nonspecific reactive change*. One may see focal or diffuse defects. Still, in many cases of inflammatory change, nodes maintain a homogeneous but "magnified" structure.[24] A similar nodal pattern can be found in some patients with lymphocytic leukemia. Still, most types of lymphoma can be distinguished from inflammatory nodes by the gradations of disease displayed in different nodal groups involved by lymphoma.[5]

Metastases from carcinoma often produce marginal deposits, which must exceed the size of a couple of lymphoid follicles in order to be recognized. In practical terms, a metastasis must be at least 5 mm in diameter to be detected in the best of circumstances. Central defects larger than 10 mm are suspect for malignancy.

Lymphomas usually produce enlarged nodes with a foamy or lacy appearance or conglomerate masses with irregular or disorganized uptake of contrast material. However, up to 29% of nodes involved by Hodgkin lymphoma may not produce a classic pattern.[25] They may instead show irregular filling defects more typical for carcinoma. In other patients, lymphatic flow may be obstructed to the degree that the affected nodes do not opacify at all.

Because flow patterns provide information about the presence or absence of neoplastic disease, early lymphangiographic radiographs are critical for interpretation. An obstructive pattern is manifested by collateral vessel filling, delayed flow (channels should not retain contrast material at 24 hours in most healthy people), dermal backflow, or opening of lymphaticovenous anastomoses.[25] Channels may be displaced about enlarged, nonopacified nodes. Small filling defects are much more likely to represent tumor metastases when they are associated with obstructed flow.

If the patient's primary diagnosis is in doubt, surgical or needle biopsy of abnormal nodes is warranted. The differential diagnosis of the patterns described here is a large one, including such varied conditions as inflammation from leaking abdominal aortic aneurysm or spinal osteomyelitis, Whipple's disease, Waldenström's macroglobulinemia, sarcoidosis, syphilis, tuberculosis, and collagen vascular diseases.[26]

CONCLUSION

Despite the use of cross-sectional imaging techniques, lymphography maintains a limited place in staging Hodgkin lymphoma and various other neoplasms. It is the best study for thoracic duct injuries causing chylothorax unresponsive to conservative treatment. The use of lymphography is probably best confined to major cancer referral and treatment centers, where the volume of procedures is sufficient to maintain the operator's technical expertise as well as the radiologist's interpretive skills.

REFERENCES

1. Weissleder R, Thrall JH: The lymphatic system: Diagnostic imaging studies. *Radiology* 1989; 172:315–317.
2. Dixon AK: The current practice of lymphography: A survey in the age of computed tomography. *Clin Radiol* 1985; 36:287–290.
3. Pera A, Capek M, Shirkhoda A: Lymphangiography and CT in the follow-up of patients with lymphoma. *Radiology* 1987; 164:631–633.
4. Dooms GC, Hricak H: Radiologic imaging modalities, including magnetic resonance, for evaluating lymph nodes. *West J Med* 1986; 144:49–57.
5. Castellino RA, Billingham M, Dorfman RF: Lymphographic accuracy in Hodgkin's disease and malignant lymphoma with a note on the "reactive" lymph node as a cause of most false-positive lymphograms. *Invest Radiol* 1974; 9:155–165.
6. Enig B, Bjerregaard Jensen B, Hjøllund Madsen E, et al: Detection of neoplastic lymph nodes in Hodgkin's disease and non-Hodgkin lymphoma: Comparison between tomography and lymphography. *Acta Radiol* 1985; 24:491–495.
7. North LB, Wallace S, Lindell MM, et al: Lymphography for staging lymphomas: Is it still a useful procedure? *Am J Roentgenol* 1993; 161:867–869.
8. Strijk SP: Lymphography and abdominal computed tomography in the staging of non-Hodgkin lymphoma. *Acta Radiol* 1987; 28:263–269.
9. Von Eschenbach AC, Jing BS, Wallace S: Lymphangiography in genitourinary cancer. *Urol Clin North Am* 1985; 12:715–723.
10. Lien HH, Kolbenstvedt A, Talle K, et al: Comparison of computed tomography, lymphography, and phlebography in 200 consecutive patients with regard to retroperitoneal metastases from testicular tumor. *Radiology* 1983; 146:129–132.
11. Deprez-Curely JP: Lymphography in testicular tumours. *Prog Clin Biol Res* 1985; 203:243–252.

12. Marks LB, Shipley WU, Walker TG, Waltman AC: Role of lymphangiography in staging testicular seminoma. *Urology* 1991; 38:264–266.
13. Heiken JP, Forman HP, Brown JJ: Staging neoplasms: Neoplasms of the bladder, prostate, and testis. *Radiol Clin North Am* 1994; 31:81–98.
14. Flanigan RC, Mohler JL, King CT, et al: Preoperative lymph node evaluation in prostatic cancer patients who are surgical candidates: The role of lymphangiography and computerized tomography scanning with directed fine needle aspiration. *J Urol* 1985; 134:84–87.
15. Vercamer R, Janssens J, Usewils R, et al: Computed tomography and lymphography in the presurgical staging of early carcinoma of the uterine cervix. *Cancer* 1987; 60:1745–1750.
16. Feigen M, Crocker EF, Read J, Crandon AJ: The value of lymphoscintigraphy, lymphangiography and computer tomography scanning in the preoperative assessment of lymph nodes involved by pelvic malignant conditions. *Surg Gynecol Obstet* 1987; 165:107–110.
17. Smales E, Perry CM, Macdonald JS, Baker JW: The value of lymphography in the management of carcinoma of the cervix. *Clin Radiol* 1986; 37:19–22.
18. Strijk SP, Debruyne FMJ, Herman CJ: Lymphography in the management of urologic tumors. *Radiology* 1983; 146:39–45.
19. Weiner SA, Lee JKT, Kao M-S, Moon TE: The role of lymphangiography in vulvar carcinoma. *Am J Obstet Gynecol* 1986; 154:1073–1075.
20. Sachs PB, Zelch MG, Rice TW, et al: Diagnosis and localization of laceration of the thoracic duct: Usefulness of lymphangiography and CT. *Am J Roentgenol* 1991; 157:703–705.
21. Ter SE, Alavi A, Kim CK, Merli G: Lymphoscintigraphy: A reliable test for the diagnosis of lymphedema. *Clin Nucl Med* 1993; 18:646–654.
22. Weissleder H, Weissleder R: Interstitial lymphangiography: Initial clinical experience with a dimeric nonionic contrast agent. *Radiology* 1989; 170:371–374.
23. Staton R: Lymphography. *Radiol Technol* 1984; 55:233–238.
24. Wiljasalo M: Lymphographic differential diagnosis of neoplastic diseases: Roentgen anatomy and roentgen pathology of the lymph glands. *Acta Radiol* 1965; 247:S12–S19.
25. Koehler PR, Salmon RB: Lymphographic patterns in lymphoma, with emphasis on the atypical forms. *Radiology* 1966; 87:623–629.
26. Parker BR, Blank N, Castellino RA: Lymphographic appearance of benign conditions simulating lymphoma. *Radiology* 1974; 111:267–274.

17

Needle Biopsy

KEY CONCEPTS

1. Percutaneous needle biopsy can be used to diagnose primary or metastatic malignancy, tumor recurrence, or infection.
2. Diagnostic yield is lower for lymphoproliferative disorders and benign disease, but can be increased by the use of larger cutting needles.
3. Pneumothorax can be avoided if aerated lung is not traversed by the biopsy needle. Placing the puncture site down may minimize any pneumothorax that does arise.
4. Bowel can be traversed with relative impunity by needles that are 20 gauge or smaller.
5. The mortality rate is extremely low with fine-needle biopsy, the greatest hazards being air embolism, pancreatitis, and pulmonary or hepatic hemorrhage.

Percutaneous needle biopsy has been applied for many years to superficial, palpable masses or in an undirected manner to liver parenchyma. However, the diagnostic potential of needle biopsy was not fully appreciated until the 1970s, when cross-sectional imaging became available. Presently, fine-needle techniques allow the great majority of soft tissue abnormalities to be sampled safely, with good prospects of obtaining diagnostic material.

Major indications include suspicion of primary or metastatic malignancy, confirmation of tumor recurrence or metastasis in a patient with known primary tumor, and diagnosis of infection.

COMMON PRINCIPLES

The success and risk of a needle biopsy procedure depend critically on a number of factors. The patient must be able to cooperate with the physican obtaining the sample; in many cases the patient's respiration must be suspended during needle placement. The organ or lesion to undergo biopsy must be identifiable on fluoroscopy, ultrasound (US), or computed tomography (CT) imaging (needles have also been designed for use with magnetic resonance imaging). The operator should be skilled at directing the needle accurately, and avoiding major vessels, bowel, and other potential intervening hazards, where possible. Once obtained, the specimen must be handled correctly: either examined on the spot by a cytopathologist or taken immediately, with relevant history and any special instructions, to the surgical pathologist. If infection is suspected, samples should be obtained for culture and appropriate staining. Accuracy of diagnosis is quite dependent on the experience and interest of the pathologist examining needle specimens.

There is no strong correlation of diagnostic accuracy or incidence of complications with needle size. However, mortality is a real risk with the use of large cutting needles (14 gauge). Fatality rates have been reported as 0.5% for hepatic and as high as 3.8% for pancreatic biopsies with use of such needles.[1]

Multiple Samples

Multiple samples increase accuracy. Sampling the periphery of a lesion is quite valuable, particularly for large masses that may have central necrosis. The negative predictive value of a biopsy is much lower than its positive predictive value. As a consequence, it is often necessary to repeat a biopsy in the face of negative results.[2,3] The low morbidity and cost of needle biopsy make a second or third biopsy procedure preferable to thoracotomy or laparotomy for diagnosis.

Nonmalignant Lesions

Needle biopsy is most diagnostic for malignant neoplasms (see the section on Site-Specific Considerations later in this chapter for accuracy in specific sites). A definitive positive diagnosis of benign lesion can rarely be made in more than 65% of patients in even the best of circumstances.[4,5] For suspected infection, the situation is somewhat better. Sensitivity of needle aspiration has been 76% in 46 cases of pulmonary infection reported by Conces and colleagues.[6] Needle biopsy of lymph nodes has also proved useful in diagnosing mycobacterial infection in patients with acquired immune deficiency syndrome.[7] If suspicion of infection is strong, but no material is obtained from a suspected fluid collection through a fine needle, it is often wise to use an 18-gauge needle or to place a 5 Fr to 8 Fr catheter for aspiration (see Chapter 18 entitled Percutaneous Drainage of Abscesses and Other Fluid Collections). Although needle biopsy has its limitations in making a positive diagnosis of benign conditions, it very rarely results in a false-positive diagnosis of malignancy.[8]

Approach
If it can be avoided, multiple tissue planes should not be crossed. For example, many adrenal biopsies can be performed by a posterior approach, staying entirely within the retroperitoneum. The diaphragm and pleural space are best avoided for liver biopsies. The number of pleural reflections traversed in a pulmonary procedure may affect the likelihood of pneumothorax. In a parenchymal organ such as liver, it is wise to traverse some normal parenchyma to reach an abnormality. Puncture of a vascular lesion at a free surface can result in peritoneal hemorrhage and death.[9]

Patient Preparation
Before any biopsy procedure, the patient's history, clinical status, and radiographic studies are reviewed to determine if needle biopsy is possible and appropriate. Hematocrit, platelet count, and coagulation studies should be obtained. Those with thrombocytopenia or abnormal coagulation can be prepared with platelet transfusions or fresh frozen plasma. Pulmonary function tests may be helpful in assessing risk of lung biopsy in a given individual.[10] As a precaution, oral intake should be restricted to clear liquids in the 4 to 6 hours preceding biopsy.

The procedure, its purpose, the attendant risks, and alternatives are explained to the patient before consent is obtained. It should be made clear that multiple needle passes are customarily needed to obtain adequate material. Most biopsies can be performed on an outpatient basis; however, those undergoing biopsy must understand the possibility of hospital admission for complications, as well as the potential necessity of repeat biopsy if results are negative or unsatisfactory. Outpatients should be prepared to spend several hours in the radiology department or other designated area for observation. They should be accompanied by a family member or friend who can drive the patient home, observe symptoms, and provide assistance, should any problems be encountered during the trip.

It is advisable to place an intravenous line prior to percutaneous needle biopsy. In many cases premedication is not necessary, but very apprehensive patients may be given midazolam (1 to 3 mg intravenously in doses of 0.5- to 1-mg increments) for sedation and fentanyl (50 to 200 µg intravenously in doses of 25- to 50-µg increments) for pain. Oxygen, naloxone, and other resuscitative drugs and equipment should be at hand for any emergency.

Biopsy Guidance

The size, location, and depth of a lesion, as well as its detectability by a given imaging modality, determine the best method for guidance. Many abdominal lesions can be approached equally well with CT or US; instrument availability and operator preference are often determining factors. Fluoroscopy is most commonly used for pulmonary, pleural, and osseous lesions. Lymph nodes opacified by lymphographic contrast material can be sampled percutaneously under fluoroscopic direction. Rarely, a bone lesion may be detected (and marked on the skin for needle biopsy) by radionuclide scanning.[11]

When an approach is chosen, the skin is prepared and anesthetized with lidocaine, and a small incision made. For fine-needle biopsy, a short, larger needle, such as an 18-gauge thin-wall vascular puncture needle, may be placed through the incision into subcutaneous tissues to stabilize the trajectory of the fine needle introduced coaxially.

No matter what imaging technique is employed, use of tandem needles can save time. When one needle is either in or near the target, a second can be placed adjacent to it, to mark the depth and angle of approach for further sampling when the first needle is removed. With a tandem technique, a fine needle can be placed with whatever number of passes necessary. A larger needle can then be advanced safely alongside to obtain a core for histologic sampling.

Fluoroscopy

When fluoroscopy is used, a C-arm helps enormously, both for detecting a lesion and for targeting. When the tube and image intensifier are lined up with the skin entry site, the needle hub and tip can be superimposed over the lesion. Changing to the lateral projection then confirms when the tip has been advanced to the proper depth for sampling (Fig.17-1). If a true lateral projection cannot be obtained, rotating the tube through various obliquities can determine if the needle tip "stays" with the target during rotation. In many cases the target can be felt as a change in resistance when it is encountered by the advancing needle. Oblique or lateral fluoroscopy

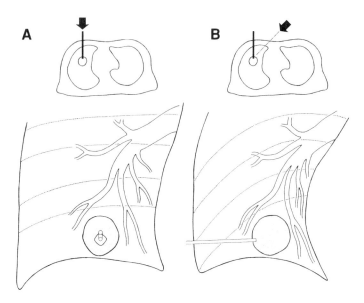

Fig. 17-1 Use of fluoroscopic C-arm for the placement of a lung biopsy needle. **A,** The needle is superimposed over the target in one projection. **B,** Needle advancement is then observed in an oblique (or lateral) projection to determine depth of advancement. With proper beam collimation, this also allows continuous fluoroscopy without direct exposure of the operator's hands.

during actual sampling can also confirm accurate placement by the observation of lesion motion with needle penetration.

Ultrasound
With US, the skin site is determined and marked, and the angle of approach and depth noted. The needle can then be placed without direct observation. Alternatively, a biopsy guide can be employed, or the needle placed freehand with simultaneous sonographic monitoring. If placement is to be monitored, the scanning head should be covered with a sterile sheath, sonographic contact being maintained by sterile gel. If a sterile sheath is unavailable or deemed cumbersome, scrupulous cleansing of the scanning head with povidone-iodine and absolute alcohol has been shown to be safe.[12] The cable connecting the head to the rest of the sonographic unit can be draped with towels secured by sterile clips.

The availability of electronic delineation of the tract of a US biopsy guide is most helpful, for it is often quite difficult to image the needle tip. Jiggling the needle, sliding its stylet in and out rapidly six or seven times, and injecting a small amount of saline are ways of increasing its sonographic visibility. Reading and colleagues have described the use of a screw stylet to greatly enhance the echogenicity of biopsy needles.[13] Electronic transponder stylets permitting precise depiction of the needle tip have been developed for some sonographic units,[14] but such electronic localizers have not gained wide application. Overall, US has produced good results in guiding biopsies in even very small abdominal lesions.[12] It has also been valuable in approaching pleural lesions.[15]

Computed Tomography

Computed tomography is well suited to approaching small, deep lesions, especially those surrounded by large vessels or bowel. The needle tip can be unequivocally demonstrated, and depiction of surrounding structures is not hindered by the presence of gas or bone. Biopsy is most readily performed when the approach can be made in an axial plane; off-axis biopsy trajectories are much more problematic.

Another difficulty with CT is the amount of time expended with needle placement, scanning, and repositioning. Rapid image reconstruction is indispensable for CT biopsy to be practical. Catheters or other radiopaque markers may be placed on the patient during localization scans to help plan an approach. Spiral scanning speeds recognition of needle course and tip position, particularly for upper abdominal biopsies in which inconstant respiratory excursions may cause difficulties. A CT stereotactic device developed for percutaneous needle biopsy can greatly decrease the number of needle passes needed and can accurately guide nonaxial trajectories.[16]

Biopsy Needles

A dazzling variety of needles are commercially available. Aspiration needles differ chiefly in tip and trocar configuration. Tips may be beveled, pencil- or diamond-shaped, blunt, hooked, spiraled, notched, or trephinated (see Fig. 17-2). Some are supplied with attached aspirating syringes or have a specially designed self-aspirating mechanism. Larger needles may have an inner notched trocar, over which a cutting cannula is slipped. Some needles are adapted to particular sites, such as bone, lung, and pleura (see the section on Site-Specific Considerations later in this chapter). Coaxial systems have been fabricated to allow multiple samples to be obtained with a single needle placement.[17] A blunt-tip needle has been designed by Hawkins and associates to deflect from, rather than puncture, muscular arteries, thus minimizing the possibility of major bleeding.[18] More recently, various vendors have produced self-contained biopsy gun needles, generally using notched inner shafts and sharp outer cutting cannulas, that automate specimen retrieval by the firing of a spring-loaded mechanism.[19–21]

In general, larger needles obtain larger specimens, and one needle of a given size has no great advantage over another in terms of material

Tru-cut   Turner   Franseen   Shark Jaw

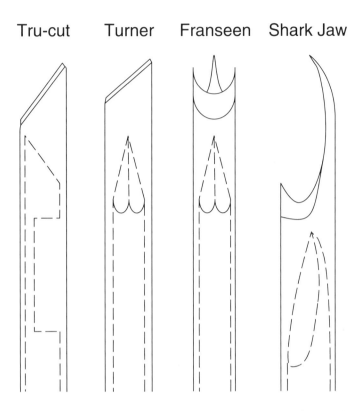

Fig. 17-2 Four of the many types of biopsy needles available (not drawn to scale). The Tru-Cut is a cutting-gap needle, the Franseen is trephined, and the other two represent beveled cutting needles.

obtained, particularly for cytologic study. Histologic analysis is more dependent on sample size. In this regard, in vitro experiments by Andriole and associates have indicated some benefit related to the degree of bevel in an instrument.[22] Their studies also found that cutting-gap and trephined needles, such as the Lee and Franseen needles, tended to give larger samples for their size, whereas screw-stylet needles obtained smaller amounts of tissue.

The length and bore of a needle should correspond to the depth of a lesion, clearance considerations (CT gantry, image intensifier), and the anticipated ease of hitting a target. A biopsy gun without a removable handle may be difficult to place if imager clearance is limited. A large superficial mass can be easily entered with a short, large-gauge needle. However, the vascularity of a lesion must also be taken into consideration. For example, an abnormality suspected to be a cavernous hemangioma or metastatic renal cell carcinoma should be approached gingerly, usually with a needle no larger than 20 gauge. Fine (22-gauge or smaller) needles, particularly those with beveled stylets, may not follow a straight course if directed through any great length of soft tissue. The particular equipment chosen for the task at hand depends on the operator's experience and personal preference.

Sampling Technique

For simple aspiration or cutting needles, a syringe can be attached directly to the hub. A Luer-Lok makes coupling more secure. The larger the syringe, the greater the suction that can be generated. With suction applied, the needle is advanced into the target, either in a single motion or with a 1- to 2-cm to-and-fro excursion. Rotation may be helpful with cutting needles. When an 18-gauge or smaller needle is used with a 50-ml syringe, no more than 10 ml of suction is needed to obtain maximal samples.[23] Suction should be maintained or slowly released during withdrawal.

After needle removal, the syringe can be detached and used to draw up several milliliters of heparinized saline (nonbacteriostatic, if infection is a consideration). The saline is injected through the needle into a sterile sample cup or tube. The stylet or trocar can be reinserted to expel any remaining material. At the time the needle is being cleared, single drops can applied to slides and spread immediately for air-drying or alcohol fixation.

If two people are available to perform an aspiration, attaching the syringe to a length of connecting tubing is more convenient. The operator can then use two hands to make the needle pass, while the assistant provides suction. The syringe can be filled with 5 to 10 ml of heparinized saline, so that suction is efficiently generated and the sample can be immediately expelled from the needle by injection.

Needles with syringes premounted, such as the Menghini Surecut, make it possible to conduct a biopsy easily with one hand. However, the added length and weight of such devices may make checking needle position by CT scan or fluoroscopy more difficult. For more complicated biopsy devices, the manufacturer's instructions should be consulted prior to use.

A nonaspiration technique can be employed with very fine needles (such as 22- or 23-gauge Chiba needles) to obtain material for cytologic analysis. By this method, the needle is advanced to the lesion, and sampling performed with the stylet removed (no syringe or suction applied), followed by rapid to-and-fro excursions until blood is noted at the needle hub.[24] Although nonaspiration needle biopsy has its proponents, its practice has not been widely adopted.

Automated biopsy with disposable gun devices has become quite popular. These devices have several advantages:[20,21] Relatively large cores of tissue can be obtained for the needle size used, the cores obtained show little crush artifact when compared to conventional needles, and once the biopsy gun is in place, it can be triggered simply and removed immediately. In our practice, we have noted that the speed of sampling minimizes pain and improves patient acceptance. We now prefer biopsy guns for those procedures in which their placement is practical.

Aspiration versus Core, or Cytology versus Histology
In addressing the relative merits of cytologic and histologic study in needle biopsy, it may be helpful to define a few terms. *Fine-needle biopsy* can be rather arbitrarily defined as that performed with needles of 1 mm diameter or less.[1] In practical terms, this means needles smaller than 19 gauge (Table 17-1). *Cutting needles* are those designed to procure a core of tissue, and cores can be obtained with needles as small as 22 gauge. Many authors, however, imply larger cutting devices (14 to 19 gauge) when they refer to cutting needles.[4,25] Very fine-bore needles are used to aspirate aggregates of cells for cytologic examination. Histologic study depends on the preservation of tissue architecture. In many cases, material obtained with a needle can be submitted for both cytologic and histologic review.

Cytologic study is highly sensitive for detection of carcinoma, but histologic study is more reliable in the diagnosis of lymphoma, thymoma, or benign lesions.[4] For lymphoma, needle biopsy is of greatest value in the event of recurrence; histologic slides on file can be compared with the needle specimen.[26] Hodgkin lymphoma is especially difficult to diagnose percutaneously. At our institution, Lieberman and associates found histologic workup more useful for various types of malignancy (sensitivity of 83% versus 62% for cytology), particularly in determining tissue of origin, but the addition of cytologic study can improve accuracy.[27] Others have confirmed the increased accuracy of combined histologic and cytologic examination of specimens.[28,29]

Table 17-1   Conversion of Needle Gauge to Diameter Equivalents

Needle Gauge	Millimeters	Inches
23	0.64	0.025
22	0.71	0.028
21	0.81	0.032
20	0.89	0.035
19	1.07	0.042
18	1.24	0.049
17	1.47	0.058
16	1.65	0.065
15	1.83	0.072
14	2.11	0.083

Sample Handling and Evaluation

One's colleague in pathology should be consulted for the preferred handling of specimens at a given institution. Immediate placement of a specimen in buffered formalin prevents its use for immunohistochemical studies or for touch preparations. The same holds true if an entire core is submitted for frozen section review.

The attendance of a cytopathologist at the time of biopsy or the preparation of frozen sections can determine not only the adequacy of the specimen but also, in many instances, the diagnosis. If more tissue is needed, it can be obtained immediately. Repeating a biopsy at another time increases cost and is inconvenient for both patient and physician.

The pathologist should be given all pertinent clinical history, including any previous malignancy and its treatment, so that special stains can be used when needed. For suspected infection, both culturing and staining should be done, for one or the other may be negative for disease in nearly half of cases.[6] Special media may be needed to transport specimens for anaerobic, fungal, viral, and mycobacterial culture, and these must be obtained before needle aspiration.

Potential Complications

Needle biopsy can be complicated by bleeding, local infection, pneumothorax, air embolism, bile leakage, peritonitis, pancreatitis, or tumor seeding of the biopsy tract. Malignancy growing along the biopsy tract is a small but real risk, with an incidence up to 1:1000 in abdominal biopsies.[30] For this reason one should be circumspect about sampling potentially curable tumors for which the likelihood of a malignant diagosis is high and surgical resection is already planned. All in all, use of fine needles (20 gauge or smaller) is extraordinarily safe, with severe complications reported in 0.04% to 0.05% and a mortality rate of 0.004% to 0.008% in two large reviews, including a combined total of more than 65,000 abdominal biopsies.[1,31] For cutting needles, severe complications are twice as common as for fine aspiration needles (but still quite unusual), and a mortality of 0.027% has been reported for more than 11,000 abdominal procedures.[31] A multihospital survey of biopsies using 19-gauge or smaller needles by Smith found a virtually identical mortality rate (0.031%).[32]

A prospective study of nearly 400 procedures by Yankaskas and colleagues showed that 13% of patients had pain requiring analgesics after abdominal or pelvic biopsy with standard needles.[33] A drop in hematocrit felt to represent post-biopsy bleeding was found in nine patients. The fall in hematocrit was noted from 3 to 72 hours after the procedure and appeared more likely in those with cancer. Even so, most of the patients described had clinically silent bleeding, and the incidence of minor complications is a function of how closely patients are observed.

SITE-SPECIFIC CONSIDERATIONS

Thoracic Biopsy

For primary lung tumors, a primary goal of biopsy is to distinguish small cell from other malignancy, a distinction important for therapy. This determination is usually possible with needle sampling. The sensitivity of needle aspiration for primary or metastatic carcinomas in lung is over 90%.[5,26,34] Bronchoscopy is preferred for central endobronchial lesions, but most other thoracic masses can be safely approached by percutaneous needles.

Needle biopsy has also been quite useful for inflammatory lesions. More than two thirds of patients with tuberculosis who have had at least four sputum samples negative for acid-fast bacilli on microscopic examination have immediate diagnostic confirmation made possible by percutaneous biopsy.[35] This avoids the weeks of delay before sputum cultures become positive, and in some cases needle biopsy is the only means of obtaining a firm diagnosis. Needle aspiration can guide antibiotic treatment in patients with lung abscess. Cultures show mixed organisms in many cases, and anaerobic organisms are quite common. One must not forget that lung abscesses can be caused by central obstructing tumors. Carcinoma was found by Griñan and associates in 8 of 32 patients for whom cytologic examination was performed in addition to staining and culture for microorganisms.[36]

If a lesion is suspected to be an arteriovenous malformation or a peripheral pulmonary arterial aneurysm or is adjacent to large vessels in the hilum, dynamic contrast material–enhanced CT scan is warranted prior to biopsy. Mediastinal biopsies generally call for CT guidance. As noted earlier, large cutting needles may be needed to enable a diagnosis of thymoma or lymphoma.[4] Small lesions near the heart or great vessels are best approached with fine needles. For pleural biopsy, the Cope needle can be used when no discrete mass is detected and has been valuable in the diagnosis of mesothelioma, tuberculosis, and lymphoma.[15] This needle should be placed immediately superior to the rib, and avoid the inferior course of the neurovascular bundle.

Pneumothorax

Whether pneumothorax is considered a complication or an anticipated adverse side effect of pulmonary needle biopsy is semantic. The incidence of pneumothorax after biopsy is correlated with the depth of the lesion and number of needle passes made, but it is not related to the size of the needle.[37] A rate of 10% to 35% can be expected when fluoroscopy is used for guidance.[34–38] The incidence is higher when the procedure is performed with CT (43% to 57%), related perhaps to the longer duration of the procedure or to the smaller size or increased difficulty of lesions referred for CT-guided biopsy.[5,39] Also at greater risk are those patients with abnormal pulmonary function tests. Fish and colleagues showed a pneumothorax rate of 46% in those with FEV-1 (1-second forced expiratory volume) less than 70% predicted, compared to an incidence of only 19% for those with normal pulmonary tests.[10] In the latter group, pneumothorax was almost always inconsequential.

Various measures have been proposed to avoid pneumothorax or to minimize any pneumothorax that does arise. Care must be taken that the needle administering lidocaine does not violate the pleural space; otherwise, a pneumothorax can be created before biopsy is even attempted.[38] If a lesion can be reached without traversing aerated lung, the risk of pneumothorax is practically nil.[40] Certain lesions within 8 mm of the pleural surface can be approached by subpleural injection of 20 to 40 ml of saline, which produces a bulge displacing aerated lung from the needle path. Klose biopsied 27 patients with 14-gauge needles using such a CT-guided procedure without a single instance of pneumothorax.[41] Others have used pleural effusions or even existing pneumothoraces as "windows" to reach mediastinal lesions without puncturing visceral pleura and causing an air leak.[42]

When aerated lung must be violated, Hill and associates have been able to decrease the pneumothorax rate to less than 20% in patients with even advanced lung disease by using CT guidance routinely and avoiding any bullae found.[43] The use of a "blood-patch" (injection of autologous clot during removal of a guiding needle) has not been proved an effective preventive measure.[38] Immediate postbiopsy placement of a patient with the biopsy site down also does not necessarily diminish the rate of pneumothorax, but it can greatly decrease the need for chest tube placement by allowing the air leak to seal quickly.[44] The patient should be instructed to maintain the position for 1 to 2 hours without coughing or talking, if possible.

Upright inspiratory and expiratory chest radiographs are obtained immediately after the biopsy procedure, and repeat films from 1 to 4 hours later; outpatients should be observed for about 4 hours. If the biopsy-site-down recommendations of Moore and colleagues are followed, the first postbiopsy chest radiographs can be delayed for 1 or 2 hours, as long as the patient does not have symptoms or other early evidence of large pneumothorax.[44] When pneumothorax occurs, 90% of instances are evident immediately, and only 2% first appear more than 1 hour later.[45] If a patient develops delayed symptoms, radiographs should be obtained without hesitation.

Chest Tube Placement

The necessity of intervention for pneumothorax has been reported in 3% to 20% of all thoracic biopsies,* and the operator must always be prepared

*References 5,10,26,36,39,44,45.

to insert a chest tube. Criteria for placement include any pneumothorax associated with dyspnea or distress or any pleural air collection shown to be increasing in size on serial chest films. Many small apical pneumothoraces do not need aspiration, but the size at which intervention is warranted in the absence of symptoms is a matter of judgment.

A Heimlich chest tube is small, effective, and easy to insert. With the patient upright, the tube and its trocar are introduced anteriorly through the second or third intercostal space at the midclavicular line. The catheter is fed off the trocar when loss of resistance signals entry into the pleural space. The tube then can be attached to the one-way valve supplied, to suction, or to a three-way stopcock for immediate aspiration with a large syringe. Care must be taken that all connections are secure and that any stopcock included in the line cannot be accidentally opened to atmospheric pressure.

Other Pulmonary Complications

Other hazards of lung biopsy include air embolism and pulmonary hemorrhage, both potentially fatal. Biopsy on deep inspiration or with Valsalva should be avoided, and the patient should be instructed to suppress coughing as much as possible. All increase the possibility that air may enter pulmonary veins from the lung.[46] Air embolism should be treated by placing the patient in a left lateral decubitus and Trendelenburg position. The patient may need transfer to an institution with a hyperbaric chamber. Hemoptysis is seen to a minor degree in many patients, but massive bleeding is fortunately quite unusual; it has been reported with 18-gauge or larger needles. The patient should be given oxygen and placed with the involved lung dependent. In severe cases, selective intubation of the uninvolved lung may be required for tamponade of the hemorrhage.

Bone

Biopsy of osseous lesions has been traditionally performed with very large trephines or boring needles, such as the Turkel, Ackermann, Craig, and Jamshidi. However, smaller needles have been developed that can be used with a motorized drilling attachment.[47] Most bone lesions presenting for needle biopsy are lytic, and if enough destruction is present, standard fine needles can be used without difficulty.[48] One point to keep in mind: about one third of patients with known cancer and a solitary bone lesion have a benign lesion.

Diagnostic accuracy with large trephine needles has been 81% to 95%, while major bleeding has been encountered in 2%.[11] The number of passes into a vertebral body should be limited to two, and a smaller needle should be used, if possible, for the risk of neurologic complication is not negligible (8%).[11] Access to thoracic spine lesions can be attained with needle placement between vertebral pedicle and the adjacent rib; this avoids the intercostal nerves and pleura.[49]

If blood returns through the needle, about 5 ml should be aspirated and allowed to clot. This blood can be submitted as a tissue specimen, with both sections and smears prepared. Clot examination may be more sensitive for metastatic carcinoma than the study of bone tissue. Hewes and colleagues found that in those cases of osseous neoplasm from which both tissue and clot had been obtained, only 39 of 54 would have been positive for malignancy had examination of blood been omitted.[50]

Disk space biopsy is indicated for patients with narrowing or destruction in conjunction with pain, fever, leukocytosis, or elevated erythrocyte sedimentation rate. Use of a large trephined needle can be diagnostic in 68%, with infection the most common finding.[51]

Abdomen and Pelvis

Ileus may occasionally be encountered after needle placement through peritoneum. Frank peritonitis has been described as complicating 0.3% of biopsies performed with 18- and 19-gauge cutting needles.[25]

Liver

Hepatic percutaneous needle biopsy has greater than 90% sensitivity for tumor.[26] The presence of ascites has long been considered a relative contraindication, but it has recently been shown not to pose any additional hazard.[52]

Although most hepatic hemangiomas can be diagnosed by noninvasive means, occasional lesions cannot be distinguished from possible malignancy without biopsy. As long as needles no larger than 20 gauge are used and care is taken to traverse normal parenchyma in reaching the lesion, percutaneous biopsy of hemangioma is safe.[53] The presence of endothelial elements in an aspirate supports the diagnosis. However, the pathologist must be alerted to the possibility that the lesion is a hemangioma for a positive diagnosis to be made.

Hemorrhage and bile leakage are the greatest potential problems associated with hepatic biopsy. Hepatocellular carcinoma and various metastatic lesions may be very vascular, and bleeding from such tumors is a prime cause of death due to cutting needle biopsy.[31,32,54] Bleeding risk is elevated in the presence of cirrhosis and hepatic dysfunction, both common conditions in those referred for diagnosis.

One method of preventing hemorrhage is to plug the biopsy tract. Chuang and Alspaugh have performed embolizations of the hepatic tract of high-risk patients by preloading a 6 Fr sheath over the cannula of a 14-gauge Tru-Cut needle.[55] Serial injections of gelatin sponge (Gelfoam) during withdrawal prevented significant bleeding in all 22 patients undergoing the procedure.

At the University of Wisconsin–Madison, we have modified this technique by placing a 16-gauge short venous catheter into the biopsy cannula after specimen (but not cannula) removal.[56] In this manner, gelatin foam or embolic coils can be introduced without a preloaded sheath in place.

Alternative approaches to hepatic biopsy include the use of a percutaneous transjugular venous needle, which can be guided into hepatic veins, and placement of sheathed needles, brushes, biopsy forceps, or Simpson atherectomy catheters through existing percutaneous biliary drainage tracts.[2,57]

Pancreas

Fine-needle biopsy can provide a positive diagnosis of pancreatic carcinoma in 69% to 85% of cases.[2,3,58,59] This compares favorably with surgical biopsy, which may have a sensitivity of 65% to 76%.[2,60] Use of an 18-gauge biopsy gun in 50 pancreatic biopsies was associated with 92% sensitivity for carcinoma in a report by Elvin and associates.[61] Although no major complications arose in that study, further experience is needed to determine the safety of routine use of such devices in the pancreas.

False-negative studies can be related to the marked desmoplastic character of many pancreatic malignancies. This fibrotic reaction may be responsible for the lower incidence of pancreatitis after needle biopsy of larger lesions. In the series described by Mueller and associates, all five patients who developed severe pancreatitis after fine-needle biopsy had lesions smaller than 3 cm in diameter.[62] In fact, those with normal pancreatic tissue may be at greater risk for this severe and occasionally fatal complication. Thus, caution should be exercised in pursuing biopsy in patients with questionable pancreatic abnormalities.

Adrenal Glands

Incidentally discovered adrenal masses are not rare, and they may present problems in the staging of extraadrenal neoplasms. Because benign adrenocortical masses commonly contain lipid, this feature can be used to differentiate them from primary or metastatic malignancies by CT or MRI examinations.[63] Needle biopsy is indicated for those lesions not displaying typical characteristics. Adrenal biopsy can be very accurate, with sensitivity for malignancy of over 90% in larger series.[64,65] Pitfalls include the inability to distinguish normal adrenal from adenoma microscopically or to distinguish primary adrenal carcinoma from metastatic renal cell carcinoma. Successful needle biopsy of pheochromocytoma has been performed, but premedication with α- and β-blockers (phenoxybenzamine and propranolol) is advisable.[66] A small but real risk of adrenal biopsy is pneumothorax, particularly for left-sided lesions in which the posterior sulcus cannot be avoided.

Other Sites

Needle biopsy has not been widely used for the diagnosis of renal neoplasm, although renal cyst aspiration was in vogue for a number of years. Renal biopsy can be used to confirm the diagnosis of renal cell carcinoma in patients who have disseminated disease or who are not candidates for nephrectomy.[67] Aspiration cytologic study can be extremely useful for making the diagnosis of renal tuberculosis in those patients without acid-fast bacilli detected in their urine.[68] However, the main function of renal biopsy at present is to diagnose diffuse parenchymal disease or renal transplant rejection. In these cases, large cutting needles are generally needed. Biopsy guns can ease the biopsy procedure and can provide more than adequate specimens.[21] Ultrasound is commonly used to direct biopsy toward the lower pole of the kidney, avoiding major vessels.

Percutaneous biopsy has been used extensively for masses or lymph nodes suggesting recurrent gynecologic, genitourinary, or colonic tumor after surgical resection. Stereotactic mammographic needle placement is widely employed for the diagnosis of breast cancer. Masses involving or extending into inferior vena cava can be sampled by long intravenous needles or biopsy forceps introduced through vascular sheaths.[57,69] Presently, rectal sonographic probes are being used to guide needle aspiration of focal prostatic lesions. The potential benefits and place of prostatic biopsy have yet to be defined in the wider population suffering prostatic enlargement.

REFERENCES

1. Livraghi T, Damascelli B, Lombardi C, Spagnoli I: Risk in fine-needle abdominal biopsy. *J Clin Ultrasound* 1983; 11:77–81.
2. Cohan RH, Illescas FF, Braun SD, et al: Fine needle aspiration biopsy in malignant obstructive jaundice. *Gastrointest Radiol* 1986; 11:145–150.
3. Teplick SK, Haskin PH, Kline TS, et al: Percutaneous pancreaticobiliary biopsies in 173 patients using primarily ultrasound or fluoroscopic guidance. *Cardiovasc Intervent Radiol* 1988; 11:26–28.
4. Goralnik CH, O'Connell DM, El Yousef SJ, Haaga JR: CT-guided cutting-needle biopsies of selected chest lesions. *Am J Roentgenol* 1988; 151:903–907.
5. Van Sonnenberg E, Casola G, Ho M, et al: Difficult thoracic lesions: CT-guided biopsy experience in 150 cases. *Radiology* 1988; 167:457–461.
6. Conces DJ Jr, Clark SA, Tarver RD, Schwenk GR: Transthoracic aspiration needle biopsy: Value in the diagnosis of pulmonary infections. *Am J Roentgenol* 1989; 152:31–34.
7. Bottles K, McPhaul LW, Volberding P: Fine needle aspiration biopsy of patients with the acquired immunodeficiency syndrome (AIDS): Experience in an outpatient clinic. *Ann Intern Med* 1988; 108:42–45.
8. Welch TJ, Sheedy PF, Johnson CD, et al: CT-guided biopsy: Prospective analysis of 1,000 procedures. *Radiology* 1989; 171:493–496.

9. Terriff BA, Gibney RG, Scudamore CH: Fatality from fine-needle aspiration biopsy of a hepatic hemangioma. *Am J Roentgenol* 1990; 154:203–204.

10. Fish GD, Stanley JH, Miller KS, et al: Postbiopsy pneumothorax: Estimating the risk by chest radiography and pulmonary function tests. *Am J Roentgenol* 1988; 150:71–74.

11. Mink J: Percutaneous bone biopsy in the patient with known or supected osseous metastases. *Radiology* 1986; 161:191–194.

12. Reading CC, Carboneau JW, James EM, Hurt MR: Sonographically guided percutaneous biopsy of small (3 cm or less) masses. *Am J Roentgenol* 1988; 151:189–192.

13. Reading CC, Carboneau JW, Felmlee JP, James EM: US-guided percutaneous biopsy: Use of a screw biopsy stylet to aid needle detection. *Radiology* 1987; 163:280–281.

14. Perrella RR, Kimme-Smith C, Tessler FN, et al: A new electronically enhanced biopsy system: Value in improving needle-tip visibility during sonographically guided interventional procedures. *Am J Roentgenol* 1992; 158:195–198.

15. Mueller PR, Saini S, Simeone JF, et al: Image-guided pleural biopsies: Indications, technique, and results in 23 patients. *Radiology* 1988; 169:1–4.

16. Onik G, Cosman ER, Wells TH Jr, et al: CT-guided aspirations for the body: Comparison of hand guidance with stereotaxis. *Radiology* 1988; 166:389–394.

17. Frederick PR, Miller MH, Bahr AL, Longson FW: Coaxial needles for repeated biopsy sampling. *Radiology* 1989; 170:273–274.

18. Hawkins IF Jr, Akins EW, Mladinich C, et al: Transvisceral access using a blunt needle: Technical note. *Semin Intervent Radiol* 1988; 5:149–151.

19. Quinn SF, Demlow T, Dunkley B: Temno biopsy needle: Evaluation of efficacy and safety in 165 biopsy procedures—technical note. *Am J Roentgenol* 1992; 158:641–643.

20. Hopper KD, Abendroth CS, Sturtz KW, et al: Blinded comparison of biopsy needles and automated devices in vitro: 1. Biopsy of diffuse hepatic disease. *Am J Roentgenol* 1993; 161:1293–1297.

21. Hopper KD, Abendroth CS, Sturtz KW, et al: Blinded comparison of biopsy needles and automated devices in vitro: 2. Biopsy of medical renal disease. *Am J Roentgenol* 1993; 161:1299–1301.

22. Andriole JG, Haaga JR, Adams RB, Nuñez C: Biopsy needle characteristics assessed in the laboratory. *Radiology* 1983; 148:659–662.

23. Hueftle MG, Haaga JR: Effect of suction on biopsy sample size. *Am J Roentgenol* 1986; 147:1014–1016.

24. Fagelman D, Chess Q: Nonaspiration fine-needle cytology of the liver: Technique for obtaining diagnostic samples. *Am J Roentgenol* 1990; 155:1217–1219.

25. Berger H, Permanetter W, Steiner W, Markl A: Feinnadel- und schneidebiopsietechnik in der perkutanen punktion abdomineller raumforderungen. *Radiologe* 1988; 28:265–268.

26. Koss LG: Aspiration biopsy: A tool in surgical pathology. *Am J Surg Pathol* 1988; 12:43–53.

27. Lieberman RP, Hafez GR, Crummy AB: Histology from aspiration biopsy: Turner needle experience. *Am J Roentgenol* 1982; 138:561–564.

28. Dekker A, Reyna EL, Fuhrman C: Usefulness of a near-total fine-needle aspiration biopsy retrieval method: A study of its use in 85 consecutive patients. *Diagn Cytopathol* 1991; 7:308–316.
29. Dock W, Grabenwoeger F, Schurawitzki H, et al: Technik der Nebennierenbiopsie: Ultraschall versus CT als Zielmethode. *Rofo* 1992; 157:344–348.
30. Lundstedt C, Stridbeck H, Andersson R, et al: Tumor seeding occurring after fine-needle biopsy of abdominal malignancies. *Acta Radiol* 1991; 32:518–520.
31. Weiss H, Düntsch U, Weiss A: Risiken der feinnadelpunktion: Ergebnisse einer umfrage in der BRD (DEGUM-umfrage). *Ultraschall Med* 1988; 9:121–127.
32. Smith EH: Complications of percutaneous abdominal fine-needle biopsy. *Radiology* 1991; 178:253–258.
33. Yankaskas BC, Staab EV, Craven MB, et al: Delayed complications from fine-needle biopsies of solid masses of the abdomen. *Invest Radiol* 1986; 21:325–328.
34. Ariza MAD, Aguirán ERA, Atance JLV, et al: Transthoracic aspiration biopsy of pulmonary and mediastinal lesions. *Eur J Radiol* 1991; 12:98–103.
35. Yew WW, Kwan SYL, Wong PC, Fu KH: Percutaneous transthoracic needle biopsies in the rapid diagnosis of pulmonary tuberculosis. *Lung* 1991; 169:285–289.
36. Griñan NP, Lucena FM, Romero JV, et al: Yield of percutaneous needle lung aspiration in lung abscess. *Chest* 1990; 97:69–74.
37. Westcott JL: Percutaneous transthoracic needle biopsy. *Radiology* 1988; 169:593–601.
38. Herman SJ, Weisbrod GL: Usefulness of the blood patch technique after transthoracic needle aspiration biopsy. *Radiology* 1990; 176:395–397.
39. Harter LP, Moss AA, Goldberg HI, Gross BH: CT-guided fine-needle aspirations for diagnosis of benign and malignant disease. *Am J Roentgenol* 1983; 140:363–367.
40. Haramati LB, Austin JHM: Complications after CT-guided needle biopsy through aerated versus nonaerated lung. *Radiology* 1991; 181:778.
41. Klose K-C: CT-guided large-bore biopsy: Extrapleural injection of saline for safe transpleural access to pulmonary lesions. *Cardiovasc Intervent Radiol* 1993; 16:259–261.
42. Bressler EL, Kirkham JA: Mediastinal masses: Alternative approaches to CT-guided needle biopsy. *Radiology* 1994; 191:391–396.
43. Hill PC, Spagnolo SV, Hockstein MJ: Pneumothorax with fine-needle aspiration of thoracic lesions: Is spirometry a predictor? *Chest* 1993; 104:1017–1020.
44. Moore EH, LeBlanc J, Montesi SA, et al: Effect of patient positioning after needle aspiration lung biopsy. *Radiology* 1991; 181:385–387.
45. Perlmutt LM, Braun SD, Newman GE, et al: Timing of chest film follow-up after transthoracic needle aspiration. *Am J Roentgenol* 1986; 146:1049–1050.
46. Cianci P, Posin JP, Shimshak RR, Singzon J: Air embolism complicating percutaneous thin needle biopsy of lung. *Chest* 1987; 92:749–751.

47. Hauenstein KH, Wimmer B, Beck A, Adler CP: Knochenbiopsie unklarer knochenläsionen mit einer neuen 1,4 mm messenden biopsiekanüle. *Radiologe* 1988; 28:251–258.
48. Bennett JD, Yacyshyn BJ, Haddad RC, Lefcoe MS: Fine-needle aspiration of bone lesions. *J Can Assoc Rad* 1990; 41:65–68.
49. Brugieres P, Gaston A, Heran F, et al: Percutaneous biopsies of the thoracic spine under CT guidance: Transcostovertebral approach. *J Comput Assist Tomogr* 1990; 14:446–448.
50. Hewes RC, Vigorita VJ, Freiberger RH: Percutaneous bone biopsy: The importance of aspirated osseous blood. *Radiology* 1983; 148:69–72.
51. Armstrong P, Chalmers AH, Green G, Irving JD: Needle aspiration/biopsy of the spine in suspected disc space infection. *Br J Radiol* 1978; 51:333–337.
52. Murphy FB, Barefield KP, Steinberg HV, Bernardino ME: CT- or sonography-guided biopsy of the liver in the presence of ascites: Frequency of complications. *Am J Roentgenol* 1988; 151:485–486.
53. Tung GA, Cronan JJ: Percutaneous needle biopsy of hepatic cavernous hemangioma. *J Clin Gastroenterol* 1993; 16:117–122.
54. McGill DB, Rakela J, Zinsmeister AR, Ott BJ: A 21-year experience with major hemorrhage after percutaneous liver biopsy. *Gastroenterology* 1990; 99:1396–1400.
55. Chuang VP, Alspaugh JP: Sheath needle for liver biopsy in high-risk patients. *Radiology* 1988; 166:261–262.
56. Crummy AB, McDermott JC, Wojtowycz M: Technical note: A technique for embolization of biopsy tracts. *Am J Roentgenol* 1989; 153:67–68.
57. Krieves D, Keller FS, Dotter CT, Rösch J: Percutaneous intravenous biopsy. *Diagn Imaging* 1980; 49:297–302.
58. Tudway DC, Newman J, Chard MJ: Ultrasound-guided fine-needle histological biopsies in the abdomen. *Clin Radiol* 1988; 39:377–380.
59. Hall-Craggs MA, Lees WR: Fine-needle aspiration biopsy: Pancreatic and biliary tumors. *Am J Roentgenol* 1986; 147:399–403.
60. Parsons L Jr, Palmer CH: How accurate is fine-needle biopsy in malignant neoplasia of the pancreas? *Arch Surg* 1989; 124:681–683.
61. Elvin A, Andersson T, Scheibenpflug L, Lindgren PG: Biopsy of the pancreas with a biopsy gun. *Radiology* 1990; 176:677–679.
62. Mueller PR, Miketic LM, Simeone JF, et al: Severe acute pancreatitis after percutaneous biopsy of the pancreas. *Am J Roentgenol* 1988; 151:493–494.
63. Mitchell DG, Crovello M, Matteucci T, et al: Benign adrenocortical masses: Diagnosis with chemical shift MR imaging. *Radiology* 1992; 185:345–351.
64. Tikkakoski T, Taavitsainen M, Päivänsalo M, et al: Accuracy of adrenal biopsy guided by ultrasound and CT. *Acta Radiol* 1991; 32:371–374.
65. Wadih GE, Nance KV, Silverman JF: Fine-needle aspiration cytology of the adrenal gland: 50 biopsies in 48 patients. *Arch Pathol Lab Med* 1992; 116:841–846.
66. Koenker RM, Mueller PR, van Sonnenberg E: Interventional radiology of the adrenal glands. *Semin Roentgenol* 1988; 22:314–322.

67. Niceforo JR, Coughlin BF: Diagnosis of renal cell carcinoma: Value of fine-needle aspiration cytology in patients with metastases or contraindications to nephrectomy. *Am J Roentgenol* 1993; 161:1303–1305.
68. Das KM, Vaidyanathan S, Rajwanshi A, Indudhara R: Renal tuberculosis: Diagnosis with sonographically guided aspiration cytology. *Am J Roentgenol* 1992; 158:571–573.
69. Withers CE, Casola G, Herba MJ, Viloria J: Intravascular tumors: Transvenous biopsy. *Radiology* 1988; 167:713–715.

18

Percutaneous Drainage of Abscesses and Other Fluid Collections

KEY CONCEPTS

1. Most intraabdominal and pelvic abscesses can be drained by percutaneous catheters.
2. Abscesses with fistulae can also be treated but need a longer period of drainage.
3. If a patient does not improve within 24 to 48 hours of drainage, the reason for inadequate response must be found and corrected.
4. Catheters can be removed when the patient is afebrile, leukocytosis has resolved, and tube output is negligible.
5. A fistula should be suspected if drainage continues to be more than 50 ml/day after the first few days.

INDICATIONS

Any abdominal, pelvic, or other soft-tissue abscess that cannot be readily treated by simple incision and drainage may be initially approached by percutaneous catheters. Untreated abdominal abscesses are almost invariably fatal, and mortality even with surgery may be quite high, from 17% in single abdominal abscess to 43% to 80% in patients with multiple abscesses.[1-3] Various other noninfected fluid collections can also be managed by percutaneous techniques.

CONTRAINDICATIONS AND CAUTIONS

There are no absolute contraindications to percutaneous catheter drainage, but care must be taken to avoid bowel, spleen, major vessels, and the diaphragm during tube placement. Transgression of the diaphragm is likely to lead to pleural empyema. Severe coagulopathy is a relative contraindication to catheter placement. Multiloculated or multiple abscesses require multiple drains. Foreign bodies must be removed if present, for they serve as foci of infection. Abscesses around infected vascular grafts must be managed surgically. Infected hematomas or other collections containing very viscous or debris-laden fluid are less likely to respond. Some small collections resolve with intravenous antibiotics alone, and amebic liver abscesses almost invariably respond to conservative therapy. When a catheter is placed and no clinical improvement is seen within 24 to 48 hours, surgery or other percutaneous measures must be vigorously pursued.

CHOOSING AN ENTRY SITE

Percutaneous drainage has been made possible by the advent of cross-sectional imaging, allowing not only the earlier detection of infected fluid collections but also fine-needle aspiration for diagnosis and the planning for percutaneous catheter approach. Ideally, the site of entry should allow the most direct approach (extraperitoneal if possible), and avoid vessels and viscera.

As noted, the diaphragm should not be traversed. Posteriorly, the pleural reflection is at the level of the twelfth rib; in the mid-axillary line, pleura extends to the tenth rib.[4,5] For subphrenic lesions, sharply cephalad angulation may be needed. Alternatively, a subxiphoid approach can be used. Pleural transgression does not inevitably lead to spread of infection, but empyema is a real risk.[6,7]

At times, it may be necessary to place catheters transgluteally to treat pelvic abscess.[8] In such cases, the route chosen should be low in the greater sciatic foramen, close to the sacrum above the sacrospinous ligament. In this fashion the sacral plexus and sciatic nerve can be avoided. The transgluteal approach tends to be more painful for the patient, and because of the amount of muscle being traversed, a stiffening cannula may be required for catheter insertion.

Another approach to deep pelvic abscesses is by transrectal catheter. In the procedure described by Carmody and colleagues, the abscess is drained with the patient in a left lateral decubitus position on a fluoroscopy table.[9] The initial diagnostic computed tomography (CT) is used for reference, and the rectosigmoid is filled with water-soluble contrast medium to guide a sheath needle advanced through an enema tube. A self-retaining drain is inserted over a guidewire and through a peel-away sheath. Transvaginal drains have been placed in a similar fashion.[10]

Although catheters have been placed through stomach or bowel in order to reach an abscess,[11] this placement is usually inadvertent and not planned. One exception is the transgastric drainage of pancreatic pseudo-cysts.[12] Recognition of unintended bowel transgression may take several days, but, fortunately, most such cases are managed successfully by catheter alone. One must avoid manipulating for at least 2 weeks (to allow a fibrous tract to form), and the catheter should be slowly withdrawn over 2 to 3 days. If the stomach is violated, the patient should have nothing by mouth for 24 hours prior to catheter removal.

A transhepatic approach for otherwise inaccessible abscesses of the lesser sac has been used successfully and without complication by Mueller and associates.[13] Precautions in such cases have included avoidance of central portions of the liver, restriction of catheter size to 9 Fr or smaller, and gradual catheter withdrawal over a period of days after clinical resolution of the abscess. Patients with cirrhosis, portal hypertension, bleeding disorder, or biliary obstruction should be treated surgically.

In choosing a site for percutaneous drainage, physical factors and patient comfort should be kept in mind. A drain is best placed in the most dependent portion of an abscess in order to have gravity assist in its evacuation. However, a direct posterior approach is seldom optimal because the catheter does not allow the patient to lie supine comfortably, and kinking of the tube can result.

PLACING THE CATHETER

Before draining a fluid collection, it is best to place a diagnostic needle (often 20 or 18 gauge, if 22-gauge needle yields no aspirate) in order to determine is the fluid is infected. If the fluid is not obviously purulent, Gram staining should be performed immediately, and samples sent for culture, sensitivity, and special stains (e.g., acid-fast bacilli and potassium hydroxide preparations). Some sterile fluid collections, hematomas in particular, are better left alone; introducing a catheter may complicate the condition by allowing bacteria access.

Patients referred for suspected abscess are almost invariably receiving intravenous antibiotics. However, if none has been given, a broad-spectrum antibiotic covering gram-negative and anaerobic organisms should be started before proceeding. Any anticoagulation should be stopped, and recent prothrombin and partial thromboplastin time values should be available.

There are two basic methods for placing a drainage catheter percutaneously: trocar technique and Seldinger technique. The former is generally reserved for large, relatively superficial lesions with no critical intervening structures. The catheter is threaded over a matched trocar, and, after appropriate sterile preparation of the skin, local anesthesia, and small incision, it is advanced until pus can be aspirated through the trocar or until imaging determines that the tip is well into the fluid space (Fig. 18-1). The trocar is then stabilized while the catheter is slipped over it to curl into the

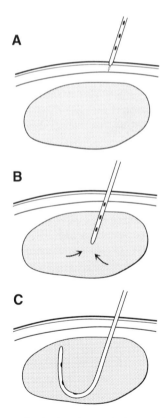

Fig. 18-1   The trocar method of catheter drainage. **A,** Placement of the trocar catheter through the skin and into the fluid collection. **B,** After removal of the trocar (but not the stiffening cannula), fluid is aspirated to confirm position. **C,** The catheter is advanced off the cannula to curl within the collection.

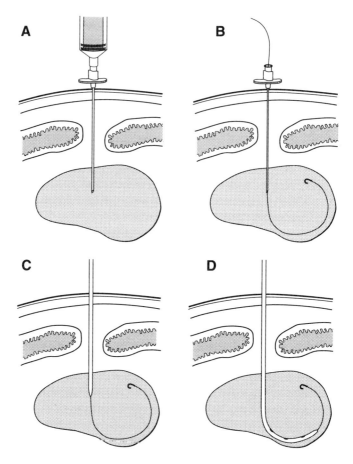

Fig. 18-2 The modified Seldinger method of catheter drainage. **A,** A hollow needle is guided into the fluid collection and gentle suction is applied. **B,** After fluid is obtained, a guidewire is passed through the needle. **C,** The tract is dilated. **D,** The drainage catheter is introduced over the guidewire.

abscess. With Seldinger technique, a needle is first placed into the fluid, a guidewire is coiled into the abscess, and serial dilators are used before the drainage catheter is introduced over the wire (Fig. 18-2).

In general, catheters should be no smaller than 8 Fr to ensure drainage of infected fluid, and it is clear that 5 Fr and 6 Fr tubes are inadequate.[3] Larger sump tubes, such as the 12 Fr to 14 Fr van Sonnenberg catheters, have much to recommend them, although a catheter with a single large lumen may be just as effective. When blood clots or necrotic debris must be evacuated, even larger tubes may be introduced.

After as much purulent material as possible is aspirated, a sinogram can be performed. No more than 30 ml of contrast material should be injected at the time of initial drainage, to avoid the risk of bacteremia and sepsis. Contrast injection may demonstrate fistulous communication with biliary ducts, pancreatic duct, or bowel. This sinogram also serves as a baseline for future studies. If an abscess is large and contains septations or a large amount of debris, a curved catheter may be rotated gently or a soft-tipped guidewire curled within the cavity to break up any loculations.

The catheter may be sutured directly to the skin. As an alternative, an enterostomy stoma ring can be applied to the entry site, and the catheter secured to the ring by sutures.[14] Connecting tubing should be secured with tape to make transmission of inadvertent tension to the catheter less likely.

CATHETER MANAGEMENT AND END POINTS

The management of drainage catheters is an area in which there is no great consensus. Many put catheters to dependent drainage or low intermittent suction. Depending on the viscosity of the draining material, the catheter and sump port can each be flushed with 5 ml of saline every day or every nursing shift. Strict records of tube input and output are mandatory. Care must be taken that a stopcock is not the limiting factor in draining thick fluid. If a constant drip infusion through one port or catheter is elected (with suction through another), input-output observation becomes critical. The amount infused should never exceed the volume drained. Antibiotics are chosen according to the sensitivity of the organisms cultured, and clinical response is measured by the return to normal of the patient's temperature and leukocyte count within several days. The use of acetylcysteine (Mucomyst) or antibiotic infusion is controversial, and no consistent benefit has been demonstrated.[3] In certain collections, such as pleural empyema or infected hematoma, intermittent instillation and aspiration of thrombolytic agents has been helpful.[15–17]

The net output of the catheter should quickly drop to less than 50 ml/day; otherwise, a fistula should be suspected. Serial sinograms are obtained every several days to confirm optimal catheter placement, determine decrease in cavity size, and detect any fistula. When tube output approaches zero and the cavity is essentially collapsed about the drain, the catheter may be removed. If the abscess is associated with fistula, clamping the drainage tube for several days is advised to detect any reaccumulation of fluid. In complicated abscesses or when there is any doubt about the efficacy of percutaneous drainage, a CT examination should be performed before drain removal.[18] If the lesion is deep, the catheter may be slowly withdrawn over several days. Successful drainage is usually accomplished within 1 to 2 weeks in uncomplicated cases. Those individuals able to care adequately for their catheters may be discharged and followed as outpatients until tube removal is deemed appropriate.

FISTULAE

In the past, an underlying fistula was considered a contraindication to percutaneous drainage, but experience at many centers has shown that an abscess with fistula can be managed just as successfully as an uncomplicated abscess.[19–21] In the great majority of cases, a fistula is not suspected and not found until several days after catheter placement. If it is demonstrated, an additional catheter should be placed as close as possible to the communication (Fig. 18-3). Bowel rest or biliary diversion (in the case of biliary fistulae) may be appropriate. Fistulae associated with bowel or biliary obstruction do not resolve until the obstruction is relieved. Laboratory

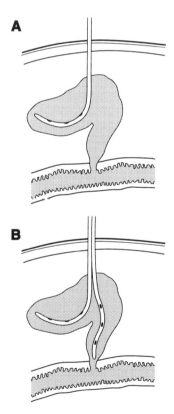

Fig. 18-3 **A,** Abscess found to communicate with bowel lumen. **B,** A second catheter is introduced to the site of communication to divert enteric leakage and allow the fistula to seal.

analysis for fluid amylase or bilirubin may confirm pancreatic or biliary communication. Somatostatin or its synthetic analog, octreotide, may speed healing by diminishing fluid secretion.[22] Successful management of fistulae with percutaneous catheters usually requires twice as much time as simple abscess drainage, often longer than 1 month. Failure to appreciate a fistula is a prime cause of treatment failure.[18–23]

CONSIDERATIONS BY ABSCESS LOCATION

Liver and Spleen

Catheter drainage has been quite effective in the treatment of liver abscess, and complete resolution can be expected in more than 80% of patients. However, Stain and associates reported a series in which 23 of 29 patients recovered after treatment by intravenous antibiotics alone.[24] Diagnostic aspiration was very important in guiding antibiotic therapy; they found one fourth of their patients had different organisms found in the aspirate than had been cultured from their blood, and many abscesses were polymicrobial. Percutaneous or surgical drainage was reserved for the few who had not shown improvement with at least 1 week of conservative management.

Others have reported similar experiences in treating abscesses of the liver and spleen. Schwerk's group at Marburg, Germany, treated 42 patients (including 6 with splenic abscesses) with attempted total aspiration by needle, often repeated at 2- to 6-day intervals, and had 95% success.[7] The only 4 patients undergoing drainage catheter placement had abscesses larger than 10 cm in diameter. When multiple abscesses were present, only the largest were aspirated. In another report 8 patients with splenic abscesses were cured, 4 by aspiration with a 19-gauge needle and 4 by catheter drainage without any major complications.[25]

When catheter drainage is clearly needed, poor clinical response may be due to the presence of multiple loculations, devitalized tissue, and other debris. Morettin has described the use of a 24 Fr Malecot cystostomy catheter modified by the extension of the slits along the shaft.[26] By retracting the obturator, a propellerlike device is created that allows the percutaneous debridement of devitalized tissue. It was used only in patients with pyogenic liver abscess who had persistent leukocytosis and indication of retained debris upon CT scan after at least 2 weeks of standard drainage. Debridement was performed through well-formed tracts with the patients heavily sedated. Although bacteremia and moderate bleeding were encountered, open surgery was avoided and all abscesses that were debrided healed within another 2 weeks.

When dealing with liver abscess, the source of infection must be sought. The gastrointestinal or biliary tract is often responsible, and the possibility of an occult colonic carcinoma must not be dismissed without clinical investigation.

Amebic liver abscesses generally need neither aspiration for diagnosis nor percutaneous drainage.[27] They are almost invariably cured by treatment with metronidazole or chloroquine alone. Only those lesions superinfected with pyogenic organisms require any further intervention.

Percutaneous drainage has been considered contraindicated in echinococcal cyst of the liver because of the risk of soilage of the peritoneum and possible anaphylaxis. However, Khuroo and colleagues have successfully treated 12 patients with hydatid cysts by catheter placement and instillation of hypertonic saline.[28] Only one patient developed limited urticaria, and none had anaphylaxis.

Pancreas

There continues to be controversy about the role of percutaneous techniques in treating pancreatic fluid collections. It is clear that drainage of complicated pancreatic collections is not as successful as for abscesses elsewhere in the abdomen, but surgical treatment often is followed by the need for reoperation or subsequent percutaneous drainage.[23,29,30] Even in the case of uncomplicated pseudocysts, surgical indications are changing.

Noninfected Pseudocysts

Until recently, the standard recommendation for dealing with symptomatic pancreatic pseudocyst was conservative treatment for 4 to 6 weeks, followed by internal drainage if the pseudocyst did not resolve. This was predicated by the observation that the incidence of life-threatening complications increased with time and that spontaneous late resolution was unlikely. This approach is being reconsidered by many surgeons after the report of Vitas and Sarr concerning 68 patients with pseudocysts and no factors predisposing to recurrent pancreatitis (such as alcoholism) who were treated nonoperatively.[31] Although many patients had large and chronic collections, 59% had resolution of symptoms and decrease or disappearance of their pseudocysts without any drainage procedure. Over more than 4 years of follow-up, only 9% developed severe complications needing urgent intervention, while the rest had elective surgery.

Simple percutaneous aspiration of pseudocysts is limited by a high rate of recurrence.[12] Catheter placement has improved outcome, with complete resolution in 63% to 86% of patients.[12,29,32–34] Many pseudocysts communicate with the pancreatic duct, but percutaneous drainage is just as likely to be successful as long as the catheter is kept in place for a more extended period of time (averaging 1 month).[33,34] Despite this experience with percutaneous drainage, many clinicians are reluctant to have catheters placed into noninfected collections for fear of introducing bacteria.

Catheter intervention is probably best reserved for those pseudocysts continuing to produce symptoms despite a prolonged trial of conservative management.

Infected Pseudocysts and Pancreatic Abscesses

Many times the clinical distinction between infected and noninfected pseudocyst is difficult to make; both may present with pain, fever, and leukocytosis. For this reason, diagnostic needle aspiration is indispensable for evaluation. In those with infection, there is little question that catheter drainage is indicated; it has been curative in 78% to 94% of patients so treated.[29,34,35] Pancreatic abscess, which commonly contains considerable debris, may be less responsive. Even so, most patients have palliation, if not complete resolution.[29,32] Phlegmons should be surgically debrided. In difficult situations, surgery and percutaneous drainage are often complementary procedures, one following the other. As is to be expected, the outcome of any intervention has correlated with the severity of illness as gauged by APACHE II (Acute Physiology and Chronic Health Evaluation) scores.[35]

Other Abdominal, Pelvic, and Retroperitoneal Abscesses

Percutaneous drainage has been as successful as surgery in treating abdominal and pelvic abscess.[6,36] Fluid collections associated with diverticulitis and appendicitis respond quite well to catheter therapy, allowing what might be a two- or three-stage surgical approach to become a single-stage elective operation after resolution of the acute inflammatory process.[6,23,37–39] Tuberculous abscesses have also been treated successfully.[40]

Crohn disease patients are prone to develop abscess complicated by fistula (usually to the ileum). Catheter drainage may be appropriate for palliation, although fistulae tend to recur despite adequate drainage, treatment with parenteral nutrition, and bowel rest.[41] The diseased segment of bowel must be resected for definitive therapy. Those without bowel fistulae respond well to percutaneous drainage alone.[41,42]

Percutaneous catheter drainage alone has been successful in treating 67% to 91% of abdominal and pelvic abscesses in several large series.* Morbidity and mortality are related to the severity of underlying illness and the presence of multiorgan failure. Catheter therapy resolves fistulae in 77% to 86% of cases, as long as the presence of a fistula is recognized.† If an abscess recurs after catheter removal, a second percutaneous drainage is very often successful, but a second recurrence must be treated surgically.[20,23]

---

*References 2,6,8,23,36,43–46.
†References 8,9,20,44,47,48.

Lung Abscesses and Pleural Empyema

Lung abscess does not commonly require catheter or open drainage because there is often communication with the tracheobronchial tree and a combination of intravenous antibiotics and postural drainage is effective. Nevertheless, if such measures fail, percutaneous drainage is a low-morbidity alternative to open thoracostomy. In three published series, abscesses were cured in 27 of 30 patients, often with resolution of associated pleural fluid.[49–51] Although bronchial connection was commonly present, in no instance did a chronic bronchopleural fistula develop.

Computed tomography is invaluable for planning the drainage route. Only those abscesses contiguous with pleura should be selected, and aerated lung must not be traversed during catheter placement. The affected lung should be dependent at the time of drainage, to minimize the risk of aspiration of infected fluid into the opposite lung. The following criteria are recommended for selecting patients for percutaneous catheter drainage: sepsis does not abate with 5 to 7 days of antibiotic treatment, abscess is greater than 4 cm in diameter and causes mediastinal shift, enlarging abscess, or the patient is ventilator-dependent.[49]

There has been good success in resolving thoracic empyema by percutaneous chest tube placement, as long as fluid has been present less than 1 month.[52,53] As already mentioned, instillation of fibrinolytic agents can accelerate drainage of viscous fluid and has led to success in more than 90% of patients.[15,16] In the protocol of Moulton and associates, 80-ml aliquots of urokinase (1000 units/ml) are instilled, and the catheter is clamped for 1 to 2 hours.[15] The tube is then placed on suction for at least 1 hour before repetition of the procedure. Outcome is gauged by tube output and follow-up CT scans. Use of urokinase or streptokinase should be avoided in the presence of recent hemorrhage or bronchopleural fistula.

COMPLICATIONS AND FAILURES

Complications of drainage procedures include bacteremia, unintended enterostomy, infection of previously uninfected sites, and hemorrhage. Drainage of pancreatic fluid collections tends to produce the most morbidity, with major complications arising in 9% to 16% of patients.[29,30] Bleeding is much more common in patients with pancreatitis, and special care must be taken that a suspected abscess is not actually a pseudoaneurysm consequent to the pancreatic disease.[30] Cases of massive bleeding may be amenable to arterial embolotherapy.

Transgression of the pleural space may produce either pneumothorax or pleural empyema. Inadvertent placement of catheters through bowel can usually be treated by catheter repositioning and delayed removal.[6,11,30]

Percutaneous catheter drainage of abscess may fail from a complication of entry, such as hemorrhage; premature removal of catheter; inadequate size or number of catheters; poorly liquefied necrotic debris; or failure to recognize a fistula. Fistulae associated with radiation therapy, tumor, regional enteritis, foreign bodies, or bowel obstruction are not cured by percutaneous drains, although catheters may play a temporizing role in such patients. Drainage of infected tumors is usually avoided, but catheter placement may still provide substantial palliation in selected patients.[54] Infected hematomas have been notoriously difficult to drain, but infusion with thrombolytic agents shows some promise in improving evacuation.[17,55] If a patient does not respond positively within 2 days of tube placement, a technical problem should be sought immediately. If no remediable probem is uncovered, surgery should not be delayed.

CATHETER TREATMENT OF OTHER FLUID COLLECTIONS

Related transcatheter techniques have been applied to a variety of noninfected fluid collections causing problems. Pleurodesis through radiologically placed catheters has been a less traumatic method of treating intractable malignant effusions.[56] Large-volume paracentesis of malignant ascites, up to 4 or 5 L removed at one time, can provide substantial palliation.[57] When large volumes of fluid are removed at one sitting, vital signs must be watched carefully, and patients should have intravenous access.

We have used catheters to decompress pneumatoceles producing respiratory compromise.[58] Intracavitary instillation of amphotericin B via catheter can control recurrent hemoptysis caused by aspergillomas.[59]

Percutaneous aspiration has been used to treat lymphoceles with some success.[60] Because of problems with recurrence, catheter drainage, especially combined with sclerotherapy, is more likely to result in cure. Sclerotherapy may be performed with repeated instillation of povidone-iodine or tetracycline solutions.[61,62]

Large hepatic cysts may cause abdominal pain or fullness. Placement of a catheter and sclerosis with absolute ethanol or hypertonic saline have produced excellent results with minimal morbidity.[63–66] Fluid aspirated should be sent for cytologic examination, and contrast medium should be injected prior to sclerotherapy to detect any biliary communication, which is an absolute contraindication to injection of a sclerosing agent. When absolute ethanol is used, 20 ml to 100 ml is injected after evacuation of the cyst, the injected volume depending on the size of the cyst. The ethanol is left within the cavity for 20 minutes while the patient rolls into various positions to allow treatment of all walls of the cyst. After the ethanol is completely aspirated, the procedure may be repeated two or three times at one sitting. The patient may experience mild to moderate pain, but the procedure should be terminated and all the sclerosant immediately removed if severe pain arises.

REFERENCES

1. Van Waes PFGM, Felberg MAM, Mali WPTM, et al: Management of loculated abscesses that are difficult to drain: A new approach. *Radiology* 1983; 147:57–63.
2. Serrano A, Dahl EP, Rubin RH, et al: Eclectic drainage of subphrenic abscesses. *Arch Surg* 1984; 119:942–945.
3. Pruett TL, Simmons RL: Status of percutaneous catheter drainage of abscesses. *Surg Clin North Am* 1988; 68:89–105.
4. Nichols DM, Cooperberg PL, Golding RH, Burhenne HJ: The safe intercostal approach? Pleural complications in abdominal interventional radiology. *Am J Roentgenol* 1984; 141:1013–1018.
5. Neff CC, Mueller PR, Ferrucci JT Jr, et al: Serious complications following transgression of the pleural space in drainage procedures. *Radiology* 1984; 152:335–341.
6. Hemming A, Davis NL, Robins RE: Surgical versus percutaneous drainage of intra-abdominal abscesses. *Am J Surg* 1991; 161:593–595.
7. Schwerk WB, Görg C, Görg K, et al: Perkutane drainagen von leber- und milzabszessen. *Z Gastroenterol* 1991; 29:146–152.
8. Butch RJ, Mueller PR, Ferrucci JT Jr, et al: Drainage of pelvic abscesses through the greater sciatic foramen. *Radiology* 1986; 158:487–491.
9. Carmody E, Thurston W, Yeung E, Ho C-S: Transrectal drainage of deep pelvic collections under fluoroscopic guidance. *Can Assoc Radiol J* 1993; 44:429–433.
10. vanSonnenberg E, D'Agostino HB, Casola G, et al: Percutaneous abscess drainage: Current concepts. *Radiology* 1991; 181:617–626.
11. Mueller PR, Ferrucci JT Jr, Butch RJ, et al: Inadvertent percutaneous catheter gastroenterostomy during abscess drainage: Significance and management. *Am J Roentgenol* 1985; 145:387–391.
12. Grosso M, Gandini G, Cassinis MC, et al: Percutaneous treatment (including pseudocystogastrostomy) of 74 pancreatic pseudocysts. *Radiology* 1989; 173:493–497.
13. Mueller PR, Ferrucci JT Jr, Simeone JF, et al: Lesser sac abscesses and fluid collections: Drainage by transhepatic approach. *Radiology* 1985; 155:615–618.
14. Schoenfeld RB, Lecky D, Ring EJ, et al: Stabilization of percutaneous catheters. *Am J Roentgenol* 1982; 138:972.
15. Moulton JS, Moore PT, Mencini RA: Treatment of loculated pleural effusions with transcatheter intracavitary urokinase. *Am J Roentgenol* 1989; 153:941–945.
16. Aye RW, Froese DP, Hill LD: Use of purified streptokinase in empyema and hemothorax. *Am J Surg* 1991; 161:560–562.
17. García-Vila J, Sáiz-Pachés V, Doménech-Iglesias MA, et al: Infected intraabdominal hematomas: Percutaneous drainage. *Abdom Imaging* 1993; 18:313–317.
18. Lang EK, Springer RM, Glorioso LW, Cammarata CA: Abdominal abscess drainage under radiologic guidance: Causes of failure. *Radiology* 1986; 159:329–336.

19. Schuster MR, Crummy AB, Wojtowycz MM, McDermott JC: Abdominal abscesses associated with enteric fistulae: Management by percutaneous methods. *J Vasc Interv Radiol* 1992; 3:359–363.
20. Ercoli FR, Milgrim LM, Nosher JL, Brolin RE: Percutaneous catheter drainage of abscesses associated with enteric fistulae. *Am Surg* 1988; 54:45–49.
21. Berger H, Winter T, Pratschke E, Sauerbruch T: Perkutane drainagebehandlung fistelassoziierter abszess und biliärer fisteln. *Rofo* 1989; 150:342–345.
22. Spiliotis J, Vagenas K, Panagopoulos K, Kalfarentzos F: Treatment of enterocutaneous fistulas with TPN and somatostatin, compared with patients who received TPN only. *Br J Clin Pract* 1990; 44:616–618.
23. Brolin RE, Flancbaum L, Ercoli FR, et al: Limitations of percutaneous catheter drainage of abdominal abscesses. *Surg Gynecol Obstet* 1991; 173:203–210.
24. Stain SC, Yellin AE, Donovan AJ, Brien HW: Pyogenic liver abscess: Modern treatment. *Arch Surg* 1991; 126:991–996.
25. Hadas-Halpren I, Hiller N, Dolberg M: Percutaneous drainage of splenic abscesses: An effective and safe procedure. *Br J Radiol* 1992; 65:968–970.
26. Morettin LB: Percutaneous debridement of complex pyogenic liver abscesses: Technique and results. *Eur Radiol* 1992; 2:247–251.
27. Ralls RW, Barnes PF, Johnson MB, et al: Medical treatment of hepatic amebic abscess: Rare need for percutaneous drainage. *Radiology* 1987; 165:805–807.
28. Khuroo MS, Zargar SA, Mahajan R: Echinococcus granulosus cysts in the liver: Management with percutaneous drainage. *Radiology* 1991; 180:141–145.
29. Lang EK, Paolini RM, Pottmeyer A: The efficacy of palliative and definitive percutaneous versus surgical drainage of pancreatic abscesses and pseudocysts: A prospective study of 85 patients. *South Med J* 1991; 84:55–64.
30. Lee MJ, Rattner DW, Legemate DA, et al: Acute complicated pancreatitis: Redefining the role of interventional radiology. *Radiology* 1992; 183:171–174.
31. Vitas GJ, Sarr MG: Selected management of pancreatic pseudocysts: Operative versus expectant management. *Surgery* 1992; 111:123–130.
32. Stanley JH, Gobien RP, Shabel SI, et al: Percutaneous drainage of pancreatic and peripancreatic fluid collections. *Cardiovasc Intervent Radiol* 1988; 11:21–25.
33. Karnel F, Gebauer A, Jantsch H, et al: Perkutane katheterdrainage von pankreaspseudozysten. *Rofo* 1991; 155:242–245.
34. vanSonnenberg E, Wittich GR, Casola G, et al: Percutaneous drainage of infected and noninfected pancreatic pseudocysts: Experience in 101 cases. *Radiology* 1989; 170:757–761.
35. Adams DB, Harvey TS, Anderson MC: Percutaneous catheter drainage of infected pancreatic and peripancreatic fluid collections. *Arch Surg* 1990; 125:1554–1557.
36. Malangoni MA, Shumate CR, Thomas HA, Richardson JD: Factors influencing the treatment of intra-abdominal abscesses. *Am J Surg* 1990; 159:167–171.
37. vanSonnenberg E, Wittich GR, Casola G, et al: Periappendiceal abscesses: Percutaneous drainage. *Radiology* 1987; 163:23–26.
38. Mueller PR, Sainai S, Wittenburg J, et al: Sigmoid diverticular abscesses: Percutaneous drainage as an adjunct to surgical resection in 24 cases. *Radiology* 1987; 164:321–325

39. Neff CC, vanSonnenberg E, Casola G, et al: Diverticular abscesses: Percutaneous drainage. *Radiology* 1987; 163:15–18.
40. Pombo F, Martín-Egaña R, Cela A, et al: Percutaneous catheter drainage of tuberculous psoas abscesses. *Acta Radiol* 1993; 34:366–368.
41. Lambiase RE, Cronan JJ, Dorfman GS, et al: Percutaneous drainage of abscesses in patients with Crohn disease. *Am J Roentgenol* 1988; 150:1043–1045.
42. Casola G, vanSonnenberg E, Neff CC, et al: Abscesses in Crohn disease: Percutaneous drainage. *Radiology* 1987; 163:19–22.
43. Olak J, Christou NV, Stein LA, et al: Operative vs percutaneous drainage of intra-abdominal abscesses. *Arch Surg* 1986; 121:141–146.
44. Kerlan RK Jr, Jeffrey RB Jr, Pogany AC, Ring EJ: Abdominal abscess with low-output fistula: Successful percutaneous drainage. *Radiology* 1985; 155:73–75.
45. vanSonnenberg E, Wittich GR, Casola G, et al: Complicated pancreatic inflammatory disease: Diagnostic and therapeutic role of interventional radiology. *Radiology* 1985; 155:335–340.
46. Gordon DH, Macchia RJ, Glanz S, et al: Percutaneous management of retroperitoneal abscesses. *Urology* 1987; 30:299–306.
47. Mueller PR, Ferrucci JT, Simeone JF, et al: Detection and drainage of bilomas: Special considerations. *Am J Roentgenol* 1983; 140:715–720.
48. Papanicolaou N, Mueller PR, Ferrucci JT Jr, et al: Abscess-fistula association: Radiologic recognition and percutaneous management. *Am J Roentgenol* 1984; 143:811–815.
49. vanSonnenberg E, D'Agostino HB, Casola G, et al: Lung abscess: CT-guided drainage. *Radiology* 1991; 178:347–351.
50. Ha HK, Kang MW, Park JM, et al: Lung abscess: Percutaneous catheter therapy. *Acta Radiol* 1993; 34:362–365.
51. Shim C, Santos GH, Zelefsky M: Percutaneous drainage of lung abscess. *Lung* 1990; 168:201–207.
52. Westcott JL: Percutaneous catheter drainage of pleural effusion and empyema. *Am J Roentgenol* 1985; 144:1189–1193.
53. Hunnam GR, Flower CDR: Radiologically-guided percutaneous catheter drainage of empyemas. *Clin Radiol* 1988; 39:121–126.
54. Mueller PR, White EM, Glass-Royal M, et al: Infected abdominal tumors: Percutaneous catheter drainage. *Radiology* 1989; 173:627–629.
55. Vogelzang RL, Tobin RS, Burstein S, et al: Transcatheter intracavitary fibrinolysis of infected extravascular hematomas. *Am J Roentgenol* 1987; 148:378–380.
56. Morrison MC, Mueller PR, Lee MJ, et al: Sclerotherapy of malignant pleural effusion through sonographically placed small-bore catheters. *Am J Roentgenol* 1992; 158:41–43.
57. Ross GJ, Kessler HB, Clair MR, et al: Sonographically guided paracentesis for palliation of symptomatic malignant ascites. *Am J Roentgenol* 1989; 153:1309–1311.
58. Sewall L, Franco A, Wojtowycz M, McDermott J: Pneumatoceles causing respiratory compromise: Treatment by percutaneous decompression. *Chest* 1993; 103:1266–1267.

59. Shapiro MJ, Albelda SM, Mayock RL, McLean GK: Severe hemoptysis associated with pulmonary aspergilloma: Percutaneous intracavitary treatment. *Chest* 1988; 94:1225–1231.

60. Jensen SR, Voegeli DR, McDermott JC, Crummy AB: Percutaneous management of lymphatic fluid collections. *Cardiovasc Intervent Radiol* 1986; 9:202–204.

61. Burgos FJ, Teruel JL, Mayayo T, et al: Diagnosis and management of lymphoceles after renal transplantation. *Br J Urol* 1988; 61:289–293.

62. Shokeir AA, El-Diasty TA, Ghoneim MA: Percutaneous treatment of lymphocele in renal transplant recipients. *J Endourol* 1993; 7:481–485.

63. Andersson R, Jeppsson B, Lunderquist A, Bengmark S: Alcohol sclerotherapy of nonparasitic cysts of the liver. *Br J Surg* 1989; 76:254–255.

64. Bean WJ, Rodan BA: Hepatic cysts: Treatment with alcohol. *Am J Roentgenol* 1985; 144:237–241.

65. El Mouaaouy A, Naruhn M, Lauchart W, Becker HD: Behandlung der symptomatischen nichtparasitären lebercysten mittels percutaner drainage und spülung mit hypertoner kochsalzlösung. *Chirurg* 1991; 62:810–813.

66. Kairaluoma MI, Leinonen A, Ståhlberg M, et al: Percutaneous aspiration and alcohol sclerotherapy for symptomatic hepatic cysts: An alternative to surgical intervention. *Ann Surg* 1989; 210:208–215.

19

Percutaneous Gastrostomy

KEY CONCEPTS

1. Percutaneous gastrostomy is an alternative for long-term feeding or gastric decompression.
2. Patients with gastroesophageal reflux or who are at risk for aspiration pneumonia can be fed safely by a transgastric jejunal tube.
3. Ultrasonography and fluoroscopy are used to avoid the liver and the colon during tube placement.
4. Most patients can be fed the day after gastrostomy.
5. Tubes must be carefully secured, both internally and externally, for 2 weeks to prevent the possibility of displacement before a fibrous tract has formed.

Percutaneous gastrostomy is a quick, simple, and safe method for obtaining access to the stomach. The prime indication is for long-term feeding, but it may also be used for gastric decompression or, rarely, for simplified dilation of upper gastrointestinal stricture when a per oral approach has failed.

ENTERIC NUTRITIONAL SUPPORT

Malnutrition is increasingly recognized as a problem for many hospitalized and chronically ill patients.[1–3] Those who are unable to take nourishment for themselves but who have an otherwise intact and functioning gastrointestinal tract may benefit from tube feeding. In most cases, when the need for nutritional support is of limited duration, small-bore nasoenteric feeding tubes are quite adequate. However, if tube feeding is necessary for more than 4 to 6 weeks, gastrostomy provides a well-tolerated alternative.

Nearly all patients fed through a nasal tube are distressed by nasopharyngeal irritation, mouth breathing, and feelings of limited mobility.[4] Reflux about a tube traversing the gastroesophageal junction can become a problem. Nasoenteric tubes are also prone to accidental removal and recurrent occlusion. Many of these difficulties can be avoided by gastrostomy. One factor appreciated by patients discharged with gastric feeding tubes is the ability to appear in public without feeling excessively self-conscious.

Gastrostomy as an operative procedure has been performed for over a century, in many cases with local anesthesia alone; however, its widespread acceptance has been limited by reports of up to 35% mortality and 56% morbidity.[5] More recent improvements in surgical technique and patient preparation have reduced procedure-related mortality to 1.8% or less.[5–7]

A percutaneous, trocar approach to gastrostomy was described in 1967 by Jascalevich,[8] but over a decade passed before its first clinical application.[9] About the same time, endoscopy was enrolled by a number of investigators to guide percutaneous placement.[10,11] It was soon recognized that the procedure could be simplified by use of fluoroscopy and a small nasogastric tube.[12–14] The placement of long feeding tubes by a percutaneous transgastric approach has permitted the extension of the technique to patients with a history of gastroesophageal reflux and aspiration pneumonia.[15,16]

PATIENT SELECTION

Those likely to benefit from percutaneous gastrostomy for feeding include individuals with impaired swallowing due to neurologic disease or obstructing oropharyngeal and/or esophageal neoplasms (or even nonobstructing neoplasms undergoing radiotherapy), burn or trauma patients, cancer patients suffering anorexia and inanition, and patients with pharyngeal or esophageal fistula. Patients with widely disseminated malignant neoplasms or cachexia from very advanced pulmonary disease are unlikely to experience any benefit.[17] The appropriateness of feeding enterostomy in a given case is a judgment to be made by the radiologist, patient, referring physician, and patient's family, after a clear delineation of the potential risks and benefits of the procedure. Percutaneous gastrostomy should *not* be performed as a mere short-cut for long-term care; debilitated patients fed through tubes need careful monitoring for potential nutritional problems and signs of aspiration.[18]

Gastrostomy for feeding is contraindicated in the presence of gastric outlet or more distal bowel obstruction (gastrostomy for decompression may be indicated in such circumstances). The severely neurologically impaired, as well as those with known gastroesophageal reflux or poor gastric emptying, should not have stomach feedings. Rather, they should have transgastric jejunal tubes, because the more distal the infusion, the less likely the occurrence of reflux and aspiration.[1,19]

A history of prior gastric surgery, including partial gastric resection, does not preclude percutaneous gastrostomy or gastrojejunostomy.[20] As long as details of the surgical procedure and present anatomy are available, tube placement can be performed safely with only slightly modified technique (use of longer needles, angulated fluoroscopy, peel-away sheaths, and nylon T-fasteners). Ascites can cause problems with external leakage of fluid around the catheter entry site, but such difficulties can be minimized by large-volume paracentesis prior to percutaneous gastrostomy.[21] Portal hypertension is a relative complication because of the increased risk of puncturing a gastric varix during tube insertion. As in any percutaneous interventional procedure, anticoagulant medication should be stopped prior to percutaneous gastrostomy, and any coagulation abnormalities must be reversed.

TECHNIQUE

The patient should be given nothing by mouth for at least 8 hours prior to gastrostomy placement. Anitbiotics are not routinely given. Care should be taken to ensure that no organ or bowel interposes itself between the anterior abdominal wall and the stomach. To that end, real-time ultrasound is used to mark the edge of the left lobe of liver on the skin. Transverse colon usually contains enough gas to be readily apparent on fluoroscopy. Dilute barium given the previous day may be helpful in delineating the colon, but in some patients it may be necessary to instill air or radiographic contrast by way of the rectum. If it is suspected that small bowel lies anterior to stomach (a very rare situation), cross-table radiographs may be obtained. A soft, small-bore nasogastric tube is inserted, if one is not already in place.

A subcostal approach to the left of midline is chosen with the assistance of fluoroscopy. The outer third of the rectus abdominis muscle should be avoided because of the course of the inferior epigastric artery. Often the site chosen overlies colon or small bowel loops, but gastric insufflation reliably creates a "window" for tube placement (Fig. 19-1). The epigastrium is sterilely prepared and draped, local anesthesia is infiltrated, and a small skin incision made. In the unusual patient in whom the colon cannot be displaced caudally, infracolonic gastrostomies have been placed, but such procedures are best performed only after bowel opacification with dilute barium or water-soluble contrast medium.[22,23]

At this point, any retained gastric fluid is aspirated by way of the nasogastric tube, which is then used to inflate the stomach with 600 to 1000 ml of air. The patient is instructed to hold the distention as well as possible. Glucagon (0.5 to 1 mg) may be given intravenously prior to insufflation in order to prevent air from escaping through the pylorus. However, some patients experience retching and vomiting with its administration, and glucagon is not absolutely necessary for successful gastrostomy.

With the stomach inflated, a 5 Fr Teflon sheath needle is advanced by a quick, sharp jab to a depth of 4 to 5 cm. Stomach wall is quite compliant,

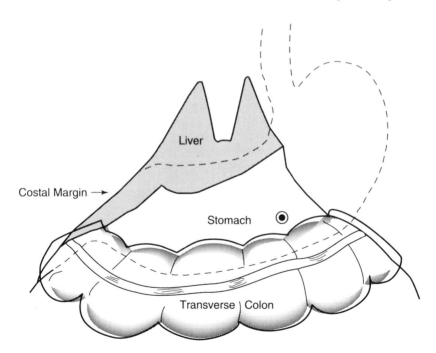

Fig. 19-1 Anatomic relationships relevant to gastrostomy placement. Dot marks an appropriate entry site.

but if distention is adequate no difficulty in entry should be encountered. Limiting the depth of the jab prevents penetration of the posterior gastric wall and possible pancreatic or splenic vessel injury. After removal of the needle trocar, water-soluble contrast is injected through the sheath. Intragastric position is confirmed by delineation of rugae and pooling in the fundus. A stiff guidewire is advanced through the sheath to make several coils within the stomach. Teflon dilators are used to prepare for placement of a locking loop catheter, such as a Cope nephrostomy catheter.

Catheter introduction is greatly assisted by a central stiffener and a tapered tip to the catheter. Cope nephrostomy catheters ordinarily are 8 Fr to 12 Fr in diameter but can be ordered in larger sizes. Fluoroscopy (with oblique angulation to avoid exposing the operator's hands) is advisable because tenting of stomach wall can be observed about dilators and catheters as they are inserted. Gastric entry of tubes is appreciated by fluoroscopy, as the tenting "gives way." Also, with fluoroscopy one can recognize any buckling and intraperitoneal looping of the guidewire immediately. If, despite these precautions, small bowel or transverse colon has interposed itself, fluoroscopic monitoring may lead to early recognition of the situation before a larger catheter is inserted.

No sedation is usually needed, and most patients have minimal, if any, discomfort from the procedure. If there are complaints of pain, peritoneal irritation from looping of guidewire should be suspected. Percutaneous gastrostomy can usually be completed within 10 to 15 minutes of gastric insufflation. If stomach tenting prevents insertion of dilators or catheter, more air should be injected through the nasogastric tube.

Once the gastric tube is in place, it must be secured both internally (locking loop) and externally by suture to the patient's skin or to a stoma ring applied to the patient's skin. The nasogastric tube may be removed. The patient is kept at bedrest with frequent monitoring of vital signs, and the gastric tube should be maintained on low suction until the next morning. If no problems arise, feedings can be initiated by graduated instillation of first saline and later nutrient solutions. Tube changes should be avoided during the first 1 to 2 weeks in order to allow a fibrous tract to form around the catheter.[24] For the same reason, gastrostomy tubes should not be removed before 2 weeks have elapsed.

VARIATIONS

Percutaneous gastrostomy can be performed by trocar-loaded catheter, avoiding intermediate dilatation of the tract.[25] Large intragastric balloons have been devised to provide a target for needle or trocar,[26] but such special devices are largely unneeded. Gastrostomy catheters can be secured internally by balloons or "mushroom" devices, as well as by locking loops.

Sheaths generally are necessary for introduction of Foley catheters or other large, soft tubes.

Placement of a transgastric jejunal feeding tube at the time of gastrostomy requires more time, skill, and exposure to radiation.[15,16] A fundal loop of wire can be used to direct the guiding catheter toward the pylorus. A curved metal cannula can serve the same purpose. Unless the stomach is secured to anterior abdominal wall during these manipulations, there is danger of wire coiling in the peritoneum and loss of gastric access. This is particularly true if a fibrous tract has not yet formed. Coaxial manipulations through a large-bore gastrostomy balloon catheter help one avoid this danger.[27] Togglelike and nylon T-anchoring devices have been used to approximate anterior gastric wall to anterior abdominal (gastropexy), facilitating introduction of large catheters as well as the maneuvers needed for small bowel intubation.[28–30]

In the presence of complete esophageal obstruction, percutaneous gastrostomy may be performed without a nasogastric tube. Under fluoroscopic or computed tomographic guidance a 22-gauge needle can be advanced percutaneously into the collapsed stomach. When the tip is confirmed to be intragastric by injection of water-soluble contrast material, air is injected through the fine needle. After sufficient gastric distention, tube placement proceeds in the manner described.

COMPLICATIONS

Complications of varying degrees have been reported in 4% to 16% of patients, with about 3% needing surgical treatment.[13,15,16,31] In their review of major published series, Ho and Yeung found a procedure-related mortality of about 1%, primarily from peritonitis or hemorrhage.[31]

Transient peritoneal signs and mild fever may be seen in 5% to 10% of patients, but symptoms usually resolve within 1 to 2 more days of tube suction and use of intravenous antibiotics. Peritoneal air is to be expected and is of no concern unless the amount of pneumoperitoneum is increasing.[32] Despite early fears that lack of gastropexy would lead to internal leakage and diffuse peritonitis, such complications are quite rare. In fact, even accidental displacement or removal of catheters up to 12 Fr in size has not been associated with serious problems.[31] External leakage of gastric contents has complicated up to 7% of surgical gastrostomies,[33] and, although much less likely, it can also occur with percutaneous gastrostomy.[34]

Patients commonly have minor hematomas of the abdominal wall or gastric mucosa.[32] Major hemorrhage requiring transfusion arises in fewer than 1% of patients,[35] an incidence comparable to hemorrhage from surgical gastrostomy.[7,36]

Subcutaneous emphysema should alert one to improper tube positioning; the catheter should have external fixation for at least 2 weeks in addition to internal retention devices.[34] If a balloon-tip catheter is used, external fixation must be maintained to prevent distal migration. Displaced balloon catheters can cause pyloric or biliary obstruction.

Catheters placed on traction may produce erosion or ulceration of the stomach wall. Those patients with transgastric jejunal tubes should have positioning checked after any episodes of vomiting. If the tube has moved proximally, danger of aspiration is increased. Infectious complications are rare after percutaneous gastrostomy, most commonly minor skin infections that respond to local care alone.

A major cause of morbidity and mortality from the use of surgical gastrostomy for feeding is aspiration pneumonia,[18,37] and one can anticipate the same consequence for percutaneous techniques. The risk of aspiration in the *immediate* periprocedural period is minimized by radiologically guided percutaneous gastrostomy because heavy sedation or general anesthesia is not needed.[31] Nevertheless, if a patient gives any indication of gastroesophageal reflux, a transgastric jejunal tube must be placed.

GASTRIC OR SMALL BOWEL FEEDING?

Although small bowel alimentation may be safer, gastric feedings are preferable for patients not at risk for aspiration. Blenderized food is much less expensive than the liquid formulas needed for jejunal infusion. Moreover, jejunal feedings may cause diarrhea and electrolyte disturbances. Another consideration is the frequent plugging of long, smaller-bore catheters that greatly increases the need for tube changes.

Radionuclide gastric emptying studies are easily performed and can reproducibly detect gastroesophageal reflux. Olson and associates used such studies to determine which type of enteral tube should be placed in their patients and found that the long-term incidence of pneumonia was lower in the group with gastrostomy feedings than in those with small bowel feedings.[38] Risk of aspiration may also be related to the method of feeding. Bolus feeding into the stomach can substantially decrease lower esophageal sphincter tone, an effect not observed with continuous infusion of the same feeding solution at 80 ml/hour.[39] The quality of nursing care is undoubtedly a factor in preventing aspiration pneumonia. Mullan and colleagues reported that the lowest rates of aspiration occurred on intensive care wards (the rates were five times higher on general medical or surgical wards!) and aspiration risk did not correlate with the location of the feeding tube.[40] If gastric rather than jejunal feeding is chosen, it is recommended that low-rate infusions be given, with the patient's head elevated and with close monitoring of gastric residual fluid volumes.

COMPARISON OF GASTROSTOMY METHODS

Percutaneous gastrostomy is as safe as surgical tube placement, and prospective studies have documented that percutaneous endoscopic gastrostomy is considerably less expensive than surgical gastrostomy.[41] Although similar prospective comparisons with fluoroscopically guided gastrostomy are lacking, it can be assumed that the nonendoscopic procedure will result in even further cost savings.

Some endoscopic techniques insert the gastrostomy tube perorally, and thus the wound is exposed to the anaerobic flora of the mouth.[42] Prophylactic use of antibiotics does not change the incidence of catheter colonization but instead selects for resistant strains. It is noteworthy that a death from necrotizing fasciitis has resulted from endoscopic gastrostomy.[43] There have also been reports of implantation metastases from tubes inserted endoscopically in patients with head and neck malignancies.[44] Other potential problems presented by endoscopic techniques arise from the heavy sedation required, as well as tubes designed to be removed or replaced only by repeat endoscopy!

Endoscopic approaches are ineffective in the face of esophageal occlusion. Radiologic gastrostomy can be performed in such patients, it can proceed at bedside, and use of fluoroscopy can also prevent the small bowel or colon perforation seen after some endoscopic procedures.[45]

These considerations suggest that percutaneous gastrostomy under radiologic guidance should be the method of choice for creating a feeding enterostomy.

REFERENCES

1. Torosian MH, Rombeau JL: Feeding by tube enterostomy. *Surg Gynecol Obstet* 1980; 150:918–926.
2. Meguid MM, Eldar S, Wahba A: The delivery of nutritional support: A potpourri of new devices and methods. *Cancer* 1985; 55:S259–S289.
3. Heymsfield SB, Bethel RA, Ansley JD, et al: Enteral hyperalimentation: An alternative to central venous hyperalimentation. *Ann Intern Med* 1979; 90:63–71.
4. Padilla GV, Grant M, Wong H, et al: Subjective distresses of nasogastric tube feeding. *J Parenter Enter Nutr* 1979; 3:53–57.
5. Kumar SS: Tube gastrostomy: A routine adjunct in major abdominal operations. *Am Surg* 1985; 51:201–203.
6. Ruge J, Vasquez RM: An analysis of the advantages of Stamm and percutaneous endoscopic gastrostomy. *Surg Gynecol Obstet* 1986; 162:13–16.
7. Shellito PC, Malt RA: Tube gastrostomy: Techniques and complications. *Ann Surg* 1985; 201:180–185.
8. Jascalevich ME: Experimental trocar gastrostomy. *Surgery* 1967; 62:452–453.
9. Preshaw RM: A percutaneous method for inserting a feeding gastrostomy tube. *Surg Gynecol Obstet* 1981; 152:659–660.

10. Gauderer MWL, Ponsky JL: A simplified technique for constructing a tube feeding gastrostomy. *Surg Gynecol Obstet* 1981; 152:83–85.

11. Russell TR, Brotman M, Norris F: Percutaneous gastrostomy: A new simplified and cost-effective technique. *Am J Surg* 1984; 148:132–137.

12. Wills JS, Oglesby JT: Percutaneous gastrostomy. *Radiology* 1983; 149:449–453.

13. Wills JS, Oglesby JT: Percutaneous gastrostomy: Further experience. *Radiology* 1985; 154:71–74.

14. Tao HH, Gillies RR: Percutaneous feeding gastrostomy. *Am J Roentgenol* 1983; 141:793–794.

15. Ho CS, Gray RR, Goldfinger M, et al: Percutaneous gastrostomy for enteral feeding. *Radiology* 1985; 156:349–351.

16. Alzate GD, Coons HG, Elliott J, Carey PH: Percutaneous gastrostomy for jejunal feeding: A new technique. *Am J Roentgenol* 1986; 147:822–825.

17. Stuart SP, Tiley EH, Boland JP: Feeding gastrostomy: A critical review of its indications and mortality rate. *South Med J* 1993; 86:169–172.

18. Campbell-Taylor I, Fisher RH: The clinical case against tube feeding in palliative care of the elderly. *J Am Geriatr Soc* 1987; 35:1100–1104.

19. Gustke RF, Varma RR, Soergel KH: Gastric reflux during perfusion of the proximal small bowel. *Gastroenterology* 1970; 59:890–895.

20. Stevens SD, Picus D, Hicks ME, et al: Percutaneous gastrostomy and gastrojejunostomy after gastric surgery. *J Vasc Interv Radiol* 1992; 3:679–683.

21. Lee MJ, Saini S, Brink JA, et al: Malignant small bowel obstruction and ascites: Not a contraindication to percutaneous gastrostomy. *Clin Radiol* 1991; 44:332–334.

22. Mirich DR, Gray RR: Infracolic percutaneous gastrojejunostomy: Technical note. *Cardiovasc Intervent Radiol* 1990; 12:340–341.

23. Ignotus P, Gray R, Pugash R: Infracolonic percutaneous gastrojejunostomy. *Radiology* 1992; 183:583.

24. Johnston WD, Lopez MJ, Kraybill WG, Bricker EM: Experience with a modified Witzel gastrostomy without gastropexy. *Ann Surg* 1982; 195:692–699.

25. vanSonnenberg E, Wittich GR, Cabrera OA, et al: Percutaneous gastrostomy and gastroenterostomy: 2. Clinical experience. *Am J Roentgenol* 1986; 146:581–586.

26. vanSonnenberg E, Cubberley DA, Brown LK, et al: Percutaneous gastrostomy: Use of intragastric balloon support. *Radiology* 1984; 152:531–532.

27. Wojtowycz M: Coaxial tube system for transgastric jejunal feeding. *J Intervent Radiol* 1989; 4:46–48.

28. Brown AS, Mueller PR, Ferrucci JT Jr: Controlled percutaneous gastrostomy: Nylon T-fastener for fixation of the anterior gastric wall. *Radiology* 1986; 158:543–545.

29. Cope C: Suture anchor for visceral drainage. *Am J Roentgenol* 1986; 146:160–162.

30. Coleman CC, Coons HG, Cope C, et al: Percutaneous enterostomy with the Cope suture anchor. *Radiology* 1990; 174:889–891.

31. Ho CS, Yeung EY: Percutaneous gastrostomy and transgastric jejunostomy. *Am J Roentgenol* 1992; 158:251–257.

32. Wojtowycz M, Arata JA Jr, Micklos TJ, Miller FJ Jr: CT findings after uncomplicated percutaneous gastrostomy. *Am J Roentgenol* 1988; 151:307–309.

33. Wilkinson WA, Pickleman J: Feeding gastrostomy: A reappraisal. *Am Surg* 1982; 80:273–275.
34. Wojtowycz M, Arata JA Jr: Case report: Subcutaneous emphysema after percutaneous gastrostomy. *Am J Roentgenol* 1988; 151:311–312.
35. Rose DB, Wolman SL, Ho CS: Gastric hemorrhage complicating percutaneous transgastric jejunostomy. *Radiology* 1986; 161:835–836.
36. Wasiljew BK, Ujiki GT, Beal JM: Feeding gastrostomy: Complications and mortality. *Am J Surg* 1982; 143:194–195.
37. Swartzendruber FD, Laws HL: The superior feeding gastrostomy. *Am Surg* 1982; 80:276–278.
38. Olson DL, Krubsack AJ, Stewart ET: Percutaneous enteral alimentation: Gastrostomy versus gastrojejunostomy. *Radiology* 1993; 187:105–108.
39. Coben RM, Weintraub A, Dimarino AJ, Cohen S: Gastroesophageal reflux during gastrostomy feeding. *Gastroenterology* 1994; 106:13–18.
40. Mullan H, Roubenoff RA, Roubenoff R: Risk of pulmonary aspiration among patients receiving enteral nutrition support. *J Parenter Enter Nutr* 1992; 16:160–164.
41. Stiegmann G, Goff J, VanWay C, et al: Operative versus endoscopic gastrostomy: Preliminary results of a prospective randomized trial. *Am J Surg* 1988; 155:88–91.
42. Jonas SK, Neimark S, Panwalker AP: Effect of antibiotic prophylaxis in percutaneous endoscopic gastrostomy. *Am J Gastroenterol* 1985; 80:438–441.
43. Greif JM, Ragland JJ, Ochsner MG, Riding R: Fatal necrotizing fasciitis complicating percutaneous endoscopic gastrostomy. *Gastrointest Endosc* 1986; 32:292–294.
44. Laccourreye O, Chabardes E, Mérite-Drancy A, et al: Implantation metastasis following percutaneous endoscopic gastrostomy. *J Laryngol Otol* 1993; 107:946–949.
45. Bui HD, Dang CV, Schlater T, Nghiem CH: A new complication of percutaneous endoscopic gastrostomy. *Am J Gastroenterol* 1988; 83:448–451.

20

Biliary Interventions

KEY CONCEPTS

1. Percutaneous transhepatic cholangiography (PTHC) is an excellent method for examining biliary anatomy, but it has largely been superseded by cross-sectional imaging and endoscopic retrograde studies with contrast material.
2. Fine-needle PTHC is successful in nearly all patients with dilated ducts and in 70% to 80% of those without ductal dilatation.
3. Success of PTHC is proportional to the number of fine-needle passes made, but complications do not increase with up to a dozen attempts.
4. Broad-spectrum antibiotics should be started at least 1 hour before cholangiography or other biliary interventions.
5. Percutaneous biliary drainage (PBD) is used primarily to palliate unresectable malignant disease, but those patients with a very limited life expectancy or with otherwise asymptomatic jaundice should not be subjected to PBD.
6. Expandable biliary endoprostheses provide excellent palliation for patients with malignant biliary obstruction, but their role in the treatment of benign strictures has not been established.
7. Percutaneous cholecystostomy is used for diagnosis and treatment of acalculous (as well as calculous) cholecystitis in high-risk patients. Gallstones may later be removed through a dilated percutaneous tract.
8. A T tube tract must mature at least 5 to 7 weeks before it can be safely used to remove retained biliary stones. Choledochoscopy can assist stone removal and possible contact lithotripsy.

The era of nonsurgical intervention in the biliary tree began with the description of percutaneous biliary drainage (PBD) by Molnar and Stockum in 1974.[1] Transhepatic needle cholangiography had been performed for years prior to this, but therapeutic measures had remained outside the scope of radiologists. In the past 20 years the application of percutaneous measures has changed dramatically and continues to do so in the face of information gained by clinical trials, the development of endoscopy, and research on shock-wave and laser lithotripsy of gallstones.

Obstructive jaundice can now be diagnosed rapidly by ultrasonography, and the level and cause of obstruction are often evident. When full morphologic definition of the biliary tree is needed, retrograde opacification by way of endoscopic cannulation has become the first-line procedure. Percutaneous transhepatic cholangiography (PTHC) is now usually reserved for failed endoscopy or for patients with previous gastrointestinal surgery whose altered anatomy makes endoscopic examination difficult. It remains to be seen what effect magnetic resonance imaging (MRI) and helical computed tomographic cholangiography may have on the diagnosis of biliary disorders, but early work is promising.[2]

Although PBD was initially proposed as a routine preoperative measure for those with severe obstructive jaundice, its application in such patients has been limited by improvements in preoperative patient preparation, surgical technique, and endoscopic biliary drainage. It is now mainly employed as a palliative measure in patients with unresectable obstructing malignancies, but it continues to play a useful role in those with biliary obstruction and suppurative cholangitis, in postoperative or posttraumatic biliary leakage, and in selected patients with cholelithiasis. It is well suited for treating the complications of laparoscopic cholecystectomy.

One recent major advance has been the introduction of expandable biliary endoprostheses. Expandable stents have proved to be very useful in the palliation of malignant biliary obstruction.[3] Although most such obstructions can be stented endoscopically, the percutaneous route is an effective alternative.[4] The development of covered wire stents or removable self-expanding stents may allow the future application of these devices to the treatment of benign strictures.[5,6]

PATIENT PREPARATION

No matter what percutaneous intervention is planned (PTHC, PBD, stent insertion, percutaneous cholecystostomy), certain common principles apply. As a matter of course, the indications for the requested procedure are reviewed, the patient's medical history is obtained, and any previous studies are examined. Coagulation tests and hematocrit are ordered, if they are not already available. Medical anticoagulation must be stopped.

Impaired coagulation must be reversed by administration of vitamin K, platelets, or fresh frozen plasma, as needed. In the face of irreversible coagulopathy, ascites, or advanced cirrhosis, alternative diagnostic or therapeutic measures must be considered. When percutaneous intervention is deemed appropriate, the procedure and its indications, risks, and alternatives are explained to the patient, and consent is obtained.

Antibiotics

For needle cholangiography, PBD, and other manipulations in the biliary tree, patients take nothing by mouth for at least 8 hours, and broad-spectrum antibiotics should be started at *least 1 hour prior to* the procedure. Infected bile is present in about one third of all patients with obstruction from malignant disease and in more than two thirds of those with stones or benign strictures.[7-9] Previous biliary surgery predisposes to bacterial colonization. Despite the best of precautions, percutaneous biliary drains render bile colonized in virtually all cases by 2 to 3 weeks.[10,11] Simple tube cholangiography or mere tube changes can provoke life-threatening cholangitis and sepsis.[12,13] Antibiotics are therefore essential for adequate patient preparation!

One common antibiotic regimen is the combination of ampicillin and an aminoglycoside. *Escherichia coli* and *Klebsiella, Streptococcus,* and *Staphylococcus* species are commonly found at the time of biliary drainage, and coverage for gram-negative bacteria is necessary.[10] A single cephalosporin, such as cefazolin (1 g given intramuscularly or intravenously), may be used.[14] If acute cholangitis is present at the time of planned intervention, cefoperazone may be more appropriate because of its wider spectrum and its excretion in the bile.[14] Anaerobes are also commonly present in patients with acute cholangitis, making the addition of metronidazole or clindamycin advisable. Because of the number of *Enterococcus* species causing sepsis that Clark and colleagues noted in their review of their case material, they have recently altered their antibiotic prophylaxis regimen to include mezlocillin (4 g given intravenously).[9] In the presence of penicillin allergy, they use a combination of cefotetan 1 g and vancomycin 1 g or aztreonam 1 g, vancomycin 1 g, and metronidazole 500 mg. Because of the emergence of antibiotic resistance in many bacteria, periodic consultation with infectious disease specialists for specific recommendations is advised.

Anesthesia

A prerequisite for any percutaneous procedure is adequate anesthesia. Much of the pain produced from percutaneous biliary manipulations appears to be mediated primarily by intercostal somatic nerves.[15] Visceral neural receptors are implicated in acute nausea from distention of the bile ducts by injection of contrast medium or by the mechanical effects of wires and catheters, but they otherwise do not seem to contribute substantially to the pain from transhepatic procedures.

Generous local anesthesia with lidocaine and intravenous administration of benzodiazepines and opiates (such as midazolam and fentanyl) are usually sufficient for simple diagnostic fine-needle cholangiography. In some patients this combination of medications may allow the insertion of drainage catheters or dilatation of strictures without undue discomfort. However, many drainage procedures or extended manipulations can be quite painful, and other measures are called for.

For dilating and stenting benign biliary strictures, Lee and colleagues have routinely used general anesthesia, allowing what has usually been a multistage procedure to be accomplished in a single session.[16] Vogelzang and Nemcek have described several other alternatives, including intercostal nerve block and epidural anesthesia.[15] Pleural block is another anesthetic technique of demonstrated value in percutaneous biliary drainage.[17] Epidural anesthesia and pleural block are best administered and monitored by an anesthesiologist.

Intercostal Nerve Block

Intercostal block is performed after the approach for biliary drainage is chosen, with injection of a mixture of bupivacaine 0.75% and epinephrine 1:200,000 in the intercostal space being traversed, as well as in the intercostal spaces immediately cephalad and caudad.[15] Puncture is made with a 25-gauge needle adjacent to the inferior rib margin about 10 cm posterior to the catheter entry site. Approximately 5 ml of the local anesthetic is infiltrated about the neurovascular bundle, while intravascular injection is carefully avoided. Local effectiveness persists for 8 to 12 hours, and the nerve block procedure may be repeated later in the day and on succeeding days for residual pain.[15]

Pleural Block

Injection of bupivacaine 0.5% through an epidural needle or catheter into the right pleural space has been found quite effective in preventing pain from percutaneous biliary drainage. In the method described by Rosenblatt and associates, after administration of local anesthesia and with the patient in a left lateral decubitus position, an 18-gauge epidural needle is attached to a 5-ml air-filled glass syringe and the needle is advanced into the pleural space.[17] When the pleural space is entered, the resistance at the needle tip drops, and the plunger of the syringe falls. A total of 30 ml of bupivacaine is then injected. After instillation of the medication, the patient is turned to a right lateral decubitus position for 10 minutes.

The anesthetic diffuses through the parietal pleura to produce multiple intercostal nerve blocks. As with intercostal nerve block, pleural block effectiveness is checked by pinprick. When an epidural-type catheter is left in place, additional bupivacaine can be administered at any time. The anesthetic effect lasts 4 to 8 hours.[17] Because of the potential for toxicity (cardiac arrhythmia, hypotension, or seizures), an anesthesiologist should be present.

Epidural Anesthesia
An epidural catheter is placed in the mid-thoracic spine, and it may be left in place for hours to days. Injection of an opiate produces a sensory blockade, with relatively little effect on motor fibers. However, if the anesthetic level reaches higher than anticipated, respiratory arrest is a risk. Although it is expensive (on the order of $500), epidural anesthesia eliminates all but mild pain in more than 90% of patients.[18] It is recommended for particularly involved procedures, such as cannulation and dilatation of tight strictures or percutaneous removal of stones. Only a certified anesthesiologist should perform this technique.

PERCUTANEOUS TRANSHEPATIC CHOLANGIOGRAPHY

Indications
As noted earlier, PTHC is now often a procedure of last resort. When a contrast study of the biliary ducts is desired, it is more often accomplished endoscopically. However, one large category of patients for whom PTHC remains quite valuable is those with previous gastrointestinal surgery and endoscopically inaccessible bilioenteric anastomoses. Fine-needle cholangiography can uncover the cause of jaundice or other symptoms related to stones, benign strictures, malignant tumors, or parasitic infection. Also, PTHC is highly accurate in making the diagnosis of malignant obstruction, as well as for determining the resectability of hilar neoplasms.[19,20]

Technique
With the patient supine on a tilting table, fluoroscopy is used to examine the depth of the lateral costophrenic sulcus. A needle placed through the eighth intercostal space (or below) at the midaxillary line is unlikely to puncture lung in most patients, although punctures above the tenth rib traverse the pleural space.[21] The level chosen depends on individual factors, such as presence of obstructive lung disease and size of the liver. When the appropriate entry point is chosen, anesthesia is given. Any intravenous sedation should be carefully administered to avoid oversedation. Automatic blood pressure monitoring and pulse oximetry should be used routinely. The patient must be able to cooperate by suspending respiration as directed.

Although ultrasonic guidance is feasible, it is not routinely needed for diagnostic cholangiography, especially if intrahepatic ductal dilatation is present. Rather, fluoroscopy is used to observe advancement into the liver of the long (15-cm or 20-cm) 21-gauge needle. For practical purposes, aiming toward the pedicle of the twelfth thoracic vertebral body while staying in the midaxillary plane places the needle through hepatic parenchyma near the hilum. The needle is advanced in a smooth motion during suspended respiration until it nearly reaches midline. Advancement should be stopped if a course toward the diaphragm or toward other extra-hepatic structures is noted. When redirection or repeat puncture is required, the needle must be withdrawn to a point near the hepatic capsule without actually removing it from the liver.

With the needle in position, the stylet is removed, and a 20-ml syringe and connecting tubing filled with dilute water-soluble contrast medium are connected to the hub. Small, intermittent injections are then made through the needle as it is withdrawn a few millimeters at a time under continuous fluoroscopic observation. Radiation exposure is minimized by appropriate "tight" collimation. If parenchyma is injected, a small, irregular stain results. Different flow patterns are evident if the needle tip encounters hepatic artery or vein, portal vein, or lymphatic channels. The arteries and veins characteristically exhibit a rapid "washout" of the contrast agent. Injection of a bile duct, however, shows contrast material easily flowing from the needle tip to persistently fill branching tubular structures.

As soon as biliary filling is recognized, it is sometimes useful to measure biliary pressure or to allow 10 to 20 ml of bile to drain before further injection. However, if it appears that the needle position is precarious or if the intrahepatic ducts are not dilated, it is best to proceed directly with cholangiography. Full-strength (300 mg iodine or more/ml) contrast material is now injected, in order to maximize the opacification obtained while keeping the injected volume to a minimum. Undiluted contrast material is not used for needle placement because intense parenchymal staining from multiple passes may prevent recognition of ductal filling during a later needle pass.

Because of the risk of bacteremia and septic shock, only enough contrast material to establish the diagnosis should be injected. Spot films are exposed in multiple projections. Because iodinated contrast material is heavier than bile, gravity can be used to fill the common hepatic and common bile ducts. For this reason, a tilt table should always be used for PTHC. If the left hepatic ducts fill poorly, the patient may be placed prone to assist in opacification of these vessels.

If the gallbladder is inadvertently entered during needle placement, its contents should be aspirated as completely as possible. The needle can then be withdrawn and redirected. However, it is also possible to inject contrast medium to obtain a diagnostic cholecystogram and (if the cystic duct is unobstructed) a full cholangiogram. If this maneuver is elected, the gallbladder must again be drained before removal of the needle.

The success rate of PTHC can be anticipated to be between 95% and 100% in the presence of intrahepatic ductal dilation and from 67% to 80% in the absence of dilation.[22–24] Success is proportional to the number of needle passes made, and at least 12 to 15 passes are recommended before one abandons the procedure. Fortunately, such a number of passes is not accompanied by a higher complication rate, as long as 20-gauge or smaller needles are employed.

Findings
Stones
Stones appear as persistent filling defects on multiple films, usually distinguishable from air bubbles by their irregular or faceted shapes. The effects of gravity may be helpful in difficult cases, but it is not always possible to make the distinction. Blood clots, polypoid tumors, and biliary debris can also cause diagnostic problems. Unlike stones or air bubbles, polypoid tumors are fixed in location and show mural attachment in at least one projection.

Neoplasms
Most tumors affecting the biliary tree are not polypoid. They produce obstruction by ductal compression (as by hilar nodes or hepatic metastases) or infiltration. Typical of a pancreatic or biliary carcinoma is a short and irregular stricture, often producing a rat-tail appearance with gross dilation of the proximal ducts. Adenomas and other benign neoplasms are quite rare, and any tumor encountered should be considered malignant unless proved otherwise by histologic study.

Focal and Diffuse Strictures
Ampullary stenosis or inflammatory stricture from pancreatitis may be difficult to separate from malignant tumor, and endoscopic or percutaneous needle biopsy is indicated in such cases. Postoperative strictures tend to be longer and smoother than those of malignant neoplasms. Many such strictures are accompanied by ductal calculi.

Diffuse intrahepatic and extrahepatic stricture may represent advanced sclerosing cholangitis or infiltrating cholangiocarcinoma. Biopsy sampling of such lesions is also warranted, particularly because sclerosing cholangitis may be complicated by carcinoma.[25] When diffuse narrowing is found confined to the intrahepatic ducts, primary biliary cirrhosis also becomes a consideration.

Primary Sclerosing Cholangitis
Sclerosing cholangitis has been said to invariably involve the extrahepatic ducts, but cases have been described in which changes are confined with-

in the liver.[26,27] Most patients, however, have diffuse disease. Focal strictures tend to be short and alternate with normal-sized duct to produce
"beading." About half have "shaggy" mural irregularities, and ductal
bands and diverticula may be seen.[26] Although bands and diverticula have
been thought pathognomonic of primary sclerosing cholangitis, Gulliver
and colleagues have described them in patients with a variety of other
inflammatory or posttraumatic conditions.[28] Patients developing a superimposed cholangiocarcinoma commonly show marked and progressive
ductal dilation, progressive stricture, and intraductal masses.[25,29] Some of
these findings become evident only with time. Any patient with a history
of primary sclerosing cholangitis experiencing sudden clinical deterioration should be suspected to have malignancy.

Other Forms of Cholangitis
In acute suppurative cholangitis, the ducts are filled with debris, and there
may be abscesses of various size in communication with the ducts.
Chronic recurrent cholangitis tends to produce multiple branch strictures
with proximal areas of dilation often containing stones. There are similar
findings in those with Caroli's disease, congenital dilation of the intrahepatic ducts, which may be a variant of congenital hepatic fibrosis-polycys-
tic liver disease. Parasitic worms and flukes within the bile ducts appear as
linear defects on cholangiography.

Risks
Fine-needle transhepatic cholangiography is accompanied by a 3% rate of serious complications,[23] most due to sepsis or postprocedural bile leakage and
peritonitis. Major bleeding arises in only 0.3% of patients, and overall mortality has been reported as 0.2%.[23] Other hazards include vasovagal reactions and
pneumothorax. The risk of hypersensitivity reaction to contrast material is
always present, but low. Although multiple passes are not correlated with a
higher number of complications, the total amount of contrast medium injected
during needle passes should be watched carefully in patients with renal insufficiency. Use of 18-gauge sheath needles for diagnostic cholangiography
should be avoided, for the number of complications and the mortality risk
increase up to sixfold.[23] In patients with severely disturbed coagulation, transjugular needle cholangiography (using needles similar to those employed for
transjugular intrahepatic portosystemic shunt placement) should be considered.

PERCUTANEOUS BILIARY DRAINAGE

Indications and Cautions
Percutaneous biliary drainage is a primary palliation for patients with
unresectable malignant obstruction producing pruritus or infection. Some

forms of chemotherapy are contraindicated in the presence of jaundice, and drainage may be used to prepare for treatment in selected cases.[30] The procedure also provides a route of administration for internal radiation therapy.[31] With these specific exceptions, PBD should *not* be performed in those with otherwise asymptomatic jaundice because of the risks involved. Also, drainage must be avoided in those with diffuse hepatic metastases, liver failure, and a life expectancy measured in only days to weeks. Complication rates are considerably higher in such patients, canceling any potential benefits.[7] Other relative contraindications to PBD are the presence of significant ascites, advanced cirrhosis, and impaired coagulation. The first two conditions pose great technical difficulties for catheter introduction, and all three increase the possibility of serious complication.

Percutaneous drainage is the best nonoperative approach for treating postoperative strictures that cannot be cannulated endoscopically. Balloon dilatation and stent placement can follow drainage. The same holds true for patients suffering from primary sclerosing cholangitis, who may have focal strictures responsible for recurrent episodes of infection.[32] When the nature of a stricture is in doubt, the percutaneous tract provides access for brush, needle, or bioptome biopsy, if cytologic examination of collected bile is nondiagnostic.[33–35] Postoperative biloma with continuing leakage calls for percutaneous diversion of bile flow, in addition to drainage of the fluid collection itself.[36]

The role of PBD for the preoperative correction of jaundice has been debated from the onset. At present, available data indicate that PBD is *not* routinely indicated before biliary surgery, but it can be a helpful adjunct in certain situations (see the following section). Acute suppurative cholangitis is one such situation because emergency surgery carries a high mortality rate, and PBD can reliably stabilize patients with sepsis or shock.[37 39]

Advances in extracorporeal and contact lithotripsy and in solvent therapy have expanded the indications for percutaneous biliary catheter placement in selected patients with complicated stone disease.[40–42]

Preoperative Drainage

It had long been taught that severe obstructive jaundice poses high risks for surgery. Those with serum bilirubin levels above 10 mg/dl have suffered 15% to 25% surgical mortality and morbidity as high as 40% to 60%.[43] Jaundice, malignancy, and anemia have been demonstrated to be independent risk factors.[8] Moreover, glomerular filtration rate and renal function are adversely affected by jaundice, and the risk of postoperative renal failure is increased.[8,44]

In the late 1970s and early 1980s, multiple reports suggested improved surgical results with routine preoperative drainage.[45–47] However, these studies were in part skewed by selection consequent to PBD and cholangiography; patients found to be unresectable or dying during the preoperative period were excluded from subsequent surgery. Historical controls were misleading, so prospective and randomized studies were especially important. Hatfield and colleagues and Pitt and colleagues randomized 57 and 79 patients, respectively, either to PBD followed 11 to 12 days later by operation or to surgery alone.[43,48] Both groups found that when the complications of PBD were included in analysis, there was no clear benefit to preoperative drainage.

Although percutaneous drainage is no longer considered a routine preoperative measure, its benefit in the face of active cholangitis has already been mentioned. Huang and Ker treated 41 patients by PBD, including 10 in septic shock, without a single death.[39] Immediate surgery in such circumstances is associated with mortality of 15% to 64%.[39] In Klatskin tumors (cholangiocarcinoma involving the confluence of ducts), a percutaneously placed drain can guide surgical resection. There are limited well-controlled reports suggesting that routine preoperative biliary decompression by endoscopic means *can* decrease overall mortality and morbidity, by virtue of a lower complication rate from endoscopic drainage.[49,50] Problems with sepsis and bleeding are decreased, and the very low risk of tumor seeding of the transhepatic drainage tract is avoided.

A point needing emphasis is that preoperative cholangiography (whether percutaneous or endoscopic) can accurately predict which biliary tumors are unresectable.[19] Many patients found not to be candidates for curative surgery may be spared an operation, as long as a drainage catheter can be placed. Up to 90% of patients submitting to surgery for malignant obstructive jaundice are treated by palliative bilioenteric bypass alone when the true extent of tumor is appreciated.[19,46]

Palliative Drainage for Tumor
The established indications for nonsurgical palliative treatment of malignant neoplasms are in flux, with hepatic transplantation now being offered to some patients, and aggressive resection or drainage for even deeply infiltrating carcinomas to others. Some surgeons have railed against PTHC or PBD for hilar tumors, citing anecdotal evidence supporting peripheral bilioenteric surgical drainage.[51] Lacking in their appraisal is any unbiased statement of the short-term and long-term problems with such operations.[12] In fact, a combined percutaneous transhepatic-endoscopic-laparoscopic technique has been devised for forming a left biliogastric anastomosis, which may avoid the morbidity and mortality of standard peripheral bilioenteric surgery.[52] At Johns Hopkins, surgical placement of large stenting catheters for hilar tumors is preferred for those patients who are able to undergo palliative surgery.[53] Even so, they have found prior PBD extremely helpful for guiding operative dissection.

Despite recent changes in approach, there remain patients suffering debilitating pruritus or infectious complications of biliary obstruction who are not considered suitable for surgical palliation. Among factors to be considered before choosing PBD are whether the risks of drainage outweigh the likely palliation, the ability of the patient or those supplying chronic care to deal adequately with an internal-external catheter, and the patient's psychological capacity to adjust to such a tube. An endoprosthesis may be an alternative for those experiencing problems with tube acceptance and care, and the advent of expanding metallic stents has decreased the need for repeated interventions for stent obstruction (see the section entitled Endoprostheses later in this chapter). Percutaneous drainage may be used alone or in collaboration with endoscopy when endoscopic methods fail, or it may be the initial intervention for hilar tumors.[54–56]

When PBD is used for palliation, problems with catheter plugging, displacement, external bile leakage, and cholangitis are to be anticipated. By the nature of the patients being treated, complications and early mortality are higher. Hilar tumors often cause separate obstruction of right and left hepatic ducts. Although drainage of only one side may reverse jaundice, undrained segments are likely to become infected, and bilateral drainage is recommended.[55,57] Slow-growing tumors, such as cholangiocarcinoma, may require multiple tube changes over the course of months to years, and plastic endoprostheses are best avoided in such cases.

Technique
Patient preparation with antibiotics and local, epidural, or other regional anesthesia is identical to that described for PTHC. Fine-needle cholangiography is performed in a standard fashion, but whenever PBD is planned, greater care should be taken to avoid traversing the pleural space. When a catheter is placed above the tenth rib at the midaxillary line, the pleural space is almost invariably crossed.[21] If a catheter can be directed into the liver from a lower approach, uncommon but very serious pleural complications may be prevented. However, when the diaphragm is elevated or if the liver is small, crossing the right pleural reflection may be unavoidable.

Catheter Introduction Using a Fine Needle
In many cases the position of the cholangiographic needle may be suitable for placement of a fine mandril wire into the biliary system. The wire directs an exchange dilator mounted on a stiffening cannula into the ducts. The dilator and stiffener are advanced over the wire until the point of ductal entry is reached. The wire and cannula are then held stationary as the dilator is passed well into a major duct. A heavy-duty 0.035- or 0.038-inch guidewire is then used for further manipulations. Several coaxial introducers that permit a second guidewire to be passed through an endhole sheath

are available from various manufacturers. When the Cope catheter introduction system is used, the larger wire must exit a sidehole near the tip of the dilator, and a J-tip guidewire is required for this maneuver. If the wire supplied with this kit does not exit the sidehole, a 1.5-mm J Rosen wire is recommended.

If the cholangiogram needle enters a left-sided bile duct, makes an acute or awkward angle of entry, enters very near the point of obstruction, or has engaged an extrahepatic duct, it should *not* be used for drain placement. Instead, the needle should be left in place and contrast medium injected to direct a second needle toward a more appropriate spot. Should the gallbladder be inadvertently entered, contrast material may be injected for opacification of intrahepatic bile ducts to guide conventional percutaneous transhepatic catheter placement.[58] The best method for directing a needle toward an opacified duct is to use a fluoroscopic C-arm to superimpose the needle perfectly (looking "down the barrel") upon the target. The C-arm is then rotated 90°, and the needle advanced to the proper depth. With fluoroscopy one can often observe the duct move or recoil when entered by the needle.

Sheath Needles
A 5 Fr Teflon sheath needle can be used for biliary access instead of the 21-gauge needle in the technique just described. It has the advantage of allowing immediate placement of a heavy guidewire without dilator exchanges. A larger needle can also be more easily directed toward an opacified duct. In a hard, cirrhotic liver, a sheath needle may be the only alternative for successful percutaneous drainage. However, a larger needle increases the risk for significant bleeding or bile leakage, and its routine use is not recommended.

Passage of the Obstruction
Once a duct has been securely cannulated, the obstruction may be gently probed with a straight or curved-tip catheter and soft-tipped guidewire (Fig. 20-1). Steerable wires or "slippery" wires with a hydrophilic polymer coating are especially useful for passing obstructions. The lumen can usually be engaged in even extremely tight lesions. However, if the patient has long-standing distal common bile duct obstruction and the extrahepatic duct is markedly dilated, both wire and catheter may merely curl within the obstructed duct. For these patients a repeat attempt to pass the obstructing lesion frequently succeeds after several days of external drainage of bile.

When a guidewire passes through the common bile duct and into the duodenum, a straight-tapered 5 or 6 Fr catheter should be passed over it, well beyond the lesion. The initial guidewire is then replaced with a heavier one, such as an Amplatz Super-Stiff or Coons wire. Teflon dilators are advanced through the transhepatic tract and stricture or tumor. In very tight

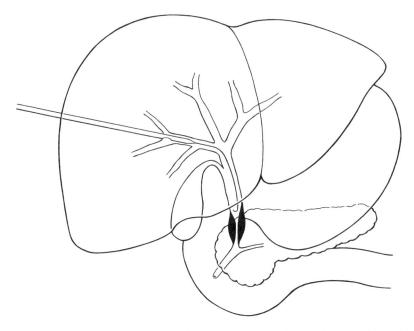

Fig. 20-1 Transhepatic catheter placement into a right intrahepatic duct with guidewire advancement to the point of distal common bile duct obstruction. (Modified from Cope C, Burke DR, Meranze S: *Atlas of interventional radiology.* Philadelphia, Mosby–Year Book, 1989; with permission.)

lesions, a tapered van Andel catheter may be introduced and then replaced with a balloon catheter for dilatation. Pigtail-tip, 8 to 10 Fr Teflon multi-sidehole catheters, such as the Ring biliary catheter, are easier to introduce at the time of initial passage. Sideholes should be present both proximal to the obstruction and distally within duodenum. There should be no side-holes in hepatic parenchyma. After the tract has been allowed to dilate and mature around this catheter for several days, a larger and softer tube can be introduced. Soft catheters are prone to "accordion" when they are advanced against heavy resistance.

Internal Drainage
Passage beyond the tumor or stenosis is desirable for several reasons. First, internal drainage of bile is made possible, eliminating the need for the patient to wear a bile bag, while preserving the enterohepatic circulation of bile salts and digestive physiology. However, if catheter passage is not possible, it is not normally necessary to replace bile salts orally. What is needed is fluid replacement, should the patient experience biliorrhea while on external drainage.

A catheter placed into duodenum is also less likely to be inadvertently displaced or removed than one with its tip in the biliary tree. A final advantage of internal drainage is that the full extent of an obstructing tumor is better appreciated by injection of a catheter traversing it.

Securing and Caring for the Catheter

Proper securing of the catheter is a critical step in percutaneous biliary drainage. Catheter displacement can be fatal![59,60] Not only is emergency replacement mandatory but also it is frequently more difficult than the initial procedure. Introduction of a wire through the tract is rarely successful after the drain has been removed, and the bile ducts are decompressed by free leakage into the peritoneum or pleural space. For this reason catheters are best secured both internally and externally.

Internal fixation is provided by a loop-retaining suture in a Cope drainage catheter. The loop does not allow withdrawal unless the suture is released, cut, or broken. Other catheter designs allowing positive retention are also available. Surgeons should be aware of the self-retaining nature of the drain, for forced intraoperative removal has been known to produce hepatic laceration and fatal hemorrhage.[61] For external fixation, two sutures are placed at the catheter entry site. An alternative to skin sutures is placement of an adhesive stoma ring over the site, with several sutures securing the catheter to the plastic ring.[62] Wrapping a 6- to 8-cm length of cloth adhesive tape about a (meticulously dried) segment of the catheter, forming projecting tags or wings with the tape, allows sutures to be passed through the tape and looped about the catheter multiple times. This procedure makes catheter crimping, constriction, and other accidental injury less likely. Additional adhesive, such as a methyl methacrylate glue, prevents the tape from slipping when wet. Finally, a gauze dressing is placed over the skin entry site.

After initial catheter placement, drainage is best left to an external bag for at least a few days, even if the obstruction has been passed. Catheter output must be carefully monitored, and any fluid loss over 500 ml in 24 hours must be replaced with intravenous electrolytes. External drainage assures biliary decompression and resolution of any cholangitis, while tube patency is continually confirmed by maintained output. After several days, an internal-external catheter may be capped for internal drainage as long as the patient is afebrile, the bile is clear and free of major debris, and there are no major abdominal symptoms to confuse clinical assessment of catheter-related problems.

A PBD catheter should be flushed daily with 5 to 10 ml of sterile saline. The patient or home care provider must be instructed in clean technique and provided materials for this routine. A phone number arranging for emergency attention for any catheter-related problems should be given to the patient before hospital discharge. Routine catheter changes are scheduled as an outpatient procedure at 4- to 6-week intervals. Patients may be prescribed oral antibiotics to be started 1 day before routine tube changes.

Problems to Watch For
As already mentioned, the catheter must be firmly secured to prevent displacement. Hemobilia often is noted in the first days after PBD, but clots in the bile ducts lyse without intervention, as long as the catheter is maintained patent by regular flushing and drains externally. If hemobilia persists or recurs, catheter position must be checked to ensure that a sidehole is not located in parenchyma. Major bleeding is sometimes tamponaded by exchange for a larger catheter, but if it is refractory to conservative measures, arteriography is indicated. Mitchell and associates found severe hemobilia complicating 3% of percutaneous biliary drainages, and they were able to control most by catheter embolization of the affected vessel (see Chapter 12 entitled Embolotherapy).[63] Arteriovenous fistulas and pseudoaneurysms are not rare after PBD, but they do not usually produce symptoms.

In the first days after drainage, a small number of patients experience biliorrhea, daily output of 1 to 8 L. This is especially dangerous if it is not recognized early and fluid replacement falls short. Improper management has led to dehydration, renal failure, and death.[48,59] Biliorrhea may resolve with conversion to internal biliary drainage.[64]

Patients showing signs of cholangitis should have their tubes opened to an external bag. If there is adequate flow of clear bile, a tube cholangiogram and ultrasound are indicated to uncover any segmental biliary blockage or hepatic abscess. Such lesions need separate drainage, except for the case of multiple segmental blocks in a patient suffering the terminal throes of cancer.

Leakage of bile or fluid from the skin entry site can present recurrent difficulties. If the patient has substantial ascites, leakage may be irremediable, and a stoma device and collection bag may need to be placed about the catheter. If bile leaks back along the catheter, tube patency must be checked. Placement of a larger catheter sometimes resolves the problem. Another option may be placement of an expanding metal stent. However, certain patients have increased duodenal pressure leading to functional biliary obstruction or back-drainage of enteric contents. In such cases specially modified longer tubes with distal sideholes confined to the tip (placed beyond the gastroduodenal ligament and into jejunum) may be tried.[65] Prior gastrointestinal surgery seems to predispose to duodenal pressure elevation.[59]

Left-sided and Bilateral Drainage
Percutaneous drainage through the left lobe is indicated in the presence of separate ductal obstruction. However, there are advantages to a left-sided

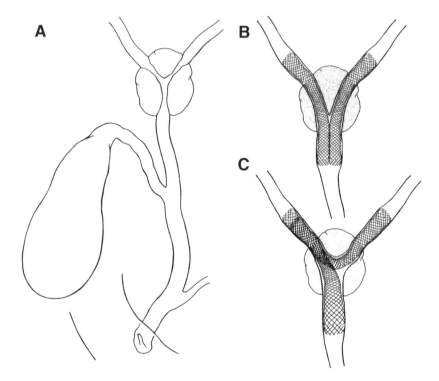

Fig. 20-2 **A,** Tumor at the liver hilum obstructing both right and left hepatic ducts. **B,** Side-by-side placement of Wallstent. **C,** Y-configuration of Wallstents, one passing through the wall of the other to bridge the two sides.

approach, even for distal biliary obstructions. Subxiphoid catheter placement avoids the pleural space and its attendant risks. The left-sided approach is often less painful. In hilar obstructions, the left lobe drainage is more likely to remain intact because the main left hepatic duct is longer than its counterpart on the right. For drainage to succeed, the left lobe must be of sufficient size, it must be accessible, and at least 10 cm of dilated duct should be present.[15] The left ducts may be opacified by placing a fine needle from the right side in the standard fashion, or ultrasound may be used to direct subxiphoid needle placement.

Patients suffering hilar ductal obstruction may need bilateral percutaneous drainage. This generally means separate entry sites, but one may be able to pass a catheter across an obstructed ductal confluence, from right lobe to left, or vice versa. If this is possible, I have found that a coaxial tube arrangement—with a central 7 Fr catheter passing through a custom-cut sidehole to the opposite duct and with the larger 12 Fr outer catheter passing into duodenum in a conventional course—provides acceptable drainage.

An O-ring and Y-adaptor allow each tube to be flushed separately. A more workable alternative at present is insertion of Wallstents in a Y configuration, one passing down the common bile duct and the other placed through its wall across the hilum into the contralateral duct (see Fig. 20-2).[66]

Risks of Percutaneous Biliary Drainage

Among the possible complications of PBD are tube obstruction, displacement, cholangitis, sepsis, bile peritonitis, hemobilia or other bleeding. If the pleural space is crossed, patients are at risk for pneumothorax, malignant effusion, and a biliopleural or biliobronchial fistula.[67] Serum amylase elevation has been noted in up to 9% of patients, but clinical pancreatitis is, fortunately, rare.[63] Even so, tube-induced pancreatitis can be severe and fatal.[61,68] Tumor seeding of the drainage tract has been an uncommon problem, complicating fewer than 1% of drainages, but in individual patients it can produce serious morbidity.[69,70] As already mentioned, unusually high flow of externally draining bile can precipitate dehydration, hypotension, and renal failure.[48] Average tube output from a completely obstructed biliary system is under 600 ml/day.[45] Any volume exceeding this amount should be replaced with intravenous electrolytes. In properly selected patients, more than 80% respond to drainage with a significant drop in serum bilirubin, and at least a 50% decrease in bilirubin is to be expected within 10 days.[57] However, supervening liver failure negates any benefits of PBD.

Quoted incidence of complications and mortality from PBD varies widely, but it is clear that the risks of the procedure are substantially higher in malignant disease.[7,13,71] Whereas 30-day mortality in those treated with palliative drainage for cancer ranges from 22% to 43%, many series have reported no deaths when PBD was done for benign obstruction.[7,11,45,71–73] Deaths directly attributable to percutaneous drainage have been cited in 0.7% to 4% of patients.* In one review of more than 600 procedures performed at a single institution, operative intervention for a complication of PBD was necessary in 1.5%.[61]

Taking both early and late complications into account, their incidence in patients with malignant tumors may be as high as 54% to 69%, mostly from minor and severe episodes of cholangitis.[7,13,69] Still, this is several times the incidence of cholangitis in patients with benign strictures or stones. The difference may seem paradoxic in that at the time of drainage, bacteria are more often cultured from the bile of those with benign lesions than from patients with carcinomas. However, external biliary catheters become uniformly colonized within several weeks, and patients with malignant tumors often have impaired immunologic function. Curiously,

---

*References 7, 38, 57, 61, 69, 71, 72.

Carrasco and colleagues have reported more problems with cholangitis in those patients whose catheters were kept closed to internal drainage than in those on external drainage.[59]

In order to put the complications of patients with PBD for malignant disease in perspective, those of surgical intervention must be taken into account. A review by Lai and colleagues of 97 patients with proximal biliary carcinoma showed that nearly 80% were grossly unresectable at operation.[74] Of all patients treated surgically, 26% did not survive their initial hospitalization, and the incidence of postoperative cholangitis varied from 15% to 37%, depending on the procedure performed. Morbidity and mortality were considerably higher for patients undergoing hepatic resection. Excluding hospital deaths, mean patient survival was slightly longer than 1 year. Palliative surgical intubation, without any attempt at resection, is recommended for those with tumor found unresectable at surgery.[74]

RELATED BILIARY INTERVENTIONS

Once percutaneous access to the biliary ducts could be established, it was not long before methods were developed for treating stones, strictures, and malignancy, as well as for obtaining additional diagnostic information through biopsies and perfusion studies.

Endoprostheses

Endoprostheses are designed to provide completely internal stenting of biliary strictures. They are most frequently applied in terminal palliative care. Because of the potential for stent occlusion over the long term, they are not indicated for benign strictures unless they can be exchanged endoscopically. The advantages of endoprostheses include absence of an external tube or drainage bag (an overriding psychological factor in some patients), avoidance of entry site pain and bile leakage, and perhaps some protection against recurrent cholangitis. Internal stents should be placed only if serum bilirubin levels fall substantially after PBD. Percutaneous drainage and stenting should be reserved for patients in whom endoscopic cannulation has failed or is not possible.

Plastic Stents

Although Szabo and associates did not observe any significant difference in the incidence of cholangitis between those with plastic biliary endoprostheses and those with internal-external drains (33% and 38%, respectively), they did find that episodes arose much later after placement (at a mean of 4 months versus 6 weeks for conventional percutaneous tubes).[75] In the case of high common bile duct obstruction, suprapapillary placement of the distal tip has been advocated as a means of decreasing the risk of cholangitis. However, a protective effect has not been observed universally by those investigators leaving endoprostheses completely above the sphincter of Oddi.[76]

Tube patency can be related to diameter, and larger stents may be placed percutaneously than can be placed by unaided endoscopy. Nonexpanding stents up to 14 Fr in size can be introduced percutaneously, but this requires at least several days for tract maturation, followed by serial dilations of the tract, a procedure that can be quite painful. Endoscopic stenting is generally limited to introduction of catheters no larger than 10 Fr, but Kerlan and colleagues have described a combined percutaneous-endoscopic technique allowing peroral placement of large-bore stents in a single session.[77] By grasping a long guidewire placed percutaneously into the duodenum, an endoscope operator pulls the wire back through the mouth. The large stent and a pusher are loaded on from above, while a balloon catheter helps pull the stent into its final position.

Overall, percutaneous stent placement succeeds in more than 90% of patients for whom it is attempted.[78,79] Tubes 12 Fr or larger are usually patent at least 6 months.[30] Reported rates of obstruction have varied from 1% to 23%.[78–80] Still, one of the great disadvantages of internal stents is that their replacement requires de novo percutaneous biliary drainage or endoscopy. Endoprosthesis occlusion does not necessarily mean that replacement is warranted. With renewed percutaneous access, a brush or dilator passed into the tube may reopen it, allowing months of subsequent effective drainage.[81]

Whenever a stent is placed, whether solely percutaneously or combined with endoscopy, a drainage catheter should be left above it for several days to ensure that blood or debris does not immediately occlude the endoprosthesis. A "safety" wire, a second guidewire within the biliary ducts, is advised for secure performance of the maneuvers necessary for stent insertion. A coaxial Lieberman sheath is advanced over the first wire, the inner dilator removed, and the second wire placed alongside the first before further manipulations are undertaken. If bilateral endoprostheses are desired for high biliary obstruction, both stents must be placed simultaneously. Otherwise, insertion of the second may displace the first!

Numerous different endoprosthesis designs have been tried. Some are straight catheters with a tapered leading end, as well as a trailing retaining suture and plastic "button" to be affixed subcutaneously.[80] Others have Mallecot "mushrooms," barbs, or other internal fixation strategies. Some are meant to remain completely above the papillary sphincter. In one review of 100 patients treated with plastic stents of various types, Dick and colleagues observed stent occlusion in 12%, usually about 6 to 7 months after placement.[82] Some have found the combination of ursodeoxycholic acid and antibiotics helpful in prolonging stent patency.[83]

Problems with migration have been described in 3% to 16%, depending on the type of endoprosthesis placed and the experience of the radiologist.[76,78–80] If migration occurs early, it may be remedied by use of a deflecting wire or balloon catheter.[80] When a balloon catheter is used to reposition or remove an endoprosthesis, the balloon is passed into the lumen of the device and inflated until the balloon catheter and stent move securely as a unit. Other uncommon complications of biliary stent placement (plastic or metal) have included acute cholecystitis and duodenal ulceration.

Expandable Metal Stents
Expandable stents are used in the palliation of malignant biliary obstruction. They should not be inserted into patients for whom surgical resection or biliary bypass procedures are contemplated, for after a matter of days the presently available metallic stents become embedded and cannot be removed from the duct. The application of metallic stents in benign biliary disease is controversial and subject to cautious study (see discussion later in this section). At present, it is recommended that metal stents not be employed for benign obstruction, except in unusual and difficult circumstances.

Although several different stents are available, the greatest experience has been reported for the self-expanding Wallstent. It is easily placed through a standard percutaneous transhepatic tract. The obstruction is passed in a conventional manner. The lesion can then be dilated with a balloon, or the Wallstent may be inserted directly by advancing the introducer sheath through the obstruction. When the carrier catheter and stent are positioned appropriately, the introducer sheath is withdrawn. The stent is then deployed according to the manufacturer's instructions. Expansion may be assisted by balloon inflation, or the stent may be allowed to open on its own, generally reaching its full diameter within 1 or 2 days. Stent deployment is aided by the use of an 8 Fr sheath with a sideport permitting injection of contrast medium to define the level of obstruction precisely. Usually Wallstent insertion follows PBD by several days, but in the absence of infection or other complications, percutaneous drainage and stenting may be performed in a single session.[84]

In one randomized study comparing 10-mm diameter Wallstents with 10 Fr polyethylene stents introduced endoscopically in patients with malignant obstruction, the median length of time to stent occlusion was significantly better in the group treated with Wallstents (9 months versus 4 months).[3] In a large retrospective comparison, Adam found a substantial drop in the need for later intervention in the Wallstent group (13% versus 43%).[85] Occlusion within 3 to 5 months was encountered in only 5% in another report.[4] Migration has not been a problem with these devices. Nevertheless, in none of these cited reports did use of an expandable endoprosthesis prolong overall survival.

When reobstruction does arise, it is more commonly caused by tumor overgrowth of the ends of the stent, rather than growth through the stent mesh or stent encrustation by biliary sludge.[86] Not only must the stent placed provide adequate coverage of the tumor but also severe angulation must be avoided; otherwise, kinking and obstruction result.[3] When stent occlusion arises, it can be relieved either with coaxial placement of a plastic endoprosthesis or with another expandable stent.

Metallic stents have been placed into patients with postoperative or other benign biliary strictures who are not candidates for surgical correction and who fail to respond to repeated balloon dilatation and prolonged internal-external stenting. Longer-term palliation has been achieved in small series of such cases, but obstruction from tissue ingrowth is common.[87,88] The Rösch-Gianturco Z stent has been employed more often for cases of benign stricture; it has fewer struts than the Wallstent and may elicit less of an epithelial response, and tumor growth through the interstices is not an issue. Unfortunately, Rösch-Gianturco stents have been observed to encrust and "turn to stone" after placement in benign disease (Kozarek RA, personal communication). Short (34 mm) Wallstents have been placed in cases of common bile duct stricture caused by chronic pancreatitis with a patency rate of 90% at nearly 3 years follow-up.[89] The length of the stent was kept to a minimum in order not to interfere with any possible biliary surgery in the future.

The major obstacle to wider application is that metallic stent insertion is practically an irreversible act, undesirable for the treatment of benign disease. Preliminary work has been done with silicone-coated Wallstents.[5] They do not become buried in ductal wall, but there have been technical problems with controlled placement. Another promising development is a flat coil spring stent made from a nickel-titanium alloy (nitinol). Stents of this design have been easily removed even several months after insertion.[6]

The application of internal stents, whether expandable or plastic, depends on patient and physician preference, as well as the expected life span of the patient. For unresectable pancreatic tumors, stents usually remain open for the patient's remaining few months. However, for slow-growing tumors, such as cholangiocarcinoma, it may be best to maintain external access and regularly change an internal-external drain. As of yet, there is no good alternative for the treatment of recurrent posttraumatic or inflammatory strictures.

Biliary Cytology and Biopsy Procedures

When a biliary obstruction appears malignant but no diagnosis has been established, the percutaneous tract can be used for cytologic or histologic confirmation. Bile collected from an external drainage bag is more likely to yield positive cytology than fluid obtained at PTHC alone.[54] Cytologic study is positive in roughly 50% of patients with cholangiocarcinoma, although reported sensitivity varies widely.[19,54,90] The positive cytology rate is lower with pancreatic primary tumors.[57]

As with other diagnostic biopsy procedures, persistence produces greater accuracy. If cytologic examination is negative, percutaneous needle biopsy can be guided by tube cholangiography. Alternative approaches include brush, forceps, bioptome, or needle biopsy through a transhepatic sheath.[34,35] Repeated biopsies by various methods can attain a sensitivity of 92% for biliary carcinoma and 73% for pancreatic carcinoma.[33]

Internal Irradiation of Biliary Neoplasms

Percutaneous biliary drainage provides a route for placement of radioisotopes within or adjacent to an obstructing tumor. Very high doses of local radiation can be administered by means of iridium-192 seeds with little exposure of liver beyond the neoplasm. Survival of patients with cholangiocarcinoma has been extended to a mean of 17 months from diagnosis, compared to 3 months for patients with untreated tumors.[31] These data are rather difficult to interpret because the simple act of palliative drainage can produce similar prolongation of survival. Also, patients treated with internal radiotherapy are subject to episodes of severe cholangitis, periductal abscess, and hemobilia.[91] A potential alternative to ionizing radiation for such tumors is the application of directed laser energy, a treatment deserving further investigation.[92]

Percutaneous Cholecystostomy

Percutaneous cholecystostomy is a means of treating patients with acute cholecystitis who present with high surgical risk. Needle puncture is directed by ultrasonography, and liver parenchyma should be traversed in order to enter the gallbladder at its hepatic attachment. An 8 Fr self-retaining catheter is then placed over a guidewire after suitable tract dilatation. Acute inflammation is safely resolved by this technique in well over 90%.[58,93–95] Acalculous cholecystitis, which often arises in critically ill patients, can be effectively managed. Percutaneous cholecystostomy can even be achieved at the patient's bedside when needed. Catheters are removed after symptoms have resolved and the cystic duct is found to be unobstructed. All bile is aspirated from the gallbladder before catheter removal. When stones are present, various means for their removal can be applied through the tract (see the section entitled Biliary Stones later in this chapter), although stone removal is not absolutely necessary in the absence of persistent symptoms.

A limitation of percutaneous cholecystostomy is that gallbladder necrosis cannot be recognized, except by failure of prompt improvement in the patient's clinical status.[58] Van Sonnenberg and colleagues reported a high incidence of severe vasovagal reactions during gallbladder drainage[96]; however, other investigators have not found this to be a problem. Accidental early removal of a catheter has led to fatal peritonitis in one reported case.[97]

Verbanck and associates have treated critically ill patients with presumed acute cholecystitis by simple transhepatic needle puncture and aspiration.[98] They insert a large (14-gauge) needle to completely aspirate the gallbladder contents and then rinse the gallbladder 15 to 30 times with saline until returned fluid is completely clear. Broad-spectrum antibiotics are injected before the needle is removed. The fluid obtained is sent for cytologic and microbiologic studies. Fifteen of 16 patients treated in this fashion had confirmation of cholecystitis on Gram stain and culture. In three cases the systemic antibiotics being given were changed as a result. All but one patient recovered, and no late complications were observed.

Gallbladder puncture and tube placement can serve as an alternative to transhepatic PBD in selected patients, as long as the cystic duct is patent.[99] Even if drainage is not planned by this route, contrast medium injection into the gallbladder (after initial evacuation of bile) often provides excellent opacification of intrahepatic and extrahepatic ducts. A conventional transhepatic drain can subsequently be placed under fluoroscopic guidance.

PERCUTANEOUS INTERVENTION IN BENIGN BILIARY DISEASE

Aside from cases of acute suppurative cholangitis, PBD is not normally indicated for patients with benign disease. There are exceptions, and each case must be assessed individually. Percutaneous access is invaluable in cases of retained common bile duct stones after cholecystectomy. Stones may be removed through a T tube tract if they do not pass through an endoscopic sphincterotomy. Postoperative biliary strictures or fistulae can be treated nonoperatively by dilation or intubation. Sclerosing cholangitis presents its own set of chronic and recurrent challenges that may be addressed percutaneously. We have successfully dilated strictures and removed stones in patients with hepatic transplants, a whole new population for whom percutaneous methods are preferable to reoperation.[100] Beyond this, the place of nonsurgical stone removal, in any or all of its novel manifestations, remains to be established. Percutaneous access clearly does play an important adjunct role for a selected few.

Strictures

There is no strict consensus on which benign strictures should undergo balloon dilatation. When strictures are dilated, there is no standard on the number of balloon dilatations, the duration of balloon inflation, or the duration of postprocedural stenting. Kozicki and colleagues have surgically repaired 85 patients with bile duct injury and obstruction; at a mean follow-up of more than 12 years, only 9 patients developed recurrent stricture.[101] Because most common duct strictures are iatrogenic and respond to operative repair, percutaneous methods should be reserved for those with contraindications to surgery or failed repeat operation. A review of 35 years of experience in treating benign biliary strictures at UCLA has shown that PBD (with or without stricture dilatation) has helped improve overall clinical results by guiding, and sometimes replacing, surgical reconstruction.[102]

The response of any individual lesion is difficult to predict. Choledochoenteric anastomotic strictures have shown the best results in most series.[30,102,103] This has not held true for others.[104] Nevertheless, it is evident that focal lesions in primary sclerosing cholangitis are more likely to recur (see the section on Interventions in Sclerosing Cholangitis later in this chapter). Balloon size should match that expected for a normal duct. Although very long and repeated inflations (up to an hour at a time) have been used, immediate success can be expected with shorter-duration inflations in most lesions.[104,105] Very tough strictures may need passage of coaxial Teflon dilators to 12 or 14 Fr. Stents are left across treated lesions from weeks to months; a minimum of 3 months is recommended by some.[102] Bret and colleagues advocate soft silicone stents up to 18 Fr in size.[106]

Success of balloon dilatation for benign strictures is about 70% at 1 to 2 years of follow-up.[104,107] Longer-term follow-up is essential because surgical experience has shown that strictures can recur many years after treatment.[101] The utility of metallic endoprostheses in benign disease is as yet unproved and controversial (see the section on Expandable Metal Stents earlier in this chapter).

Biliary Strictures in Transplanted Livers

Biliary complications are a common cause of morbidity in liver transplant recipients. From 10% to 14% of patients develop biliary strictures, generally within the first year after transplantation.[108–110] Many of these strictures are hilar; although fewer than half are associated with hepatic artery thrombosis or stenosis, they are thought to result from ischemic injury during or after surgery.[108] Balloon dilatation and long-term stenting may serve as temporizing measures, but most hilar strictures return. We have observed recurrence as late as 30 months after treatment. One-year patency of all dilated strictures in transplants is about half that attained with surgical repair (45% versus 89%).[110]

In patients with early hilar strictures, ductal mucosa may slough proximal to the obstruction, leaving a cast.[108] Such debris may need removal by stone-retrieval baskets or other means. In difficult cases we have applied electrohydraulic lithotripsy to clear stones from within transplanted livers.[100]

Intrahepatic strictures are commonly multiple. They have been correlated with hepatic artery occlusion, pretransplantation primary sclerosing cholangitis, choledochojejunostomy, and the use of Euro-Collins organ preservation solution (41% incidence of strictures versus 7% in organs preserved with the University of Wisconsin solution).[111] Strictures developing on an ischemic basis must be differentiated from bacterial or viral cholangitis, rejection, or recurrent sclerosing cholangitis.[112]

Interventions in Sclerosing Cholangitis

Primary sclerosing cholangitis, a condition associated with ulcerative colitis and most commonly affecting young and middle-aged men, is characterized by extensive submucosal fibrosis. This progressive disease leads to biliary cirrhosis and hepatic failure; more than one third of patients die within 7 years of diagnosis.[113] Conventional surgical bypass results have been generally disappointing, and hepatic transplantation is being aggressively performed in some centers.[114]

Percutaneous drainage and dilatation can provide palliation for many with this disease. Focal strictures producing jaundice, pruritus, and recurrent cholangitis can be ameliorated. Those who have had such symptoms longer than 6 months are less likely to respond to balloon dilatation and stenting.[32] Even patients with a good response usually have recurrent symptoms within 2 years.[113]

Because of the long-term problems of sclerosing cholangitis, Russell and colleagues have formulated a combined surgical-radiologic approach.[115] A side-to-side biliary jejunal anastomosis is created by a Roux-en-Y limb, with jejunum tacked subcutaneously and marked by surgical clips. Access to the limb and biliary tree is obtained by percutaneous puncture at this site. Multiple balloon dilatations of biliary strictures can be performed at 2- to 6-month intervals in this fashion.[115] An unresolved issue is how such surgery might affect future transplantation, should the patient's disease progress to hepatic failure or cholangiocarcinoma.[113] Another issue is the feeling by many physicians that primary sclerosing cholangitis is a premalignant condition and that transplantation should be performed early in the course of the disease. By the time cholangiocarcinoma is detected clincally, it can very rarely be cured.

Biliary Perfusion Studies

Occasionally, the significance of ductal dilatation may not be clear, or partial biliary obstruction may be suspected in the absence of dilated ducts. In analogy to the Whitaker uroperfusion test for hydronephrosis, van Sonnenberg and associates developed a perfusion test for detecting partial biliary obstruction.[116] With the use of a manometer, perfusion pump, and three-way stopcock, biliary pressure is measured after 5 minutes of dilute contrast medium infusion through a biliary drain or needle. The initial infusion rate is 2 ml/min, increased to 4 ml/min and to 8 ml/min if obstruction is not documented at the lower rates. If pressure readings remain normal, subsequent measurements are obtained after 3 minutes of 15 ml/min and 2 minutes of 19 ml/min, as tolerated. A study is considered abnormal if biliary pressure exceeds 20 cm of normal saline at any infusion rate. Biliary manometry and perfusion are helpful for uncovering subtle ampullary stenosis, as well as for assessing the results of stricture dilatation.[116] Manometric testing can replace prolonged clinical trials of biliary catheter clamping (the catheter maintained upstream from a treated stenosis) after removal of long-term stents.[117]

Biliary Stones

Cholesterol gallstones form as a consequence of stasis and supersaturation of bile by cholesterol. "Pigment" stones contain calcium salts of carbonate, bilirubin, phosphate, and alkanoate.[118] Gallstones are quite common, affecting more than 10% of adults in Western countries, but most calculi are asymptomatic and merit "watchful waiting."[119] Intervention is usually reserved for symptomatic disease, particularly for those at high risk of developing complications, such as diabetic patients. For many years the standard treatment for stone disease was open cholecystectomy and common bile duct exploration. However, the treatment has undergone radical changes in the last few years, especially with the introduction of laparoscopic cholecystectomy. Various nonoperative options have been explored (see the concluding sections of this chapter), but they all suffer from the problems with leaving the gallbladder in situ, namely, high rates of stone recurrence and the possibility of missing (or later development of) a gallbladder cancer. Therefore, cholecystectomy, be it open or laparoscopic, remains the most definitive option for symptomatic disease, and the less invasive techniques can be employed in patients at high operative risk or refusing surgery.[120]

Laparoscopic Cholecystectomy

Laparoscopic cholecystectomy (LC) results in a shorter hospital stay, earlier return to work, lower cost, and greater patient satisfaction on average.[119] However, the dissemination of the laparoscopic technique has led to a rise in ductal injuries and other postoperative morbidity. As experience has been gained, the complication rate of LC has started to decline.[121] Still, interventional techniques may be applied to treat the complications that do occur. Simple cystic duct remnant or other bile leaks usually resolve with biliary stenting (endoscopic or percutaneous), but larger infected bilomas also need percutaneous drainage.[121,22] Most ductal injuries should be operatively repaired. Recurrent strictures may be amenable to percutaneous balloon cholangioplasty and stenting. Another problem that has been seen after LC is "dropped gallstones" from gallbladder perforation during removal. Although such stones may be innocuous if left in place, any abscess resulting might be accessible to catheter drainage. Drainage may then be followed by tract dilatation, contact lithotripsy, and percutaneous extraction of stone fragments.[123]

T Tube Manipulations
Retained ductal stones (or stones that form years after cholecystectomy) are generally first approached by endoscopic sphincterotomy. However, when a T tube is in place, percutaneous extraction is possible through the drainage tract using techniques pioneered by Burhenne.[124] The tract must be allowed to mature at least 5 weeks after surgery, and longer, if the tube is smaller than 14 Fr. Cholangiography is performed after removal of the T tube, and a sheath is introduced. A stone basket is advanced beyond the stone before it is allowed to open. The basket is withdrawn and rotated to trap the stone within (Fig. 20-3). If the stone is 8 mm in diameter or small-

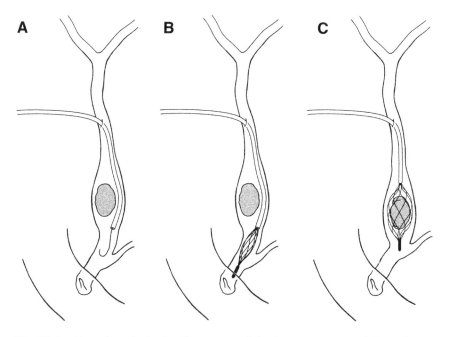

Fig. 20-3   Use of a wire basket for common bile duct stone removal through a T tube tract. **A,** Guidewire and sheath advanced beyond the stone. **B,** Basket unsheathed and opened distal to the stone. **C,** Stone trapped in the basket by means of basket rotation and withdrawal. The basket is then partially retracted into the sheath to secure the calculus, and the entire assembly is pulled out through the T tube tract.

er, the basket and sheath are completely withdrawn in a smooth motion *without* closing the basket. Closing the basket often causes fragmentation, a desirable result if a large stone is snared, but undesirable for small calculi. The procedure is repeated as many times as necessary. Stones less than 3 mm in diameter should pass spontaneously into the duodenum if no stricture is present. In difficult cases, steerable catheters, balloon catheters, safety wires, and flushing are employed.

Multiple sessions are often needed to render patients free of stones. A catheter the size of the tract should be left in place after each session, with removal only after follow-up cholangiography shows no residual stone or obstruction. With experience, success of T tube tract extraction can be as high as 95%, with complications arising in only 4%.[124] The ease of stone extraction can be enhanced by the use of small diameter choledochoscopes.[125] Choledochoscopes speed recognition of stones (with fluoroscopic guidance, bubbles and clots may present confusing filling defects) and can guide electrohydraulic lithotripsy, if needed. Laser lithotriptors can also be guided by small endoscopes, no matter what the route of access.[126]

Percutaneous Biliary Drainage for Stone Removal

In situations in which endoscopic interventions are not possible and no T tube is present, standard percutaneous techniques can be used to obtain access to the biliary tree. Berkman and associates have treated common bile duct stones by percutaneous transhepatic catheter placement, followed several days later by balloon dilatation of the ampulla of Vater.[127] They resorted to balloons only slightly larger than the largest stone present. After the dilation procedure, stones were pushed through the ampulla into the duodenum by a balloon catheter. Of the 17 patients so treated, 11 had stones larger than 10 mm in diameter, but all were successfully removed without mortality or significant complications.[127] Some endoscopists have employed similar balloon sphincteroplasty for stone removal with low morbidity,[128] but others remain skeptical.[129] Major bleeding may be less likely to occur, but pancreatitis is an acknowledged risk.

Intrahepatic stone disease, although uncommon in North America and Europe, can present particular treatment problems. At Johns Hopkins University, surgeons and interventional radiologists work closely in managing patients with multiple intrahepatic stones.[130] One or more percutaneous biliary drainage catheters may be placed, followed by tract dilatation to 16 Fr or greater. After 5 or 6 weeks allowed for tract maturation, percutaneous fragmentation and extraction procedures can be performed. Percutaneous interventions are complemented by biliary tract surgery and choledochoscopy to clear out all residual stone fragments and treat any underlying strictures. Hwang and colleagues have used similar percutaneous techniques in a large series of patients without waiting more than 1 or 2 weeks for tract maturation.[125]

Perfusion of Stones with Solvents

Whereas oral chenodeoxycholic acid and ursodeoxycholic acid may dissolve gallstones (they are commonly used to supplement electro–shock wave lithotripsy of gallstones), months to years of treatment are required for complete removal of stones, and only a minority of patients are suitable for such treatment.[118] Solvents perfused directly into the biliary ducts have been applied as a more rapid alternative for selected patients. The agents most commonly studied, glycerol-mono-octanoin (monooctanoin) and methyl-tertiary butyl ether (MTBE), both remain investigational and require an Investigation Device Exemption for use in the United States. No matter which solvent is used, pigment stones and stones showing calcification are refractory to dissolution attempts.

Monooctanoin is a very viscous fluid that must be gently heated during infusion. Outflow through a patent duct or sump catheter must be documented before starting treatment, and an overflow valve must be included in the line to prevent exceeding a pressure of 30 cm of saline.[131] Infusion for days to weeks is required for even modest success.

The agent MTBE represents a less tedious alternative but has its own peculiar hazards. It has a fairly high boiling point for an ether (55 °C), but like all ethers it must be used with meticulous ventilation and with respect for its explosive potential![132] Percutaneous cholecystostomy has been used to deliver the agent for gallbladder stones in patients refusing or at high risk for surgery. In the study of Thistle and associates, 32 of 75 patients were rendered stone free at last follow-up, and mean duration of infusion was nearly 13 hours.[42] Disadvantages of MTBE infusion include the necessity for manual instillation and aspiration of fluid over such a protracted period, sedation occurring with systemic absorption, and the risk of duodenitis and intravascular hemolysis. The efficacy of MTBE treatment may be enhanced with stone fragmentation, which increases the surface-volume ratio.[41]

Biliary Lithotripsy

Extracorporeal shock wave lithotripsy (ESWL) has been applied to both gallbladder stones and common duct calculi.[40,133] When the gallbladder is treated, common duct patency must be demonstrated by opacification on oral cholecystogram. In a series of 175 carefully selected patients, Sackmann and colleagues were able to reduce stones to fragments no larger than 3 mm in all but 20%; with adjuvant oral medication, 91% of patients had no demonstrable stones at 18 months.[133] Unfortunately, only about 7% of patients with symptomatic stones are optimal candidates for

ESWL (single radiolucent stone no larger than 20 mm diameter). Even with looser criteria, only 16% can be treated with a reasonable expectation of success.[119] Stones with calcified rims are amenable to ESWL therapy, although they are more resistant to fragmentation. Second-generation lithotripsy devices can treat patients without the need for anesthesia or sedation.[134] Bland and associates have had 74% success in clearing common duct stones by ESWL combined with endoscopic or percutaneous drainage.[40] Nevertheless, in the United States biliary ESWL has yet to obtain Food and Drug Administration approval because of high cost, as well as high residual fragment and stone recurrence rates.

Contact lithotripsy after percutaneous cholecystostomy has been employed in highly selected patients by some groups.[135–137] In the procedure used by Cheslyn-Curtis and associates, individuals are screened for contracted, nonfunctioning, or thick-walled gallbladders, which are subsequently excluded from percutaneous treatment.[136] Those selected are ideally treated in a single session under general anesthesia. Ultrasonography is initially used to guide fine-needle placement for cholecystography. The gallbladder fundus is then punctured directly (without traversing hepatic parenchyma), and telescoping dilators are employed to open the tract to 28 or 30 Fr. After electrohydraulic or ultrasonic lithotripsy and fragment removal, a Foley catheter is left in place for 10 days. They have achieved clearance of stones without affecting gallbladder function in more than 90% of patients treated.[136] Although gallstone recurrence has been noted in 35% at 3-year follow-up, this rate has been diminished with adjuvant oral bile salt therapy, and most recurrent stones have been asymptomatic.[135] This technique may be modified in the future for fragmentation of stones with smaller-diameter devices, such as laser lithotriptors or the Rotolith catheter as described by Lindberg and colleagues.[138]

REFERENCES

1. Molnar W, Stockum AE: Relief of obstructive jaundice through percutaneous transhepatic catheter: A new therapeutic method. *Am J Roentgenol* 1974; 122:356–367.
2. Stockberger SM, Wass JL, Sherman S, et al: Intravenous cholangiography with helical CT: Comparison with endoscopic retrograde cholangiography. *Radiology* 1994; 192:675–680.
3. Davids PHP, Groen AK, Rauws EAJ, et al: Randomised trial of self-expanding metal stents versus polyethylene stents for distal malignant biliary obstruction. *Lancet* 1992; 340:1488–1492.
4. Stoker J, Lameris JS, Jeekel J: Percutaneously placed Wallstent endoprosthesis in patients with malignant distal biliary obstruction. *Br J Surg* 1993; 80:1185–1187.
5. Silvis SE, Sievert CE, Vennes JA, et al: Comparison of covered versus uncovered wire mesh stents in the canine biliary tract. *Gastrointest Endosc* 1994; 40:17–21.

6. Goldin E, Beyar M, Safra T, et al: A new self-expandable and removable metal stent for biliary obstruction: A preliminary report. *Endoscopy* 1993; 25:597–599.
7. Yee ACN, Ho C-S: Complications of percutaneous biliary drainage: Benign versus malignant diseases. *Am J Roentgenol* 1987; 148:1207–1209.
8. Greig JD, Krukowski ZH, Matheson NA: Surgical morbidity and mortality in one hundred and twenty-nine patients with obstructive jaundice. *Br J Surg* 1988; 75:216–219.
9. Clark CD, Picus D, Dunagan WC: Bloodstream infections after interventional procedures in the biliary tract. *Radiology* 1994; 191:495–499.
10. Audisio RA, Bozzetti F, Severini A, et al: The occurrence of cholangitis after percutaneous biliary drainage: Evaluation of some risk factors. *Surgery* 1988; 103:507–512.
11. Olak J, Stein LA, Meakins JL: Palliative transhepatic biliary drainage: Assessment of morbidity and mortality. *Can J Surg* 1986; 29:243–246.
12. Choi TK, Fan ST, Lai ECS, Wong J: Malignant hilar biliary obstruction treated by segmental bilioenteric anastomosis. *Surgery* 1988; 104:525–529.
13. Cohan RH, Illescas FF, Saeed M, et al: Infectious complications of percutaneous biliary drainage. *Invest Radiol* 1986; 21:705–709.
14. Spies JB, Rosen RJ, Lebowitz AS: Antibiotic prophylaxis in vascular and interventional radiology: A rational approach. *Radiology* 1988; 166:381–387.
15. Vogelzang RL, Nemcek AA Jr: Toward painless percutaneous biliary procedures: New strategies and alternatives. *J Intervent Radiol* 1988; 3:131–134.
16. Lee MJ, Mueller PR, Saini S, et al: Percutaneous dilatation of benign biliary strictures: Single-session therapy with general anesthesia. *Am J Roentgenol* 1991; 157:1263–1266.
17. Rosenblatt M, Robalino J, Bergman A, Shevde K: Pleural block: Technique for regional anesthesia during percutaneous hepatobiliary drainage. *Radiology* 1989; 172:279–280.
18. Harshfield DL, Teplick SK, Brandon JC: Pain control during interventional biliary procedures: Epidural anesthesia vs IV sedation. *Am J Roentgenol* 1993; 161:1057–1059.
19. Lynn RB, Wilson JAP, Cho KJ: Cholangiocarcinoma: Role of percutaneous transhepatic cholangiography in determination of resectability. *Dig Dis Sci* 1988; 33:587–591.
20. Gibby DG, Hanks JB, Wanebo HJ, et al: Bile duct carcinoma: Diagnosis and treatment. *Ann Surg* 1985; 202:139–144.
21. Neff CC, Mueller PR, Ferrucci JT Jr, et al: Serious complications following transgression of the pleural space in drainage procedures. *Radiology* 1984; 152:335–341.
22. Keller FS, Katon RM, Dotter CT, et al: Fine needle cholangiography (FNC) in the nonjaundiced patient. *J Clin Gastroenterol* 1979; 1:125–129.
23. Harbin WP, Mueller PR, Ferrucci JT Jr: Transhepatic cholangiography: Complications and use patterns of the fine-needle technique. *Radiology* 1980; 135:15–22.
24. Teplick SK, Flick P, Brandon JC: Transhepatic cholangiography in patients with suspected biliary disease and nondilated intrahepatic bile ducts. *Gastrointest Radiol* 1991; 16:193–197.

25. MacCarty RL, LaRusso NF, May GR, et al: Cholangiocarcinoma complicating primary sclerosing cholangitis: Cholangiographic appearances. *Radiology* 1985; 156:43–46.

26. MacCarty RL, LaRusso NF, Wiesner RH, Ludwig J: Primary sclerosing cholangitis: Findings on cholangiography and pancreatography. *Radiology* 1983; 149:39–44.

27. Li-Yeng C, Goldberg HI: Sclerosing cholangitis: Broad spectrum of radiographic features. *Gastrointest Radiol* 1984; 9:39–47.

28. Gulliver DJ, Baker ME, Putnam W, et al: Bile duct diverticula and webs: Nonspecific cholangiographic features of primary sclerosing cholangitis. *Am J Roentgenol* 1991; 157:281–285.

29. Miros M, Kerlin P, Walker N, et al: Predicting cholangiocarcinoma in patients with primary sclerosing cholangitis before transplantation. *Gut* 1991; 32:1369–1373.

30. Ring EJ, Kerlan RK Jr: Interventional biliary radiology. *Am J Roentgenol* 1984; 142:31–34.

31. Karani J, Fletcher M, Brinkley D, et al: Internal biliary drainage and local radiotherapy with iridium-192 wire in treatment of hilar cholangiocarcinoma. *Clin Radiol* 1985; 36:603–606.

32. May GR, Bender CE, LaRusso NF, Wiesner RH: Nonoperative dilatation of dominant strictures in primary sclerosing cholangitis. *Am J Roentgenol* 1985; 145:1061–1064.

33. Cohan RH, Illescas FF, Braun SD, et al: Fine needle aspiration biopsy in malignant obstructive jaundice. *Gastrointest Radiol* 1986; 11:145–150.

34. Kuroda C, Yoshioka H, Tokunaga K, et al: Fine-needle aspiration biopsy via percutaneous transhepatic catheterization: Technique and clinical results. *Gastrointest Radiol* 1986; 11:81–84.

35. Terasaki K, Wittich GR, Lycke G, et al: Percutaneous transluminal biopsy of biliary strictures with a bioptome. *Am J Roentgenol* 1991; 156:77–78.

36. Berger H, Winter T, Pratschke E, Sauerbruch T: Perkutane drainagebehandlung fistelassoziierter abszess und biliärer fisteln. *Rofo* 1989; 150:342–345.

37. Nuñez D Jr, Guerra JJ Jr, Al-Sheikh WA, et al: Percutaneous biliary drainage in acute suppurative cholangitis. *Gastrointest Radiol* 1986; 11:85–89.

38. Lois JF, Gomes AS, Grace PA, et al: The risks of percutaneous transhepatic drainage in patients with cholangitis. *Am J Roentgenol* 1987; 148:367–371.

39. Huang MH, Ker CG: Ultrasonic guided percutaneous transhepatic bile drainage for cholangitis due to intrahepatic stones. *Arch Surg* 1988; 123:106–109.

40. Bland KI, Jones RS, Maher JW, et al: Extracorporeal shock-wave lithotripsy of bile duct calculi: An interim report of the Dornier US bile duct lithotripsy prospective study. *Ann Surg* 1989; 209:743–753.

41. Faulkner DJ, Kozarek RA: Gallstones: Fragmentation with a tunable dye laser and dissolution with methyl tert-butyl ether in vitro. *Radiology* 1989; 170:185–189.

42. Thistle JL, May GR, Bender CE, et al: Dissolution of cholesterol gallbladder stones by methyl-tert-butyl ether administered by percutaneous transhepatic catheter. *N Engl J Med* 1989; 320:633–639.

43. Pitt HA, Gomes AS, Lois JF, et al: Does preoperative percutaneous biliary drainage reduce operative risk or increase hospital cost? *Ann Surg* 1985; 201:545–553.

44. Smith RC, Pooley M, George CR, Faithful GR: Preoperative percutaneous transhepatic internal drainage in obstructive jaundice: A randomized, controlled trial examining renal function. *Surgery* 1985; 97:641–648.

45. Norlander A, Kalin B, Sundblad R: Effect of percutaneous transhepatic drainage upon liver function and postoperative mortality. *Surg Gynecol Obstet* 1982; 155:161–166.

46. Denning DA, Ellison EC, Carey LC: Preoperative percutaneous transhepatic biliary decompression lowers operative morbidity in patients with obstructive jaundice. *Am J Surg* 1981; 141:61–65.

47. Gobien RP, Stanley JH, Soucek C, et al: Routine preoperative biliary drainage: Effect on management of obstructive jaundice. *Radiology* 1984; 152:353–356.

48. Hatfield ARW, Tobias R, Terblanche J, et al: Preoperative external biliary drainage in obstructive jaundice: A prospective controlled clinical trial. *Lancet* 1982; 2:896–899.

49. Lygidakis NJ, van der Heyde MN, Lubbers MJ: Evaluation of preoperative biliary drainage in the surgical management of pancreatic head carcinoma. *Acta Chir Scand* 1987; 153:665–668.

50. Stanley J, Gobien RP, Cunningham J, Andriole J: Biliary decompression: An institutional comparison of percutaneous and endoscopic methods. *Radiology* 1986; 158:195–197.

51. Lewis WD, Cady B, Rohrer RJ, et al: Avoidance of transhepatic drainage prior to hepaticojejunostomy for obstruction of the biliary tract. *Surg Gynecol Obstet* 1987; 165:381–386.

52. Soulez G, Gagner M, Thérasse E, et al: Malignant biliary obstruction: Preliminary results of palliative treatment with hepaticogastrostomy under fluoroscopic, endoscopic, and laparoscopic guidance. *Radiology* 1994; 192:241–246.

53. Nordback IH, Pitt HA, Coleman J, et al: Unresectable hilar cholangiocarcinoma: Percutaneous versus operative palliation. *Surgery* 1994; 115:597–603.

54. Okuda K, Ohto M, Tsuhiya Y: The role of ultrasound, percutaneous transhepatic cholangiography, computed tomographic scanning, and magnetic resonance imaging in the preoperative assessment of bile duct cancer. *World J Surg* 1988; 12:18–26.

55. Deviere J, Baize M, de Toeuf J, Cremer M: Long-term follow-up of patients with hilar malignant stricture treated by endoscopic internal biliary drainage. *Gastrointest Endosc* 1988; 32:95–101.

56. Laméris JS, Stoker J, Dees J, et al: Non-surgical palliative treatment of patients with malignant biliary obstruction: The place of endoscopic and percutaneous drainage. *Clin Radiol* 1987; 38:603–608.

57. Günther RW, Schild H, Thelen M: Percutaneous transhepatic biliary drainage: Experience with 311 procedures. *Cardiovasc Intervent Radiol* 1988; 11:65–71.

58. Vogelzang RL, Nemcek AA Jr: Percutaneous cholecystostomy: Diagnostic and therapeutic efficacy. *Radiology* 1988; 168:29–34.

59. Carrasco CH, Zornoza J, Bechtel WJ: Malignant biliary obstruction: Complications of percutaneous biliary drainage. *Radiology* 1984; 152:343–346.

60. Nichols DM, Cooperberg PL, Golding RH, Burhenne HJ: The safe intercostal approach? Pleural complications in abdominal interventional radiology. *Am J Roentgenol* 1984; 141:1013–1018.
61. Schild H, Klose KJ, Staritz M, et al: Ergebnisse und Komplikationen von 616 perkutanen transhepatischen Gallenwegsdrainagen. *Rofo* 1989; 151:289–293.
62. Schoenfeld RB, Lecky D, Ring EJ, et al: Stabilization of percutaneous catheters. *Am J Roentgenol* 1982; 138:972.
63. Mitchell SE, Shuman LS, Kaufman SL, et al: Biliary catheter drainage complicated by hemobilia: Treatment by balloon embolotherapy. *Radiology* 1985; 157:645–652.
64. Sandborn WJ, Gross JB, Larson DE, et al: High-volume postobstructive choleresis after transhepatic external biliary drainage resolves with conversion to internal drainage. *J Clin Gastroenterol* 1993; 17:42–45.
65. Rankin RN, Vellet DA, Okelly KF: Biliary-jejunal drainage for failed biliary-duodenal drainage. *J Can Assn Radiol* 1991; 42:106–108.
66. Gordon RL, Ring EJ, Laberge JM, Doherty MM: Malignant biliary obstruction: Treatment with expandable metallic stents—follow-up of 50 consecutive patients. *Radiology* 1992; 182:697–701.
67. Joyce FS, Thorup J, Burcharth F: Bilio-bronchial fistula: A rare complication to biliary endoprosthesis. *Rofo* 1988; 148:723–724.
68. Rypins EB, Bitzer LG, Sarfeh IJ, Juler GL: The role of percutaneous transhepatic internal biliary drainage in preoperative patients. *Am Surg* 1987; 53:562–564.
69. Hamlin JA, Friedman M, Stein MG, Bray JF: Percutaneous biliary drainage: Complications of 118 consecutive catheterizations. *Radiology* 1986; 158:199–202.
70. Chapman WC, Sharp KW, Weaver F, Sawyers JL: Tumor seeding from percutaneous biliary catheters. *Ann Surg* 1989; 209:708–713.
71. Stambuk EC, Pitt HA, Pais SO, et al: Percutaneous transhepatic drainage: Risks and benefits. *Arch Surg* 1983; 118:1388–1394.
72. Schoenemann J, Willems M, Wolf G, Fromme M: Ergebnisse der perkutanen transhepatischen gallengangsdrainage. *Rofo* 1987; 147:619–623.
73. Bonnel D, Ferrucci JT Jr, Mueller PR, et al: Surgical and radiological decompression in malignant biliary obstruction: A retrospective study using multivariate risk factor analysis. *Radiology* 1984; 152:347–351.
74. Lai ECS, Tompkins RK, Roslyn JJ, Mann LL: Proximal bile duct cancer: Quality of survival. *Ann Surg* 1987; 205:111–118.
75. Szabo S, Mendelson MH, Mitty HA, et al: Infections associated with transhepatic biliary drainage devices. *Am J Med* 1987; 82:921–926.
76. Lammer J: Perkutane transhepatische gallengangsendoprothese. *Rofo* 1985; 142:243–253.
77. Kerlan RK Jr, Ring EJ, Pogany AC, Jeffrey RB Jr: Biliary endoprostheses: Insertion using a combined peroral-transhepatic method. *Radiology* 1984; 150:828–830.
78. Mueller PR, Ferrucci JT Jr, Teplick SK, et al: Biliary stent endoprosthesis: Analysis of complications in 113 patients. *Radiology* 1985; 156:637–639.
79. Mendez G, Russell E, LePage JR, et al: Abandonment of endoprosthetic drainage technique in malignant biliary obstruction. *Am J Roentgenol* 1984; 143:617–622.

80. Coons HG, Carey PH: Large-bore, long biliary endoprostheses (biliary stents) for improved drainage. *Radiology* 1983; 148:89–94.
81. Teplick SK, Haskin PH, Pavlides CA, Goldstein RC: Management of obstructed biliary endoprostheses. *Cardiovasc Intervent Radiol* 1985; 8:164–167.
82. Dick BW, Gordon RL, LaBerge JM, et al: Percutaneous transhepatic placement of biliary endoprostheses: Results in 100 consecutive patients. *J Vasc Interv Radiol* 1990; 1:97–100.
83. Barrioz T, Ingrand P, Besson I, et al: Randomised trial of prevention of biliary stent occlusion by ursodeoxycholic acid plus norfloxacin. *Lancet* 1994; 344:581–582.
84. Salomonowitz EK, Adam A, Antonucci F, et al: Malignant biliary obstruction: Treatment with self-expandable stainless steel endoprosthesis. *Cardiovasc Intervent Radiol* 1992; 15:351–355.
85. Adam A: Metallic biliary endoprostheses. *Cardiovasc Intervent Radiol* 1994; 17:127–132.
86. Boguth L, Tatalovic S, Antonucci F, et al: Malignant biliary obstruction: Clinical and histopathologic correlation after treatment with self-expanding metal prostheses. *Radiology* 1994; 192:669–674.
87. Rossi P, Bezzi M, Salvatori FM, et al: Recurrent benign biliary strictures: Management with self-expanding metallic stents. *Radiology* 1990; 175:661–665.
88. Maccioni F, Rossi M, Salvatori FM, et al: Metallic stents in benign biliary strictures: 3-year follow-up. *Cardiovasc Intervent Radiol* 1992; 15:360–366.
89. Deviere J, Cremer M, Baize M, et al: Management of common bile duct stricture caused by chronic pancreatitis with metal mesh self expandable stents. *Gut* 1994; 35:122–126.
90. Harell GS, Anderson MF, Berry PF: Cytologic bile examination in the diagnosis of biliary duct neoplastic strictures. *Am J Roentgenol* 1981; 137:1123–1126.
91. Meyers WC, Jones RS: Internal radiation for bile duct cancer. *World J Surg* 1988; 12:99–104.
92. Kubota Y, Seki T, Nakano T, et al: A case of bile duct cancer treated by laser via percutaneous transhepatic choledochoscopy. *Hepatogastroenterology* 1988; 35:213–214.
93. Larssen TB, Gothlin JH, Jensen D, et al: Ultrasonically and fluoroscopically guided therapeutic percutaneous catheter drainage of the gallbladder. *Gastrointest Radiol* 1988; 13:37–40.
94. Eggermont AM, Laméris JS, Jeekel J: Ultrasound-guided percutaneous transhepatic cholecystostomy for acute acalculus cholecystitis. *Arch Surg* 1985; 120:1354–1356.
95. Vauthey JN, Lerut J, Martini M, et al: Indications and limitations of percutaneous cholecystostomy for acute cholecystitis. *Surg Gynecol Obstet* 1993; 176:49–54.
96. vanSonnenberg E, Wing VW, Pollard JW, Casola G: Life-threatening vagal reactions associated with percutaneous cholecystostomy. *Radiology* 1984; 151:377–380.
97. Shaver RW, Hawkins IF Jr, Soong J: Percutaneous cholecystostomy. *Am J Roentgenol* 1982; 138:1133–1136.
98. Verbanck J, Baert F, Malysse I, et al: Simple gallbladder puncture as a diag-

nostic tool and therapy in critically ill patients with presumed acute chole-cystitis. *Eur J Gastroenterol Hepatol* 1991; 3:753–756.
99. vanSonnenberg E, D'Agostino HB, Casola G, et al: The benefits of percuta-neous cholecystostomy for decompression of selected cases of obstructive jaundice. *Radiology* 1990; 176:15–18.
100. Carlson P, Wojtowycz M, Crummy A, et al: Percutaneous transhepatic treat-ment of choledocholithiasis in the transplanted liver. *J Intervent Radiol* 1990; 5:57–60.
101. Kozicki I, Bielecki K, Kawalski A, Krolicki L: Repeated reconstruction for recurrent benign bile duct stricture. *Br J Surg* 1994; 81:677–679.
102. Millis JM, Tompkins RK, Zinner MJ, et al: Management of bile duct stric-tures: An evolving strategy. *Arch Surg* 1992; 127:1077–1084.
103. Martin EC, Fankuchen EI, Laffey KJ, Sibley RE: Percutaneous management of benign biliary disease. *Gastrointest Radiol* 1984; 9:207–212.
104. Gibson RN, Yeung AE, Savage A, et al: Percutaneous techniques in benign hilar and intrahepatic strictures. *J Intervent Radiol* 1988; 3:125–130.
105. Salomonowitz E, Castañeda-Zuñiga WR, Lund G, et al: Balloon dilatation of benign biliary strictures. *Radiology* 1984; 151:613–616.
106. Bret PM, Bretagnolle M, Fond A, et al: Use of large silicone catheters in patients with long-term percutaneous transhepatic biliary drainage. *Cardiovasc Intervent Radiol* 1986; 9:57–58.
107. Citron SJ, Martin LG: Benign biliary strictures: Treatment with percutaneous cholangioplasty. *Radiology* 1991; 178:339–341.
108. Ward EM, Kiely MJ, Maus TP, et al: Hilar biliary strictures after liver trans-plantation: Cholangiography and percutaneous treatment. *Radiology* 1990; 177:259–263.
109. McDonald V, Matalon TAS, Patel SK, et al: Biliary strictures in hepatic trans-plantation. *J Vasc Interv Radiol* 1991; 2:533–538.
110. Kuo PC, Lewis WD, Stokes K, et al: Comparison of operation, endoscopic retrograde cholangiopancreatography, and percutaneous transhepatic cholan-giography in biliary complications after hepatic transplantation. *J Am Coll Surg* 1994; 179:177–181.
111. Campbell WL, Sheng R, Zajko AB, et al: Intrahepatic biliary strictures after liver transplantation. *Radiology* 1994; 191:735–740.
112. Ludwig J, Batts KP, MacCarty RL: Ischemic cholangitis in hepatic allografts. *Mayo Clin Proc* 1992; 67:519–526.
113. Skolkin MD, Alspaugh JP, Casarella WJ, et al: Sclerosing cholangitis: Palliation with percutaneous cholangioplasty. *Radiology* 1989; 170:199–206.
114. Lemmer ER, Bornman PC, Krige JEJ, et al: Primary sclerosing cholangitis: Requiem for biliary drainage operations? *Arch Surg* 1994; 129:723–728.
115. Russell E, Yrizarry JM, Huber JS, et al: Percutaneous transjejunal biliary dilatation: Alternate management for benign strictures. *Radiology* 1986; 159:209–214.
116. vanSonnenberg E, Ferrucci JT Jr, Neff CC, et al: Biliary pressure: Mano-metric and perfusion studies at percutaneous transhepatic cholangiography and percutaneous biliary drainage. *Radiology* 1983; 148:41–50.
117. Savader SJ, Cameron JL, Pitt HA, et al: Biliary manometry versus clinical

trial: Value as predictors of success after treatment of biliary tract strictures. *J Vasc Interv Radiol* 1994; 5:757–763.

118. Hofmann AF: Bile, bile acids, and gallstones: Will new knowledge bring new power? *Am J Roentgenol* 1988; 151:5–12.

119. Strasberg SM, Clavien PA: Overview of therapeutic modalities for the treatment of gallstone diseases. *Am J Surg* 1993; 165:420–426.

120. Ransohoff DF, Gracie WA, Schmittner JP, et al: Guidelines for the treatment of gallstones. *Ann Intern Med* 1993; 119:620–622.

121. Woods MS, Traverso LW, Kozarek RA, et al: Characteristics of biliary tract complications during laparoscopic cholecystectomy: A multi-institutional study. *Am J Surg* 1994; 167:27–34.

122. Wright TB, Bertino RB, Bishop AF, et al: Complications of laparoscopic cholecystectomy and their interventional radiologic management. *RadioGraphics* 1993; 13:119–128.

123. Trerotola SO, Lillemoe KD, Malloy PC, Osterman FA: Percutaneous removal of dropped gallstones after laparoscopic cholecystectomy. *Radiology* 1993; 188:419–421.

124. Burhenne HJ: Percutaneous extraction of retained biliary tract stones: 661 patients. *Am J Roentgenol* 1980; 134:888–898.

125. Hwang MH, Tsai CC, Mo LR, et al: Percutaneous choledochoscopic biliary tract stone removal: Experience in 645 consecutive patients. *Eur J Radiol* 1993; 17:184–190.

126. Neuhaus H, Hoffmann W, Zillinger C, Classen M: Laser lithotripsy of difficult bile duct stones under direct visual control. *Gut* 1993; 34:415–421.

127. Berkman WA, Bishop AF, Palagallo GL, Cashman MD: Transhepatic balloon dilation of the distal common bile duct and ampulla of Vater for removal of calculi. *Radiology* 1988; 167:453–455.

128. MacMathuna P, White P, Clarke E, et al: Endoscopic sphincteroplasty: A novel and safe alternative to papillotomy in the management of bile duct stones. *Gut* 1994; 35:127–129.

129. Blackstone MG: Balloon sphincteroplasty vs endoscopic papillotomy for bile duct stones. *Lancet* 1993; 342:1314–1315 (editorial).

130. Pitt HA, Venbrux AC, Coleman JA, et al: Intrahepatic stones: The transhepatic team approach. *Ann Surg* 1994; 219:527–537.

131. Gadacz TR: The effect of monooctanoin on retained common duct stones. *Surgery* 1981; 89:527–531.

132. Lee LL, McGahan JP: Dissolution of cholesterol gallstones: Comparison of solvents. *Gastrointest Radiol* 1986; 11:169–171.

133. Sackmann M, Delius M, Sauerbruch T, et al: Shock-wave lithotripsy of gallbladder stones: The first 175 patients. *N Engl J Med* 1988; 318:393–397.

134. Ackermann C, Meyer B, Rothenbühler JM, et al: Schmerzfreie piezoelektrische extrakorporelle stosswellenlithotripsie bei gallenblasensteinen. *Schweiz med Wochenschr* 1989; 119:720–723.

135. Donald JJ, Cheslyn-Curtis S, Gillams AR, et al: Percutaneous cholecystolithotomy: Is gall stone recurrence inevitable? *Gut* 1994; 35:692–695.

136. Cheslyn-Curtis S, Gillams AR, Russell RCG, et al: Selection, management, and early outcome of 113 patients with symptomatic gall stones treated by percutaneous cholecystolithotomy. *Gut* 1992; 33:1253–1259.
137. Griffith DP, Gleeson MJ, Appel MF, et al: Percutaneous cholecystolithotomy: A minimally invasive alternative to cholecystectomy and to shock wave lithotripsy. *Arch Surg* 1990; 125:1114–1118.
138. Lindberg CG, Jeppsson B, Lundstedt C, et al: Percutaneous rotational lithotripsy of gallbladder stones: Clinical results with the Rotolith lithotriptor. *Acta Radiol* 1993; 34:273–278.

21

Genitourinary Interventions

KEY CONCEPTS

1. Percutaneous nephrostomy is indicated for most cases of obstructive hydronephrosis, if a retrograde ureteral stent cannot be placed.
2. A posterolateral approach below the twelfth rib, with entry into a posterior calyx or infundibulum, is desirable for most nephrostomies.
3. Percutaneous nephrolithotomy and lithotripsy continue to be indicated for large (over 3 cm), infected, or cystine stones, as well as those associated with ureteral obstruction that cannot be removed with retrograde ureteroscopy or extracorporeal shockwave lithotripsy.
4. Response of ureteral strictures to dilation and stenting is difficult to predict, but anastomotic ileal conduit strictures have a poor prognosis.
5. The Whitaker test, which measures the pressure gradient between renal pelvis and bladder after a perfusion challenge, determines the significance of questionable obstructions.

Percutaneous nephrostomy, first used solely for the decompression of obstructed upper urinary tracts, has fostered the development of an entirely new approach to urologic disease. The field of endourology, which makes use of both percutaneous and retrograde access to the genitourinary system, permits conditions previously needing open surgery and prolonged postoperative recuperation to be treated with decreased burden to the patient. The introduction of extracorporeal shock wave lithotripsy (ESWL) in the past decade has not eliminated the need for percutaneous access to the collecting system in patients with urinary calculi, but it has modified the application of percutaneous nephrostomy for renal stone disease.[1–3]

Percutaneous nephrostomy clearly remains the procedure of choice for sepsis consequent to ureteral obstruction, although retrograde ureteral stent placement by way of cystoscopy may be attempted first in some patients. Percutaneous nephrostomy is also a prime treatment for uremia or flank pain due to chronic obstruction, whether of benign or malignant cause. However, percutaneous drainage is of dubious value in patients with advanced and disseminated cancer.[4,5]

The access provided by nephrostomy permits ureteral strictures to be dilated and stented, flow through urinary fistulae to be diverted, and traumatic ureteral or renal pelvic perforations to heal.[6,7] Nephrostomy is a route for renal endoscopy, performance of endopyelotomy of ureteropelvic junction strictures, and topical treatment for upper tract transitional cell carcinoma.[8,9] Percutaneous methods are especially valuable in patients who have received renal transplants and experience immediate or delayed postoperative problems.[10] Diabetics or others developing fungal pyelonephritis may need urinary decompression and direct perfusion of amphotericin B to resolve infection.[11,12] Hemorrhagic cystitis refractory to conventional therapy may improve or resolve after percutaneous urinary diversion.[13]

Percutaneous lithotripsy achieved widespread application in the early 1980s, only to be superseded by ESWL for the treatment of renal stones. However, ESWL alone cannot remove staghorn calculi or other large stones, and nephrostomy is often needed in preparation for complicated stone extractions.[2,3,14] Stone dissolution therapy relies on infusion and drainage through percutaneous tubes.[15] Retrograde transvesical nephrostomy and other retrograde manipulations have been developed and present an alternative for selected patients.[16–19] No matter what clinical problem is being addressed, the patient's interests are best served by cooperation between radiologist and urologist, whose technical skills are exercised optimally in a complementary manner.

PATIENT PREPARATION

As before any invasive procedure, the patient's history and previous studies must be reviewed, and clear objectives formulated. When multiple interventions are likely, or in the case of complicated stone disease, the treatment plan and percutaneous approach should be discussed directly with the attending urologist prior to nephrostomy placement. For example, the removal of multiple stones in the renal collecting system depends critically on the point of entry of the nephrostomy tube.[20] If a patient has bilateral hydronephrosis, the bladder must be decompressed by a Foley catheter (or suprapubic cystostomy in rare instances) to eliminate the possibility of placing bilateral nephrostomies for bladder outlet obstruction! This unlikely scenario typically arises when a patient is directly referred from a nursing home or a medical ward whose staff are unaccustomed to managing urologic problems.

The patient is then seen. The procedure and its indications, alternatives, and risks are explained, and consent is obtained. Any anticoagulant medication is stopped. Prothrombin time, partial thromboplastin time, and platelet count are checked, and any evident coagulation defects are corrected, as possible. Any history of hypersensitivity to iodinated contrast medium or other medication is elicited. Note must be made of splenomegaly (for left-sided nephrostomy), severe scoliosis, or other anatomic anomalies that could affect the approach. Percutaneous nephrostomy is possible in cases of pelvic kidney or horseshoe kidney.[21] However, when renal anatomy is grossly distorted, computed tomography (CT) scanning may be needed for planning. Scanning with CT or ultrasound (US) can also be used to estimate the likelihood of restoring function to a chronically obstructed kidney by demonstrating renal size and cortical thickness.

Patients with signs of urinary tract infection need administration of intravenous antibiotics at least 1 hour prior to intervention.[22] Those undergoing drainage of pyonephrosis have a 7% incidence of septic shock, despite aminoglycoside prophylaxis.[22] Because renal stones are commonly associated with infection, premedication with antibiotics is also used routinely before nephrostomy for stone removal.[23,24] Antibiotics need not be given universally to otherwise asymptomatic patients, but if such a policy is pursued, urinalysis and urine culture are recommended before elective procedures. Simple changes of a nephrostomy tube do not normally require medication as long as the tube has not been obstructed.

Urinary tract pathogens are predominantly gram-negative bacteria, such as *Escherichia coli* and *Klebsiella, Enterococcus,* and *Proteus* species. For prophylaxis in the absence of any overt infection, cefazolin or cefoperazone may be given and continued for 48 hours.[22] When infection is present, therapy is directed toward the isolated organisms, and ticarcillin, piperacillin, and an aminoglycoside can be used to provide a broader range of antibiotic coverage.[22]

Simple nephrostomy tube placement in adults can be performed with local anesthesia, supplemented by an intravenous benzodiazepine (midazolam or diazepam) and an opiate for pain (morphine or fentanyl).[25] Only in special cases is epidural or general anesthesia needed. However, when extensive tract dilatation is planned, as for renal stone removal, regional or general anesthesia is indicated. We do not perform nephrostomy as an out-patient procedure; others have cautioned against the practice.[24] However, the initial evaluation can be performed on an outpatient basis, followed by a scheduled admission immediately after tube placement.

PERCUTANEOUS NEPHROSTOMY

Anatomic Considerations

The kidneys are normally obliquely oriented in the retroperitoneum, with their upper poles medial and posterior in respect to their lower poles. They have a medial-to-lateral posterior angulation of about 30° as measured from the coronal plane.[26] Therefore, on an anteroposterior projection, the calyces appearing to be in profile and laterally placed are the anterior calyces. Neighboring structures to be respected include the pleural space, liver, spleen, and colon. Although the pleural space may be safely traversed when necessary, it is best avoided for simple drainage procedures.[27] Tubes placed posteriorly through the eleventh intercostal space pass through pleura, and those placed above the eleventh rib may injure lung.[28] The inferior margins of the ribs must be avoided to prevent bleeding from the subcostal artery, as well as pain from periosteal irritation.

Most kidneys have their dominant segmental arterial supply distributed anteriorly, and their only posterior segmental artery passes behind the upper pole infundibulum.[20] However, variant posterior arterial branches are fairly common in both upper and lower poles, and puncture of a calyceal fornix in the midportion of kidney is least likely to produce major bleeding.[29] The posterolateral watershed of these vessels, described by Brödel as the "bloodless line of incision," provides the safest approach into the kidney.[20] However, the site of skin entry should not be placed too laterally, for as one approaches the posterior axillary line, the chances for injuring a posteriorly positioned colon or spleen increase.[30,31] Prevention of injury to an adjacent organ requires careful US or fluoroscopic observation during needle placement, tract dilatation, and tube introduction.

Technique

Nephrostomy placement can be guided by US, fluoroscopy, or both. If the kidney is unobstructed or partially obstructed and capable of excretion, intravenous iodinated contrast material is administered. In certain cases, such as for removal of nonobstructing stones, a retrograde ureteral catheter may have been placed during cystoscopy. If such a catheter is in position, it can be used to inject contrast medium. Not only iodinated contrast medium but also carbon dioxide (CO_2) may be injected through retrograde catheters. In a prone patient, CO_2 accumulates in posterior calyces, aiding in their recognition.

Both intravenous and directly injected contrast medium are valuable for defining anatomy and position, as well as for distending the renal collecting system. Distention produces fewer complications of perforation and excessive bleeding.[28] Severe hydronephrosis is easily defined by US in the great majority of cases, and needle placement is relatively simple, except in grossly obese patients.

Initial entry with a fine (21-gauge) needle is preferable. Routine use of a large sheath needle places the patient at greater risk for pseudoaneurysm, arteriovenous fistula, and major bleeding.[32] There may be little practical alternative to a sheath needle, however, if there is heavy perinephric scarring from inflammation or previous surgery or if the patient has a thick layer of perinephric fat. In obese patients it is helpful at times to place an 18-gauge arteriographic-type needle through the soft tissues of the retroperitoneum (but not entering renal capsule) to guide a coaxially placed, longer 21-gauge needle.

Except when a particular calyx must be entered in conjunction with stone removal, the needle is best directed toward a lower pole or midnephric posterior calyx from a posterolateral approach (Fig. 21-1). Puncture into an anterior calyx makes guidewire and catheter placement extremely difficult,

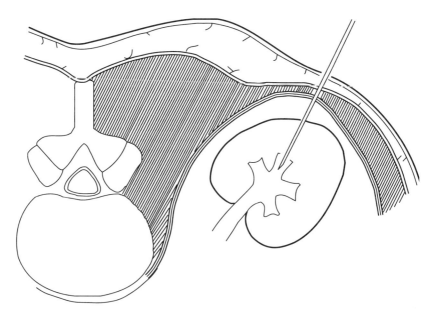

Fig. 21-1 Needle entry into a posterolateral calyx: the first step in percutaneous nephrostomy.

if not impossible, because of the acute angle that must be negotiated between entry site and renal pelvis. Ultrasound study is helpful in choosing an approach, even if the collecting system is opacified, because intervening spleen or colon can be recognized. The collecting system should be entered as peripherally as possible, avoiding the larger vessels near the renal hilum. The route taken must be made through parenchyma; otherwise, perinephric leakage of urine may result. In difficult cases it may be worthwhile to place a fine needle directly into the renal pelvis from a posterior approach. Contrast medium is injected to opacify the intrarenal collecting system in order to guide a subsequent, more peripheral needle placement.

When US is used to direct the needle, a biopsy guide is helpful. The needle is inserted to the measured depth, and its tip may be visible sonographically. Tapping the needle gently or sliding the stylet in and out may make the tip position more evident. In pregnant women with urinary tract obstruction and sepsis, the entire procedure can be performed without any fluoroscopic exposure.[33]

Needle placement with fluoroscopic guidance is greatly aided by use of a C-arm. After the entry site is selected, the calyx, fluoroscope, and needle are aligned, and the needle then is precisely superimposed over its target (looking "down the barrel"). With the patient's breathing suspended at the proper moment, fluoroscopy is interrupted, and the needle is quickly and smoothly advanced into the kidney. An increase in resistance is usually felt as the needle encounters the renal capsule. Rotation of the C-arm 90° then shows the depth of placement. To prevent major arterial injury, the needle tip should not be passed deeper than midpelvis.

Alternatively, the C-arm may be rotated after the needle is aligned but before it is advanced. In this configuration, continuous fluoroscopy during needle advancement may guide the depth of insertion, often allowing the moment of entry to be recognized. If it is clear that the needle has deviated in an undesired direction, it may be left in position while a second one is placed (the "tandem needle" technique). The direction of the first needle is a gauge by which corrections in angle can be made with the second needle.

Once the needle has been inserted, the stylet is removed. If hydronephrosis is present and the collecting system has been entered, urine returns spontaneously; otherwise, a connecting tube is used to attach a contrast-filled syringe to the needle. Gentle, intermittent aspiration is applied as the needle is slowly withdrawn. When urine returns, a small amount of contrast medium is injected to confirm proper entry. If no urine is aspirated, the needle placement procedure is repeated. Contrast medium should not be introduced in the absence of fluid return because repeated injection into the soft tissues rapidly obscures the kidney. In an obstructed collecting system, a larger volume of contrast medium is injected only after removal of a similar volume of urine. Little, if any, contrast medium should be instilled if grossly infected urine returns, for fear of inducing sepsis.

A fine (0.018-inch) guidewire is passed through the needle and should advance freely into the renal pelvis. If difficulties are encountered, repeat injection of contrast medium must confirm that the needle tip is still within the collecting system. With successful guidewire passage, a tapered dilator-stiffener combination is then passed over the wire to allow a heavier, standard (0.038-inch) guidewire to be introduced. In the Cope catheter introduction system, the standard-sized J-tip wire exits a sidehole near the tip. Other systems employ a coaxial design, which provides access through an endhole. Puncture with an 18-gauge sheath needle permits introduction of a standard guidewire without the need for an intermediate step. Teflon dilators are passed serially over the larger wire before final placement of the nephrostomy catheter.

If the course of the soft tissue tract is difficult to traverse because of local scarring or because of coiling in retroperitoneal fat, a dilator must be gingerly reintroduced into the collecting system. The wire is exchanged for another extremely stiff wire for further manipulations. At times it is prudent to employ a sheath to introduce a second "safety" wire.

A nephrostomy catheter left in place should be self-retaining, such as the Cope loop catheter. Simple pigtail catheters are displaced by respiratory motion with disconcerting frequency. An exception is made when the nephrostomy is for percutaneous nephrolithotomy. In this situation a long, straight catheter with multiple sideholes directed down the ureter is preferred. Wire introduction is easier and access is more secure for subsequent tract dilatation and insertion of the working sheath. If tract dilatation is not performed in the same session, sideholes must be present in the renal pelvis to ensure adequate drainage.

Tube Management

The catheter is sutured to the patient's skin or to a stoma ring (see Chapter 20 entitled Biliary Interventions). Vital signs must be monitored frequently for several hours to detect any possible retroperitoneal bleeding. No anticoagulation should be instituted for at least 1 day following percutaneous nephrostomy (a point to remember if the patient is undergoing hemodialysis). Some degree of hematuria is to be expected after catheter placement, but even large pelvic clots lyse rapidly, and the urine normally clears within 1 to 2 days.

The nephrostomy is left to gravity drainage. Tube output should be charted, and note must be made of any postobstructive diuresis. Regular catheter flushing is not ordinarily needed. Patients may be discharged with nephrostomy catheters in place. Tube changes may be scheduled as outpatient procedures every 4 to 6 weeks, although a few patients may need more frequent attention because of particularly high rates of catheter encrustation.

Risks

Unlike biliary drainage procedures, percutaneous nephrostomies are not as often complicated by sepsis, except when pyonephrosis is present.[22] Even renal transplant patients, with their immunosuppressive medications, do not commonly suffer infections due to nephrostomy. However, sepsis arising in transplant patients can be fatal.[10] In his multiinstitutional review of complications of percutaneous nephrolithotomy and lithotripsy (perhaps the most invasive form of percutaneous nephrostomy), Lang found that 1% of patients developed perinephric abscess, and 0.1% experienced septic shock.[28] Others, nevertheless, have reported febrile complications of varying degree in 1.9% to 6%, usually in those with struvite stones.[2,34,35] O'Keeffe and colleagues have described 9 cases of severe sepsis, 6 of them fatal, in more than 700 patients undergoing endourologic procedures for stone disease.[36] All patients had been given periprocedural antibiotics. The importance of antibiotic coverage must be stressed: in high-risk patients (those with positive urinalysis and/or culture, struvite stone, or ileal loop) it can drop the incidence of clinically evident bacteremia from nephrostomy placement from 50% to 9%.[24]

Colonic perforation has been reported in 0.2% of patients, but it does not usually need surgical repair.[28,30] In cases of stone removal, nephrostomy is complicated by hydrothorax or hydropneumothorax in up to 12% of patients when the puncture is made above the twelfth rib.[27] Ureteral or pelvic perforation is not a major problem because urothelial tears heal quickly as long as the kidney is drained. However, complete ureteral transection must be treated by stent placement or surgery.

The major risk of percutaneous nephrostomy is hemorrhage. Cope and Zeit found that nephrostomy with an 18-gauge sheath needle led to life-threatening bleeding in 1% of patients.[32] Use of the fine-needle technique has decreased this risk substantially.[23] Most deaths from percutaneous nephrolithotomy are due to hemorrhage.[28] If gross blood persists longer than 1 to 2 days in drained urine, cold saline irrigation may be helpful. Active bleeding arising from the nephrostomy tract should undergo tamponade with a larger catheter or a balloon, and several days of tamponade may be definitive treatment.[37] If bleeding does not respond to conservative measures, angiography is indicated to identify a pseudoaneurysm or arteriovenous fistula, which can then be treated by embolization.[32]

STRICTURE DILATATION AND STENT PLACEMENT

Aside from malignant obstruction and renal stone disease, one of the most common problems addressed by endourologic intervention is ureteral stricture. Stricture is commonly caused by ischemia, which may be produced by a variety of factors: radiation therapy, surgical stripping of the ureter, pressure necrosis from ureteral stone, trauma, inflammatory disease, and chronic transplant rejection.[6] A vicious cycle of ischemia, scarring, and progressive ischemia is postulated as the responsible mechanism. The observed great variability in response of strictures to balloon dilatation and ureteral stent placement may be related to the residual vascular supply to the involved segment.[6]

Prognostic Factors

Devitalized ureter does not respond to dilation, but devitalized segments are difficult to recognize a priori. Lang has described a smooth pipestem appearance of the stricture with proximal ureteral dilatation as indicative of devitalization.[6] Short strictures and those involving the upper ureter are more amenable to dilatation. If narrowing has been present for less than 3 months and there is no reason to suspect devitalization, balloon dilatation has produced lasting improvement in more than 90% of attempts.[6] Renal transplant ureteral stenoses also can be treated effectively by dilatation, and an attempt is warranted no matter how long after transplantation a lesion becomes evident.[38–40]

By contrast, benign anastomotic strictures in patients with ureteral diversion to ileal loops are quite refractory to nonoperative management. About 10% of all patients having such diversions experience obstruction.[41] Although short-term positive response after balloon dilatation is found in 40% to 60% of anastomotic strictures, Shapiro and associates have noted only 16% patency at 1 year, and even later recurrences are observed.[41] Anastomotic strictures in patients treated by radiation have an especially poor prognosis. Ureteropelvic junction obstructions are also poorly responsive to balloon dilatation, and percutaneous endopyelotomy with a mechanical or electrical pyelotome is a more appropriate intervention.[42]

Technical Points

For treating strictures, a middle- to upper-pole nephrostomy lends a mechanical advantage by allowing more of a straight-line approach. Tight strictures may be traversed by a hydrophilic polymer-coated guidewire, or a Ring-Lunderquist torque guidewire. If the character of the stricture is in doubt, cytologic material can be obtained by brush biopsy through a sheath.

Initial dilatation with a tapered Teflon catheter, such as a van Andel catheter, facilitates introduction of the balloon. If necessary, a stiffer wire can be introduced through the stricture after predilatation in this manner. In some cases when only a small catheter can be advanced through the obstruction, leaving the catheter across the stricture for 7 to 10 days aids later stent placement.[43] Especially tough strictures may yield only to coaxial Teflon dilators, which are available in sizes through 18 Fr.[44] If problems are encountered with catheter coiling in renal pelvis or in the retroperitoneal soft tissues, long Teflon sheaths allow more effective transmission of force against resistant lesions. In the future, rotational wires or catheters developed for treating vascular obstruction may be modified for recanalizing occluded ureters.[45]

In cases in which a wire successfully passes the lesion but no catheter will follow, the wire may be snared in the bladder or ileal conduit by a retrograde basket or snare (with or without the aid of cystoscopy). With both ends of a guidewire in hand and held taut, almost any stricture can be passed, dilated, and stented. If the necessity of a "through-and-through" technique can be anticipated, a long exchange guidewire is used to pass the stricture. After the wire tip is retrieved, care must be taken to protect the urethra from injury by placement of a sheath over that portion of wire traversing it.

Balloons

High-pressure balloons 4 to 8 mm in diameter are best for treating ureteral strictures. Balloons up to 10 mm in size may be applied in ureteroileal anastomoses.[6] Inflations are made for 30 to 60 seconds and repeated until residual deformity disappears. Sometimes, repeat dilatation procedures several days apart with successively larger balloons are useful.[38] At the end of dilatation, the site must be stented.

Stents

The size of the stent and its duration of placement are factors not well defined for optimal prevention of stricture recurrence. Stents of 6 to 8 Fr diameter are commonly used. Much larger stents may in themselves promote ureteral ischemia.[46] The length between renal pelvis and bladder can be measured by the "bent-wire" technique: passing a wire through a catheter placed antegrade into the bladder, making one crimp in the guidewire at the external hub when its tip is at the ureterovesical junction, and making a second bend at the hub when the wire tip has been withdrawn to the renal pelvis.

Stenting catheters are either internal-external or completely internal. The simplest internal-external device is a pigtail catheter with its tip in the bladder and sideholes in the upper collecting system. Such stents have the advantage that they can easily be removed or replaced. Other designs involve a midcatheter Cope loop or other internal fixation device meant to be positioned in the renal pelvis. Two advantages of internal-external stents are the ability to exchange an occluded stent rapidly and reliably, and the possibility of maintaining access to the upper collecting system after stent removal. The latter feature permits the adequacy of ureteral patency to be tested either with a ureteral perfusion study (see the follow-

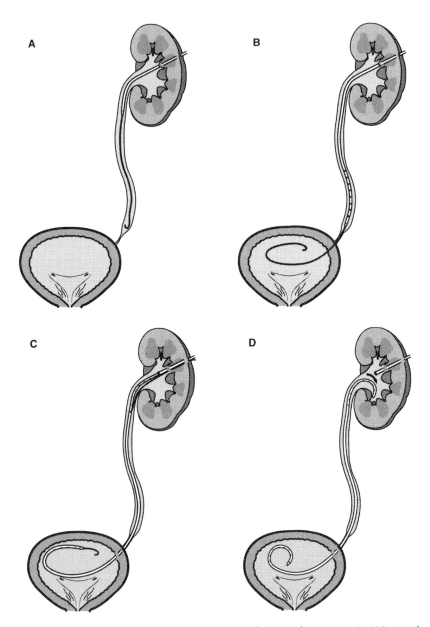

Fig. 21-2 Steps in antegrade internal ureteral stent placement. **A,** Wire and catheter are advanced through the obstruction. **B,** Guidewire is coiled within bladder and the stent is inserted (usually after balloon dilation of the stenosis). **C,** Distal portion of the stent has entered the bladder while the proximal end and pusher have reached the renal pelvis. The retaining suture is cut and removed before the guidewire is withdrawn. **D,** With removal of the inner coaxial stiffener and guidewire, the proximal stent coils in the upper collecting system, while the pusher maintains access.

ing section) or by keeping a capped nephrostomy tube in place for several days to observe if obstructive symptoms recur.

Internal stents are inserted antegrade over a guidewire with a pushing catheter (Fig. 21-2). Soft polyurethane or silicone stents are best introduced with an inner stiffener or through a sheath. Otherwise, they buckle or accordion when pushed against resistance. Some are supplied with a suture placed through the trailing end as a means of pulling the tube back if it has been advanced too far. When the leading J-tip or pigtail is in proper position, the inner stiffener is removed, but the guidewire is left in place. The suture is then cut and pulled out of the nephrostomy tract. The wire is then removed from the stent, while the pusher keeps the trailing end of the stent within the upper collecting system. As the last step, a nephrostomy tube is replaced over a second wire that is introduced either at the start of manipulations or through the pushing catheter.

The nephrostomy should be left in place for 1 to 2 days after internal stent placement to ensure that blood or debris does not cause early occlusion. Stents should not be introduced in the face of unresolved bleeding or infection. When a follow-up nephrostogram shows an absence of debris and free flow of contrast medium through the stent, the nephrostomy can be removed. Although internal stents are a lesser day-to-day burden for the patient, removal or exchange usually requires cystoscopy or repeat nephrostomy. Innovative transurethral methods may replace cystoscopy for most stent exchanges in the future (see the section on Retrograde Interventional Methods later in this chapter).

Ureteroenteric anastomotic strictures may be chronically stented by passing a wire antegrade through the stricture and out the conduit. A stenting catheter is inserted retrograde, and the end of the catheter is left in the collection bag of the conduit. In this fashion the patient's nephrostomy can be removed later, but future stent changes are easily performed over a guidewire. One must beware that repeated balloon dilatations and prolonged stent placement across an anastomotic stricture place a patient at risk for ureteroarterial fistula and massive bleeding.[47]

When used after stricture dilatation, stents are left in place for weeks to months, with 6 to 8 weeks a period often employed.[38,42] Any residual narrowing found after stent removal can be evaluated by a Whitaker test (see the following section). Stents placed for palliation of malignant obstruction are regularly changed for the duration of the patient's life. Exchanges must be performed relatively frequently (about every 4 weeks) in patients with a history of stones to prevent heavy encrustation of the stent.

Of the various materials used for plastic stents, Teflon has a low tendency for encrustation, but it is quite stiff.[48] Polyurethane is softer than polyethylene, but both materials tend to become brittle with time.[46] Silicone and Silastic stents may be difficult to introduce because of their softness and high coefficient of friction, but their long-term patency is good.[48]

Expandable metallic stents are undergoing early trials in patients with difficult-to-treat ureteral obstructions. The Wallstent has shown some promise in very tight malignant obstructions, but there is a high rate of early obstruction from edema or debris, and late overgrowth with tumor or fibrous tissue can occur.[49-51] When obstruction does arise after Wallstent placement, it is treated by coaxial placement of plastic stents. In fact, metallic stents may facilitate the insertion and subsequent exchanges of conventional plastic stents in patients with severe malignant stenoses. There is anecdotal evidence that Wallstents may provide long-term success in the nonsurgical management of narrowed ureteroenteric anastomoses, lesions notoriously resistant to simple balloon dilatation.[52] Still, until further information becomes available from well-designed studies, metallic devices should not be deployed in the ureter. As in the biliary system, such stents become embedded in mucosa and can be removed only by surgical resection.

URETERAL PERFUSION CHALLENGE (THE WHITAKER TEST)

The significance of urinary tract dilatation in a patient passing urine may be quite difficult to interpret, particularly if the patient has had previous pyeloplasty, ureteral reimplantation, or reflux. Nearly one half of all renal grafts have some degree of hydronephrosis evident in the first 3 months following transplantation.[53] Subtle obstruction may be difficult to establish, even when antegrade pyelography is performed. Residual narrowing after treatment of a ureteral stricture may or may not impede urine flow. For such situations, a urinary flow-pressure test is invaluable.

In the test formulated by Whitaker, the renal pelvis is perfused with up to 10 ml/min of fluid for 3 to 5 minutes and the pressure gradient between kidney and bladder is measured (Fig. 21-3).[54] A healthy individual shows an absolute renal pelvic pressure of less than 25 cm of water and a pressure gradient of less than 15 cm of water at maximal flow challenge. The intrarenal pressure may be measured through the infusing needle or catheter immediately after the injection ceases. Simultaneous infusion and pressure measurement require either a catheter at least 12 Fr in size or two separate needles; otherwise, the resistance within the infusing system elevates the measured pressure. To this end double-lumen needles and small double-lumen catheters have been used to provide continuous pressure monitoring.[55,56] In any event, a Foley catheter should be in place, because high absolute intrarenal pressure may simply reflect lower tract obstruction or a hypertonic bladder.[54]

Before ureteral perfusion is begun, baseline manometry is performed. If a large gradient is found at rest or if the resting pressure within the kidney

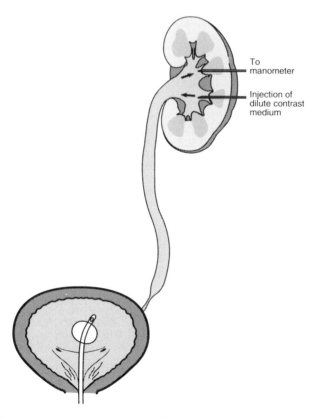

To
manometer

Injection of
dilute contrast
medium

Fig. 21-3 The double-needle ureteral perfusion (Whitaker) test. A Foley
catheter allows decompression of the bladder. One needle is used to perfuse the
kidney and the other provides constant monitoring of pressure. Ideally, bladder
pressure is also measured to determine the gradient across the ureter. When a single needle is used, the pressure is obtained immediately after injection ceases. If
a large (12 Fr or larger) nephrostomy catheter is in place, a manometer may be
used in series to measure pressures during injection.

approaches 30 cm of water, no perfusion test is needed. Normal ureteral
flow is between 0.25 and 0.50 ml/min, but the unobstructed ureter can
accommodate a much higher flow when necessary.[57] Infusion by automatic injector may be started at a low rate, such as 4 ml/min for 5 minutes,
with repeat infusion at a higher rate only if abnormal pressures are not
elicited. The fluid infused is 30% iodinated contrast medium, which allows
fluoroscopic observation of the amount of collecting system distention
present. The kidney should not be exposed to pressures above 30 cm of
water because of the risk of pyelotubular backflow and sepsis.[57] A gradient of 15 cm of water or more indicates significant obstruction. If no

obstruction is found with the bladder decompressed, the challenge should be repeated with the Foley catheter clamped to detect any functional obstruction.

It should be noted that, just as not all dilated renal collecting systems are obstructed, not all obstructed kidneys are hydronephrotic. Perhaps as many as 5% of patients with urinary tract obstruction show no dilation.[58] Lack of dilation may be due to tumor encasement or retroperitoneal fibrosis, but in some patients there is no obvious cause. A Whitaker test may be indicated when nondilated obstructive uropathy is suspected, followed by placement of a nephrostomy tube if the test is positive.

RENAL STONE REMOVAL

About 1 patient in every 1000 hospitalized is suffering from renal stone disease, but 60% of stones pass spontaneously.[59] The other 40% require intervention, which until fairly recently meant open pyelolithotomy, a major surgical procedure requiring prolonged convalescence. The first percutaneous nephrostomy for stone removal was performed in 1976.[60] Since that time, open surgery has been largely displaced by percutaneous, retrograde ureteral, and, more recently, ESWL treatments. Not only are the newer methods less invasive but also they reduce the hospitalization and recovery periods.

The ESWL procedure may now be applied to more than 80% of renal and upper ureteral stones.[60] However, percutaneous nephrolithotomy and lithotripsy are still indicated for large (over 3 cm in diameter), staghorn, infected, or cystine stones; for patients with obstructed outflow; for children; and for massively obese patients.[60] Some patients with staghorn calculi and little residual function in the affected kidney are best treated by nephrectomy.

Calcium oxalate is the sole or major component of more than 80% of urinary stones.[59,61] Other calculi are composed of apatite, struvite (magnesium ammonium phosphate), urate, cystine, or organic matrix.[61] As noted, cystine stones respond poorly to ESWL. Most staghorn calculi are composed of struvite, which forms in the presence of urea-splitting bacteria such as *Proteus mirabilis*.[62] Struvite stones are more difficult to treat and, being infected, are more likely to cause septic complications. Because percutaneous stone removal yields up to 84% stone-free rates at hospital discharge for infected calculi (a rate much better than ESWL), it is the procedure of choice for such patients.[60] Complete stone removal is important, for only 14% of patients with no residual fragments after open nephrolithotomy have recurrence, compared to a rate of 70% for those with some stone material left behind.[63] Chemolysis can sometimes be used to dissolve retained fragments (see the section on Chemodissolution later in this chapter).

The tools of percutaneous extraction include various types of wire baskets; steerable catheters; Fogarty, occlusion, and other balloon catheters; US and electromechanical lithotriptors; Randall forceps; nephroscopes; and ureteroscopes.[64] Ureteral occlusion balloons are helpful for preventing migration and impaction of intrarenal stones during manipulations. Most percutaneous procedures require dilation of the tract to 24 to 30 Fr, which can be accomplished either by passage of a set of fascial dilators or by use of a balloon catheter designed for the purpose. A large Teflon sheath is introduced, through which endoscopes and other instruments are passed. Stones nearly 1 cm in diameter can be removed through a 30 Fr sheath. Even larger stones have been removed intact through percutaneous access.[2] Tract dilation may be performed immediately after percutaneous nephrostomy or as a separate delayed procedure. Dilatation is performed with the patient under general or epidural anesthesia. After a large nephrostomy tract has been created, a catheter of appropriate size must be left in place for at least several days.

If there is a tear in the urothelium, stone fragments may be lost into the perinephric soft tissues. This occurrence is usually innocuous, but an infected fragment may cause an abscess.[28] Percutaneous nephrolithotomy and lithotripsy have a major complication rate of 3% or less in experienced hands.[2,28,65]

Stones in Calyceal Diverticula

Calyceal diverticula are uncommon, but the urinary stasis within a diverticulum promotes infection and stone formation. Symptomatic calyceal diverticula pose special problems for minimally invasive treatment. Because of the very narrow communication of diverticulum with renal collecting system, ESWL is usually not adequate for clearing stones, despite effective fragmentation.[66] Because of its low morbidity, ESWL is still recommended as the first treatment, but most patients require direct percutaneous puncture of the diverticulum. When the collection is entered, attempts should be made to find and cannulate its neck. Cannulation may be aided by injection of methylene blue through a retrograde ureteral catheter.[67] Passage of the communication not only permits more secure access to the urinary collecting system, but after stone removal the neck of the diverticulum may be dilated and stented. When this is not possible, the diverticulum may be obliterated by electrofulguration. Procedures involving calyceal diverticula not only are technically demanding but also have higher morbidity, primarily from bleeding.[66]

Ureteral Stones

Just as methods for percutaneous extraction of ureteral stones were being perfected, with removal rates of 90% to 100% attained, ESWL came into use.[68,69] Retrograde ureteroscopic techniques also developed apace, further reducing the hospitalization and recovery periods after ureteral stone removal.[70] Presently, percutaneous access is rarely needed.

When nephrostomy is performed for ureteral stones, it often must be through an intercostal approach into an upper or middle calyx.[27] This provides the closest to a straight-line approach possible to the ureter. The potential for pleural complications from high puncture must be appreciated. Because retrograde methods alone are almost uniformly effective for removing ureteral stones within the pelvis, percutaneous nephrostomy is typically applied only to mid- and upper-ureteral calculi.

The presence of a retrograde ureteral catheter greatly facilitates stone removal. The retrograde catheter can be used to push or flush the stone back into the renal pelvis. Flushing is most effective when it is performed through an occlusion balloon catheter. With a nephrostomy in place, Hunter and associates have even power-injected dilute contrast medium retrograde at rates up to 25 ml/sec for 2 seconds with no complications and good results in 31 patients![69] If flushing does not budge the stone, a flexible ureteroscope is introduced to guide the application of forceps or stone baskets.[69] Some stones become embedded in mucosa and may be very difficult to extract, but a steerable catheter or soft wire may sometimes be used to pry off such a calculus.[69] A safety wire or catheter placed past the stone interferes with retrieval attempts by means of a basket.[14] Ureteral spasm can be a difficult problem, and spasm does not respond reliably to instillation of nitroglycerin or other medications. Complications needing surgical intervention are rare.[68,69] If edema causes obstruction or if ureteral injury is suspected, a stent should be left in place.

Contact Lithotripsy
When stones are too large to be removed through a dilated percutaneous tract, they must be shattered. Shock waves may be directly applied by a variety of generators, from electrohydraulic and US lithotriptors to laser contact fibers.[59,71] Ultrasonic lithotriptors have the disadvantage of being rigid devices that cannot be directed around curves. Despite this drawback, they have gained wide acceptance and can be used with great success.

Because of the inflexibility of US lithotriptors and the limited flexibility of conventional nephroscopes, the entry site of the percutaneous tract may be critical to success. The approach to a simple renal pelvic stone is straightforward, but in many cases a calyceal stone can be removed only when that calyx is entered directly. Although some investigators prefer to "trap" a calyceal stone by entering at the infundibular junction central to it, others insist that the point of entry must be within the calyx, peripheral to the stone itself.[20,23] Upper-pole stones, multiple stones, and staghorn calculi may be best approached through a lower-pole calyx.[20] Whatever the chosen approach, a catheter should be placed down the ureter, because access is much more likely to be lost during tract dilatation if the wire cannot be advanced beyond the upper collecting system.

Because a large volume of fluid is perfused during lithotripsy, use of a sheath is imperative. A sheath allows the flush solution to be vented efficiently and keeps intrarenal pressure down.[72] It also makes hydrothorax less likely when the approach is intercostal.[27] The input-output balance of infusate must be carefully watched to prevent fluid intoxication of the patient from an unrecognized urothelial tear.[28] Rarely, decreased return of infusate may be the first indication of colonic perforation.[30]

Staghorn calculus, a prime remaining indication for percutaneous lithotripsy, presents a special challenge. Multiple nephrostomies in the treated kidney are commonly needed for effective stone removal.[62] As already mentioned, staghorn calculi are typically infected and present a higher risk of complication. Transfusion is often needed, although only 2.5% of patients have had bleeding severe enough to warrant angiography.[62] Coleman and colleagues have recommended that all patients undergoing percutaneous lithotripsy have at least 2 units of blood typed and cross-matched prior to the procedure.[20]

Contact lithotripsy can be extremely successful when performed by an experienced team as either a one-stage or two-stage procedure. Stone-free hospital discharge rates of 96% or greater have been achieved.[60,61] Serious vascular complications may arise in up to 3% and represent the primary risk of the procedure.[65] Large catheters not only allow residual fragments to be flushed from the renal collecting system but also tamponade the tract and promote healing. Because major bleeding can occur on removal of the catheter, removal should be performed only in the hospital with a safety wire in place. A balloon catheter can be expeditiously inserted over the guidewire and inflated to control hemorrhage. When such bleeding does occur, it usually resolves with replacement of a large nephrostomy catheter for several more days. If this course of action fails, arteriography and possible embolization are indicated.

Extracorporeal Shock Wave Lithotripsy

Developed in Germany in the early 1980s, ESWL sharply focuses electrically-generated shock waves onto a renal or ureteral stone. The change in impedance between soft tissue and stone results in shearing and tearing forces, which disintegrate the stone through repeated application. A maximum of 1500 to 2400 separate shocks are administered in a single treatment session.[1,73] First-generation instruments produce energy in a water bath, with a condensor discharge vaporizing water to generate the requisite shock wave.[74] Patients are immersed in the bath and are heavily anesthetized for treatment by these devices. The stone is placed in the shock wave focus under the observation of orthogonally oriented fluoroscopes, and treatment is administered with electrocardiographic (ECG) gating. Newer designs employ piezoelectrical ceramic elements, with stone positioning provided by US. Shock wave generation may be less efficient with the latter technique, but it is also less painful and freed from the constraints of a large water bath and ECG triggering.[9]

The ESWL procedure has been applied with excellent results in solitary small pelvic stones, requiring an average 4-day hospitalization and yielding a stone-free rate of more than 90%.[74] In less highly selected patients with intrarenal calculi, long-term stone-free rates of 73% are typical, and many of the remaining patients have only very small residual fragments.[63] Apatite and cystine stones, as well as calculi in the lower-pole calyces, show the worst stone-free rates after ESWL, 60% or less.[63] About 1 of every 10 ESWL patients requires retrograde ureteral manipulations, stent placement, or percutaneous nephrostomy to complete treatment.[1,14] Larger stones are prone to cause acute obstruction by forming a sandy cast of the ureter (Steinstrasse). Balloon dilatation of the ureterovesical junction, followed by forceful antegrade flushing, has been effective for alleviating such obstruction.[14] Prophylactic stent placement may be warranted for bulky stones. As noted earlier, ESWL should not be used as the first treatment for staghorn or infected calculi, but it may be indicated after a debulking session of percutaneous lithotripsy. Most proximal and mid-ureteral stones can be cleared by ESWL, but retrograde ureteroscopic techniques are quite effective for distal calculi.

An issue of some debate is the long-term effect of ESWL on renal parenchyma. Therapy with ESWL has resulted in extremely low mortality, and large series have been treated without the loss of a single kidney.[63,74] Interstitial edema and transient gross hematuria are common side effects of ESWL. Although the incidence of subcapsular hematoma has been cited as low as 0.6%, others have detected subcapsular fluid in 24% to 31% of patients.[73,75] A small, persistent drop in the percentage of effective renal plasma flow to the treated kidney has been found in patients 17 to 21 months after ESWL in one study,[76] and glomerular filtration rates dropped an average of 22% in patients with solitary kidneys followed at least 2 years post-ESWL in another.[77]

The most disturbing clinical finding has been new hypertension in 8% of patients within 1 year of stone treatment.[76] Liedl and colleagues have failed to find such an effect in hundreds of patients followed a mean of 3.6 years, with the observed incidence of new hypertension in their patients matching that expected with aging alone.[73] A possible reason for this discrepancy is the lower number of shocks administered to their patients, and they recommend that 1500 shocks be the maximum administered at a single session. In animal studies a positive correlation between the number of shocks and microscopic renal damage has been documented.[78] It should also be noted that patients with renal stone disease tend to have a higher baseline incidence of hypertension than the general population.[73]

Chemodissolution

Only a small number of renal stones can be dissolved by local perfusion of a solvent. Urate stones are amenable to treatment by sodium bicarbonate, and cystine stones have been perfused with acetylcysteine.[15] Struvite stones may respond to hemiacidrin, an electrolyte solution. Adequate outflow is essential for all forms of chemodissolution therapy. If ureteral obstruction is present, the nephrostomy tube should be a sump catheter, or a second percutaneous nephrostomy must be placed as a vent.[15] Infusion begins with a saline challenge to establish a maximum flow tolerance before pain or pressure elevation above 30 cm of water supervenes. Solvent infusion is then started at half the maximum tolerated rate and slowly increased. Dretler and Pfister have set an arbitrary goal of 120 ml/hour for hemiacidrin infusion.[15] The great majority of properly selected stones dissolve, but infusions of 20 to 30 days are typical! For this reason, chemodissolution is now limited to resolution of residual fragments after ESWL or percutaneous treatment.

URETERAL FISTULAE AND URINOMAS

Percutaneous methods are well suited to the treatment of many ureterocutaneous or ureterovisceral fistulae, as well as urinomas.[79] Fistulae may be due to trauma or surgery, and surgical repair leads to nephrectomy in 20% and mortality of 10%.[7] Simple percutaneous decompression of the upper collecting system may leave a ureteral stricture, so an internal-external stenting catheter is recommended, as long as no sideholes are located near the fistula. Long-term success has been reported as 70% in resolving fistulae of benign origin, with even better results when fistulae are treated promptly.[7] Urine leakage from renal transplants is somewhat less likely to respond, perhaps due to rejection and the possibility of ureteral necrosis.[7,10]

Leakage caused by malignant disease or related to radiation therapy is harder to treat. Balloon occlusion of the ureter has been helpful in some cases, but inflation pressure must be kept low to prevent urothelial necrosis.[14] Some investigators have resorted to electrofulguration or special methods of percutaneous clip placement to effect permanent ureteral occlusion.[80,81] In one large series Schild, Günther, and Thelen compared metallic coils combined with tissue adhesive (cyanoacrylate) to detachable balloons.[82] Although the occlusions produced by the balloons were more reliable and long-lasting, recurrent leakage was still seen in nearly one third of patients. Others have placed multiple Gianturco coils and gelatin sponge (Gelfoam) with success, but the results must be confirmed with wider experience.[83]

Bush and Mayo recently described a simple modification of a nephroureteral stenting catheter (internal-external stent) that can be used to provide total urinary diversion without placing a permanent occluding device into the ureter.[84] The ureteral portion of the catheter is heated over steam and crimped with smooth forceps. The crimped portion is cut and carefully trimmed to form a flap valve that allows exchange over a guidewire but prevents urine flow distally. Further experience is also needed to gauge the effectiveness of this approach.

RETROGRADE INTERVENTIONAL METHODS

Hawkins and associates have developed a retrograde method for nephrostomy creation with a coaxial Teflon catheter system and a long, sheathed 20- or 21-gauge needle.[16] The system is directed into a posterior calyx, and the needle—or a very sharp, stiff "rocket" wire (of an alloy developed by the National Aeronautics and Space Administration)—is advanced until it punctures skin. Caudad angulation can be created and controlled by pushing the guiding catheter cephalad. The technique is used for percutaneous stone removal and is particularly helpful in obese patients and nondilated collecting systems.[16]

Effectiveness of retrograde transvesical ureteral catheterization can be greatly enhanced through the collaboration of radiologist and urologist in difficult cases.[17] Amendola and colleagues have successfully assisted 168 of 180 attempted retrograde ureteral stent placements, ureteral dilatations, and brush biopsies by employing fluoroscopy, guidewires, and long sheaths to traverse obstructions and prevent wire or catheter from coiling within the bladder. The patient is brought to the radiologic interventional suite directly from cystoscopy with a partially placed ureteral catheter left in situ. Fluoroscopically guided retrograde interventions have been used in 5% of all patients undergoing ESWL at the University of Pennsylvania and have obviated the need for percutaneous nephrostomy in many cases.[17] Failure of such intervention is more likely in the face of distal ureteral stenosis.

Fluoroscopically guided internal stent changes are possible without cystoscopy or general anesthesia with the use of angled catheters, sheaths, and snares placed per urethra.[19] Stents are snared and carefully withdrawn, so that one end exits the urethra while the other remains within the ureter. A sheath or guidewire is used to complete the exchange. Babel and Winterkorn have published early experience with de novo catheterization of obstructed ureters by similar means.[18] Probing the lateral margin of the transureteric ridge (the crossbar of the T seen on minimal distention of the bladder with dilute contrast medium) with a hydrophilic guidewire resulted in successful catheterization in five of seven ureters approached. Because of the shorter urethra, retrograde methods are more easily applied in women.[18,19]

Related techniques can be employed for the cannulation of ureters anastomosed to an ileal conduit.[85] Only those ureters showing reflux on a loop injection of contrast medium are candidates for retrograde catheterization. A curved angiographic catheter with a guidewire advanced slightly beyond its tip is placed as far into the conduit as possible. While contrast medium is injected through a Foley catheter occluding the distal loop, the catheter is slowly withdrawn. When the ureteral anastomosis is engaged, catheter and guidewire are advanced. By means of a stiff wire, such as the Ring-Lunderquist torque guidewire, and Teflon sheaths, even stenotic ureters may be cannulated. Retrograde cannulation under fluoroscopy tends to be less tedious and frustrating than endoscopic catheterization.[85]

RENAL CYST PUNCTURE

When US and CT first provided a cross-sectional view of the kidney, there was great concern about the possible association of malignant neoplasm with renal cysts. Between 2% and 7% of cysts had been described as coexistent with carcinoma.[86] Guided percutaneous cyst puncture became a popular procedure to determine the character of a given cystic lesion. In the past decade, the imaging characteristics of uncomplicated benign renal cysts have been defined with high diagnostic accuracy, and the high incidence of cysts in the normal elderly population has become better appreciated. However, 5% to 8% of renal masses still have an indeterminate nature by noninvasive studies alone.[87] It is for such lesions, as well as for cysts causing symptoms, that percutaneous puncture is indicated.

A fine needle is guided into the lesion by US or fluoroscopic guidance (when the lesion is larger than 3 cm). Aspirated fluid should be straw-colored and crystal clear, reflecting the proximal tubular origin of a simple cyst.[87] Laboratory studies to be performed include cytologic study, culture, and lactic dehydrogenase, protein, and fat content determinations. High fat levels are characteristic of neoplasm, whereas elevated fluid protein may be the result of tumor or inflammation.[87] After fluid aspiration, iodinated contrast medium and air may be injected, with filming in cross-table prone, supine, decubitus, and upright positions for detection of any mural nodules or irregularities. Large, simple cysts do not resolve by simple aspiration, and they may be treated by injection of a sclerosing agent. This is best done through a pigtail catheter. Contrast material is injected to exclude the presence of any fluid leakage or communication with the renal collecting system. After evacuation of the cyst contents, absolute alcohol is instilled to about one quarter of the original cyst volume. The patient is rolled to expose as much of the cyst wall as possible before the alcohol is aspirated after 5 minutes.[87] Such a procedure has resulted in late recurrence in only 9%.[88] Other approaches include povidone-iodine instillation or tract dilatation to give access to urethral resectoscopes and electrofulguration.[89,90]

BALLOON DILATATION OF THE PROSTATIC URETHRA

Most men over 50 years of age have benign prostatic hypertrophy (BPH). The conventional mode of treatment has been transurethral prostatic resection. Intraurethral balloons have been investigated for the alleviation of urethral obstruction from prostatic hypertrophy.[91] Dilation is performed only after cystoscopy, voiding cystourethrography, and transrectal sonography. Retrograde urethrography is used to mark the site of the external urinary sphincter, and a 25-mm balloon dilates the urethra proximal to the external sphincter. The balloon is left inflated for 10 minutes, followed by repeat urethrography. Transient hematuria and dysuria are common, and a Council catheter is left in place for 24 hours. Early success has been good, with median lobe hypertrophy responsible for cases of failure.[91] The method does not allow histologic examination of prostatic fragments for possible carcinoma in situ. Although the technique can provide symptomatic relief with low morbidity, the effect is generally temporary, and most patients have recurrent complaints by 18 months.[92]

SELECTED RADIOLOGIC METHODS IN MALE INFERTILITY

Vasogenic Impotence

Vascular diseases have been increasingly recognized as a cause of impotence. Noninvasive tests, such as the penile-brachial systolic index; nocturnal penile tumescence; and penile rigidity have been used to search for arterial insufficiency. Duplex sonography has also been employed as a screening measure.[93] Most men with significant aortoiliac occlusive disease are impotent, and standard pelvic angiography will document this.[94] More distal occlusive disease is more difficult to demonstrate, requiring selective internal iliac arteriography.

The use of low-osmolarity contrast media and vasodilatation with intraarterial nitroglycerin (300 µg in 10 ml of saline injected slowly immediately before arteriography) with or without papaverine (30 to 50 mg) has produced much better studies than previously possible.[94] Alternatively, angiography may be performed after intracavernosal injection of papaverine 60 mg and phentolamine 1 mg with a tourniquet applied to the base of the penis until filming is complete.[93] The internal pudendal and penile arteries are best visualized with the opposite posterior oblique projection of the internal iliac being injected (i.e., left posterior oblique projection for the right internal iliac study, with the penis draped over the left thigh), using magnification technique, injection of 4 to 6 ml/seconds for 36 ml, and filming over 32 seconds.[94] Filling of the penile, cavernosal, and dorsal penile arteries should be observed. If one side is found to be entirely normal, examination of the opposite side is unnecessary. Only one side need be revascularized for the relief of arterial impotence.

Dynamic cavernosography is a means of evaluating impotence resulting from venous leakage. The corpora cavernosa are punctured with 19-gauge needles about midshaft, halfway between the dorsal and ventral surfaces.[95] Because there are communications between the corpora through the septum, only one needle need be perfused, and pressure measurements may be obtained through the other. Infusion of dilute low-osmolality contrast begins at 40 ml/min and is increased until the penis appears erect.[95] Erection is produced in a normal penis with a flow of 80 to 120 ml/min and is maintained by less than half that flow. Measured pressure should attain at least 80 mm Hg. Venous leakage is seen as filling of the veins of the prostatic plexus during erection or high infusion rates.

Direct injection of papaverine (30 to 60 mg) into the corpora cavernosa stimulates normal erectile physiology, decreasing the infusion rates needed to elicit erection.[96] Corpora cavernosography is repeated 10 minutes after injection of papaverine. Intracavernous papaverine is not absolutely necessary for the diagnosis of impotence due to venous leakage, and the use of the drug does present a risk for thrombosis and priapism.[95]

Varicoceles

Varicocele is present in 4% of adult males and in nearly 40% of men with complaints of infertility.[97] It may adversely affect fertility by elevating scrotal temperature or by poorly understood effects of stasis and hypoxia. Although subclinical varicocele may be suspected by sonography or thermography, the diagnosis is made by selective internal spermatic vein venography. The left internal spermatic vein, which empties into the left renal vein, is more likely to be incompetent than the right, which is a direct tributary of the inferior vena cava. Reflux of contrast material beyond the level of the mid-lumbar spine is abnormal, and unilateral varicocele may be responsible for diminished fertility.[98]

Definition of the venous anatomy in varicocele is important because two thirds of patients show venous duplications or communicating retroperitoneal veins.[98] Anatomic anomalies are responsible for the 15% to 20% incidence of recurrence after surgical venous ligation. Full venographic delineation of anatomy permits rational planning of treatment, including selective catheter embolization or venous sclerotherapy. Long-term follow-up has shown clinical recurrence in less than 10% of those managed by transcatheter occlusive therapy.[98,99]

REFERENCES

1. Hulbert JC: The role of endourologic procedures in relation to extracorporeal shock wave lithotripsy. *Semin Intervent Radiol* 1987; 4:50–52.
2. Ohlsén H, Kinn AC: Percutaneous extraction of upper urinary calculi under fluoroscopic control: Still a valuable complement to ESWL. *Scand J Urol Nephrol* 1993; 27:311–321.
3. Segura JW, Preminger GM, Assimos DG, et al: Nephrolithiasis clinical guidelines panel summary report on the management of staghorn calculi. *J Urol* 1994; 151:1648–1651.
4. Keidan RD, Greenberg RE, Hoffman JP, Weese JL: Is percutaneous nephrostomy for hydronephrosis appropriate in patients with advanced cancer? *Am J Surg* 1988; 156:206–208.
5. Watkinson AF, A'Hern RP, Jones A, et al: The role of percutaneous nephrostomy in malignant urinary tract obstruction. *Clin Radiol* 1993; 47:32–35.
6. Lang EK: Percutaneous management of ureteral strictures. *Semin Intervent Radiol* 1987; 4:79–89.
7. Maillet PJ, Pelle-Francoz D, Leriche A, et al: Fistulas of the upper urinary tract: Percutaneous management. *J Urol* 1987; 138:1382–1385.
8. Badlani G, Eshghi M, Smith AD: Percutaneous surgery for ureteropelvic junction obstruction (endopyelotomy): Technique and early results. *J Urol* 1986; 135:26–28.
9. Orihuela E, Smith AD: Percutaneous treatment of transitional cell carcinoma of the upper urinary tract. *Urol Clin North Am* 1988; 15:425 431.
10. Bennett LN, Voegli DR, Crummy AB, et al: Urologic complications following renal transplantation: Role of interventional radiologic procedures. *Radiology* 1986; 160:531–536.
11. Doemeny JM, Banner MP, Shapiro MJ, et al: Percutaneous extraction of renal fungus ball. *Am J Roentgenol* 1988; 150:1331–1332.
12. Bell DA, Rose SC, Starr NK, et al: Percutaneous nephrostomy for nonoperative management of fungal urinary tract infections. *J Vasc Interv Radiol* 1993; 4:311–315.
13. Zagoria RJ, Hodge RG, Dyer RB, Routh WD: Percutaneous nephrostomy for treatment of intractable hemorrhagic cystitis. *J Urol* 1993; 149:1449–1451.
14. Gordon RL, Banner MP, Pollack HM: Selected endourologic techniques. *Radiol Clin North Am* 1986; 24:633–649.
15. Dretler SP, Pfister RC: Primary dissolution therapy of struvite calculi. *J Urol* 1984; 131:861–863.
16. Hawkins IF Jr, Hunter P, Leal G, et al: Retrograde nephrostomy for stone removal: Combined cystoscopic/percutaneous technique. *Am J Roentgenol* 1984; 143:299–304.

17. Amendola MA, Banner MP, Pollack HM, Gordon RL: Fluoroscopically guided pyeloureteral interventions by using a perurethral transvesical approach. *Am J Roentgenol* 1989; 152:97–102.
18. Babel SG, Winterkorn KG: Retrograde catheterization of the ureter without cystoscopic assistance: Preliminary experience. *Radiology* 1993; 187:547–549.
19. De Baere T, Denys A, Pappas P, et al: Ureteral stents: Exchange under fluoroscopic control as an effective alternative to cystoscopy. *Radiology* 1994; 190:887–889.
20. Coleman CC, Castañeda-Zuñiga W, Miller R, et al: A logical approach to renal stone removal. *Am J Roentgenol* 1984; 143:609–615.
21. Janetschek G, Kunzel KH: Percutaneous nephrolithotomy in horseshoe kidneys: Applied anatomy and clinical experience. *Br J Urol* 1988; 62:117–122.
22. Spies JB, Rosen RJ, Lebowitz AS: Antibiotic prophylaxis in vascular and interventional radiology: A rational approach. *Radiology* 1988; 166:381–387.
23. LeRoy AJ, May GR, Bender CE, et al: Percutaneous nephrostomy for stone removal. *Radiology* 1984; 151:607–612.
24. Cochran ST, Barbaric ZL, Lee JJ, Kashfian P: Percutaneous nephrostomy tube placement: An outpatient procedure? *Radiology* 1991; 179:843–847.
25. Lind LJ, Mushlin PS: Sedation, analgesia, and anesthesia for radiologic procedures. *Cardiovasc Intervent Radiol* 1987; 10:247–253.
26. Coleman CC, Castañeda-Zuñiga WR, Amplatz K: Renal anatomy for uroradiologic interventions. *Semin Intervent Radiol* 1987; 4:1–9.
27. Picus D, Weyman PJ, Clayman RV, McClennan BL: Intercostal-space nephrostomy for percutaneous stone removal. *Am J Roentgenol* 1986; 147:393–397.
28. Lang E: Percutaneous nephrostolithotomy and lithotripsy: A multi-institutional survey of complications. *Radiology* 1987; 162:25–30.
29. Sampaio FJB, Aragao AHM: Anatomical relationship between the intrarenal arteries and the kidney collecting system. *J Urol* 1990; 143:679–681.
30. LeRoy AJ, Williams HJ Jr, Bender CE, et al: Colon perforation following percutaneous nephrostomy and renal calculus removal. *Radiology* 1985; 155:83–85.
31. Hopper KD, Chantelois AE: The retrorenal spleen: Implications for percutaneous left renal invasive procedures. *Invest Radiol* 1989; 42:592–595.
32. Cope C, Zeit RM: Pseudoaneurysms after nephrostomy. *Am J Roentgenol* 1982; 139:255–261.
33. vanSonnenberg E, Casola G, Talner LB, et al: Symptomatic renal obstruction or urosepsis during pregnancy: Treatment by sonographically guided percutaneous nephrostomy. *Am J Roentgenol* 1992; 158:91–94.
34. Hussain S, Ahmed I: Nephrostomy revisited: A cost-effective approach. *J Vasc Interv Radiol* 1994; 5:394.
35. Lee WJ, Patel U, Patel S, Pillari GP: Emergency percutaneous nephrostomy: Results and complications. *J Vasc Interv Radiol* 1994; 5:135–139.
36. O'Keeffe NK, Mortimer AJ, Sambrook PA, Rao PN: Severe sepsis following percutaneous or endoscopic procedures for urinary tract stones. *Br J Urol* 1993; 72:277–283.
37. Henriksson C, Geterud K, Pettersson S, Zachrisson BF: Use of a tamponade catheter in the bleeding nephrostolithotomy track. *Scand J Urol Nephrol Suppl* 1991; 138:15–17.

38. Voegeli DR, Crummy AB, McDermott JC, Jensen SR: Percutaneous dilation of ureteral strictures in renal transplant patients. *Radiology* 1988; 169:185–188.

39. Streem SB, Novick AC, Steinmuller DR, et al: Long-term efficacy of ureteral dilatation for transplant ureteral stenosis. *J Urol* 1988; 140:32–35.

40. Smith TP, Hunter DW, Letourneau JG, et al: Urinary obstruction in renal transplants: Diagnosis by antegrade pyelography and results of percutaneous treatment. *Am J Roentgenol* 1988; 151:507–510.

41. Shapiro MJ, Banner MP, Amendola MA, et al: Balloon catheter dilatation of ureteroenteric strictures: Long-term results. *Radiology* 1988; 168:385–387.

42. Lee WJ, Badlani GH, Karlin GS, Smith AD: Treatment of ureteropelvic strictures with percutaneous pyelotomy: Experience in 62 patients. *Am J Roentgenol* 1988; 151:515–518.

43. Gray R, Rooney M, Grosman H: Indwelling angiographic catheters to facilitate placement of ureteric stents. *Can Assoc Radiol J* 1991; 42:127–129.

44. Castañeda F, Castañeda-Zuñiga WR, Hunter DW, et al: New developments in endourology. *Semin Intervent Radiol* 1987; 4:22–25.

45. Uflacker R, Wholey MH: A new low-speed, rotational atherolytic device for ureteral recanalization. *Am J Roentgenol* 1988; 151:1157–1158.

46. Mitty HA, Train JS, Dan SJ: Placement of ureteral stents by antegrade and retrograde techniques. *Radiol Clin North Am* 1986; 24:587–600.

47. Babel SG, McDermott JC, Goldrath DE, et al: Uretero-arterial fistula after balloon dilatation and stent placement: Case report and review of the literature. *J Intervent Radiol* 1988; 3:135–138.

48. Brazzini A, Castañeda F, Castañeda-Zuñiga WR, et al: Urostent designs. *Semin Intervent Radiol* 1987; 4:26–35.

49. Lugmayr H, Pauer W: Self-expanding metal stents for palliative treatment of malignant ureteral obstruction. *Am J Roentgenol* 1992; 159:1091–1094.

50. Flueckiger F, Lammer J, Klein GE, et al: Malignant ureteral obstruction: Preliminary results of treatment with metallic self-expandable stents. *Radiology* 1993; 186:169–173.

51. vanSonnenberg E, D'Agostino HB, O'Laoide R, et al: Malignant ureteral obstruction: Treatment with metal stents. Technique, results, and observations with percutaneous intraluminal US. *Radiology* 1994; 191:765–768.

52. Reinberg Y, Ferral H, Gonzalez R, et al: Intraureteral metallic self-expanding endoprosthesis (Wallstent) in the treatment of difficult ureteral strictures. *J Urol* 1994; 151:1619–1622.

53. Kashi SH, Irving HC, Sadek SA: Does the Whitaker test add to antegrade pyelography in the investigation of collecting system dilatation in renal allografts? *Br J Radiol* 1993; 66:877–881.

54. Whitaker RH: An evaluation of 170 diagnostic pressure flow studies of the upper urinary tract. *J Urol* 1979; 121:602–604.

55. Epstein DH, Hunter DW, Coleman CC, et al: Double-lumen needle for percutaneous ureteral pressure-flow studies. *Radiology* 1989; 172:569–570.

56. Diament MJ, Koenig JC: Double-lumen central venous catheter for percutaneous ureteral perfusion studies. *Radiology* 1991; 181:286–287.

57. Jaffe RB, Middleton AW Jr: Whitaker test: Differentiation of obstructive from nonobstructive uropathy. *Am J Roentgenol* 1980; 134:9–15.

58. Spital A, Valvo JR, Segal AJ: Nondilated obstructive uropathy. *Urology* 1988; 31:478–482.
59. Dretler SP: Laser lithotripsy: A review of 20 years of research and clinical applications. *Lasers Surg Med* 1988; 8:341–356.
60. Segura JW: The role of percutaneous surgery in renal and ureteral stone removal. *J Urol* 1989; 141:780–781.
61. Segura JW, Patterson DE, LeRoy AJ, et al: Percutaneous lithotripsy. *J Urol* 1983; 130:1051–1054.
62. Lee WJ, Snyder JA, Smith AD: Staghorn calculi: Endourologic management in 120 patients. *Radiology* 1987; 165:85–88.
63. Graff J, Diedrichs W, Schulze H: Long-term followup in 1,003 extracorporeal shock wave lithotripsy patients. *J Urol* 1988; 140:479–483.
64. Castañeda-Zuñiga WR, Clayman R, Smith A, et al: Nephrostolithotomy: Percutaneous technique for urinary calculus removal. *Am J Roentgenol* 1982; 139:721–726.
65. Clayman RV, Surya V, Hunter D, et al: Renal vascular complications associated with the percutaneous removal of renal calculi. *J Urol* 1984; 132:228–230.
66. Hendrikx AJM, Bierkens AF, Bos R, et al: Treatment of stones in caliceal diverticula: Extracorporeal shock wave lithotripsy versus percutaneous nephrolitholapaxy. *Br J Urol* 1992; 70:478–482.
67. Ellis JH, Patterson SK, Sonda LP, et al: Stones and infection in renal caliceal diverticula: Treatment with percutaneous procedures. *Am J Roentgenol* 1991; 156:995–1000.
68. Bush WH, Brannen GE, Lewis GP, Burnett LL: Upper ureteral calculi: Extraction via percutaneous nephrostomy. *Am J Roentgenol* 1985; 144:795–799.
69. Hunter DW, Castañeda-Zuñiga WR, Young AT, et al: Percutaneous removal of ureteral calculi: Clinical and experimental results. *Radiology* 1985; 156:341–348.
70. Streem SB, Hall P, Zelch MG, et al: Endourologic management of upper and mid ureteral calculi: Percutaneous antegrade extraction vs transurethral ureteroscopy. *Urology* 1988; 31:34–37.
71. Dretler SP: Review: Urolithiasis. Electrohydraulic and laser lithotripsy. *J Endourol* 1993; 7:387–388.
72. Saltzman B, Khasidy LR, Smith AD: Measurement of renal pelvis pressures during endourologic procedures. *Urology* 1987; 30:472–474.
73. Liedl B, Jocham D, Lunz C, et al: Prävalenz und inzidenz der arteriellen hypertonie bei ESWL-behandelten nierensteinpatienten. *Urologe A* 1989; 28:130–133.
74. Pemberton J: Extra-corporeal shock wave lithotripsy. *Postgrad Med J* 1987; 63:1025–1031.
75. Kaude JV, Williams CM, Millner MR, et al: Renal morphology and function immediately after extracorporeal shock-wave lithotripsy. *Am J Roentgenol* 1985; 145:305–313.
76. Williams CM, Kaude JV, Newman RC, et al: Extracorporeal shock-wave lithotripsy: Long-term complications. *Am J Roentgenol* 1988; 150:311–315.
77. Cass AS: Renal function after extracorporeal shock wave lithotripsy to a solitary kidney. *J Endourol* 1994; 8:15–19.

78. Ackaert KSJW, Schröder FH: Effects of extracorporeal shock wave lithotripsy (ESWL) on renal tissue: A review. *Urol Res* 1989; 17:3–7.

79. Toporoff B, Sclafani S, Scalea T, et al: Percutaneous antegrade ureteral stenting as an adjunct for treatment of complicated ureteral injuries. *J Trauma* 1992; 32:534–538.

80. Hulbert JC: Percutaneous intrarenal endoscopic surgery. *Semin Intervent Radiol* 1987; 4:109–114.

81. Lund G, Rysavy JA, Castañeda-Zuñiga WR, et al: Techniques for percutaneous mechanical occlusion of the ureter: Experimental evaluation. *Semin Intervent Radiol* 1987; 4:73–78.

82. Schild HH, Günther R, Thelen M: Transrenal ureteral occlusion: Results and problems. *J Vasc Interv Radiol* 1994; 5:321–325.

83. Bing KT, Hicks ME, Picus D, Darcy MD: Percutaneous ureteral occlusion with use of Gianturco coils and gelatin sponge: Part II. Clinical experience. *J Vasc Interv Radiol* 1992; 3:319–321.

84. Bush WH, Mayo ME: Catheter modification for transrenal temporary total ureteral obstruction: The "occlusive" nephroureteral catheter. *Urology* 1994; 43:729–733.

85. Banner MP, Amendola MA, Pollack HM: Anastomosed ureters: Fluoroscopically guided transconduit retrograde catheterization. *Radiology* 1989; 170:45–49.

86. Emmett JL, Levine SR, Woolner LB: Coexistence of renal cyst and tumour: Incidence in 1007 cases. *Br J Urol* 1963; 35:403–410.

87. Sandler CM, Houston GK, Hall JT, Morettin LB: Guided cyst puncture and aspiration. *Radiol Clin North Am* 1986; 24:527–537.

88. Bianchi G, Cavalleri S, D'Amico A, et al: Le traitement des kystes rénaux par drainage et alcoolisation percutanés. *J Urol (Paris)* 1990; 96:185–188.

89. Gelet A, Sanseverino R, Martin X, et al: Percutaneous treatment of benign renal cysts. *Eur Urol* 1990; 18:248–252.

90. Plas EG, Hübner WA: Percutaneous resection of renal cysts: A long-term followup. *J Urol* 1993; 149:703–705.

91. Castañeda F, Letourneau JG, Reddy P, et al: Alternative treatment of prostatic urethral obstruction secondary to benign prostatic hypertrophy. *Rofo* 1987; 147:426–429.

92. Chiou RK, Binard JE, Ebersole ME, et al: Randomized comparison of balloon dilation and transurethral incision for treatment of symptomatic benign prostatic hyperplasia. *J Endourol* 1994; 8:221–224.

93. Valji K, Bookstein JJ: Diagnosis of arteriogenic impotence: Efficacy of duplex sonography as a screening tool. *Am J Roentgenol* 1993; 160:65–69.

94. Bookstein JJ, Valji K, Parsons L, Kessler W: Pharmacoarteriography in the evaluation of impotence. *J Urol* 1987; 137:333–337.

95. Delcour C, Wespes E, Vandenbosch G, et al: Impotence: Evaluation with cavernosography. *Radiology* 1986; 161:803–806.

96. Puyau FA, Lewis RW, Balkin P, et al: Dynamic corpus cavernosography: Effect of papaverine injection. *Radiology* 1987; 164:179–182.

97. Pochaczevsky R, Lee WJ, Mallett E: Management of male infertility: Roles of contact thermography, spermatic venography, and embolization. *Am J Roentgenol* 1986; 147:97–102.

98. Zeitler E, Jecht E, Richter EI, Seyferth W: Selective sclerotherapy of the internal spermatic vein in patients with varicoceles. *Cardiovasc Intervent Radiol* 1980; 3:166–169.
99. Zuckerman AM, Mitchell SE, Venbrux AC, et al: Percutaneous varicocele occlusion: Long-term follow-up. *J Vasc Interv Radiol* 1994; 5:315–319.

Index